AF861409

APIC Handbook of Infection Control and Epidemiology

THIRD EDITION

APIC
ASSOCIATION FOR PROFESSIONALS IN
INFECTION CONTROL AND EPIDEMIOLOGY, INC.

© 2002
Association for Professionals in Infection Control
and Epidemiology, Inc.

1275 K Street, Suite 1000
Washington, DC 20005-4006
Phone (202) 789-1890
Fax (202) 789-1899
E-mail APICinfo@apic.org
Internet www.apic.org

ISBN 0-9656751-6-5

EDITOR IN CHIEF

Jan Jennings, BSMT(ASCP), MS, CIC

CO-EDITOR

Joan Wideman, MT(ASCP), SLS, MS, CIC

3RD EDITION CONTRIBUTORS

Jan Jennings, BSMT(ASCP), MS, CIC
Joan Wideman, MT(ASCP) SLS, MS, CIC
Cathy Ostrowski, RN, BS, CIC
Farrin Manian, MD, MPH, FACP

3RD EDITION REVIEWERS

Marla Clifton, RN, MSN, CIC
Gayle Gilmore, RN, MA, MIS, CIC

2ND EDITION CONTRIBUTORS

Betty Bolyard, RN, MPH
Mary Brachman, RN, MS, CIC
Marla Clifton, RN, MSN, CIC
Georgia P. Dash, RN, MS, CIC
Jean Fleming, RN, MPH, CIC
Jodell Johnson, RN, MA, CIC
Pat Kulich, RN, CIC
Christine Nutty, RN, MSN, CIC
Sandy Pirwitz, RN, MS, CIC
Maureen Wild, RN, BSN, CIC

Task Force

Leader: Jan Jennings, BSMT(ASCP), MS, CIC
Members: Farrin Manian, MD, MPH, FACP
Gayle Gilmore, RN, MA, MIS, CIC
Staff Partner: Valerie Restifo, RN, MA, MS

PRODUCTION TEAM

Valerie Restifo
Project Management
Editorial Oversight

Kris Carey
Project Production

Brenda Hegedus
Editing

Amy Holcomb
Cover & Book Design

Jennifer Kerhin
Marketing Direction

TABLE OF CONTENTS

Section I

Infection Control and Epidemiology........................ 1

Program Requirements........................ 2
Principles of Epidemiology........................ 12
General Surveillance Principles........................ 18
Communicable Disease Surveillance........................ 27
Acute Care Nosocomial Surveillance........................ 67
Long-Term Care Nosocomial Surveillance........................ 86
Home Care Nosocomial Surveillance........................ 97
Environmental Surveillance........................ 112
Outbreak Investigation........................ 128

Section II

Prevention and Control........................ 131

Asepsis........................ 132
Bioterrorism and Disaster Preparedness........................ 137
Construction and Renovation........................ 152
Disinfection and Sterilization........................ 159
Environmental Maintenance........................ 171
Food Handling........................ 196
Handwashing and Hand Hygiene........................ 205
Immunizations of HCW, Children, Adult........................ 212
Isolation and Precautions........................ 249
Laundry Handling........................ 283
Reuse and Reprocessing of SUDS........................ 286
Scrubs and Surgical Apparel........................ 292
Service and Companion Animal Considerations........................ 297

Section III

Healthcare Associated Infections 299

Pressure Ulcers 300
Respiratory Tract Infections 305
Surgical Site Infections 310
Urinary Tract Infections 322
Vascular Device Related Infections 325

Section IV

Specialized Populations and Settings 343

Adult Intensive Care Units 344
Ambulatory Care Settings 352
Behavioral Health Settings 362
Correctional Settings 366
Day Care Settings, Adult and Child 380
Dentistry 387
Diagnostic Services 397
Dialysis 400
Home Care Settings 411
Immunocompromised Patients 417
Long-Term Care Facilities 421
Neonates 435
Obstetrics 447
Pediatrics 455
Rehabilitation Services 461
Surgical Services 466
Travelers 479

Section V

Employee/Occupational Health 483

Overview and Work Restrictions 484
Exposure Management 495
Immunocompromised Employees 510
Pregnant Employees 513

Section VI

Laboratory 519

Laboratory Testing 520

Section VII

Antimicrobial Agents 533

Antimicrobial Utilization 534
Common Antimicrobial Agents 538

Section VIII

Appendices 551

Glossary: Common Terms in Infection Control 553
Infection Control Resources 561

Index 595

PREFACE

Infection control is an ever evolving field that cuts across all other healthcare-related disciplines and settings. Not surprisingly, the demand for accurate information on infection control matters remains high and is likely to further increase given the changing healthcare environment. Healthcare is faced with "sicker" patients, shrinking resources, increasing emphasis on worker efficiency, emergence of multiple resistant organisms, and deployment of new technologies that may place the patient at increased risk of infection. Against this backdrop is the public demand for high-quality care, which is not likely to diminish proportionate to the expected decrease in the cost of healthcare. This demand, coupled with the desire to reduce adverse patient outcomes and protect healthcare workers, presents all healthcare workers with an unprecedented challenge. Accordingly, infection control professionals (ICPs) are compelled to assume a leadership role within their own unique healthcare organizations and to provide practical strategies in collaboration with other professionals to help reduce the risks of infection across the continuum.

The handbook is designed as a convenient, practical, portable, and up-to-date resource relating to infection control (IC) issues commonly facing healthcare workers. It is intended as a quick guide for ICPs, nursing staff, physicians, administrators, healthcare students, and other ancillary healthcare providers.

This third edition of the handbook represents many hours of hard work by dedicated members of the Association for Professionals in Infection Control and Epidemiology (APIC).

Feedback from readers of earlier editions was considered and additional content, revisions, and reorganization has greatly enhanced the final document. The handbook have been reformatted to provide a consistent chapter design and is enhanced with tables for quick information at-a-glance. This revised edition has several new chapters including: asepsis, bioterrorism and disaster planning, correctional settings, diagnostic services, environmental maintenance, environmental surveillance, food handling, immunocompromised employees, laundry handling, obstetrics, pressure ulcers, rehabilitation services, scrubs and surgical apparel, surgical services, and information for travelers. In addition, the surveillance section has been expanded and enhanced to including the addition of home care surveillance. Resources and references in each chapter provide information on where to obtain greater details including Web site addresses.

Every effort has been made to provide accurate and the most up-to-date information. However, as errors may still occur and some information may become obsolete almost overnight, the reader is encouraged to make full use of the references provided and stay in close touch with the current literature.

Jan Jennings, BSMT(ASCP), MS, CIC

Joan M. Wideman, MT(ASCP) SLS, MS, CIC

Section I

INFECTION CONTROL AND EPIDEMIOLOGY

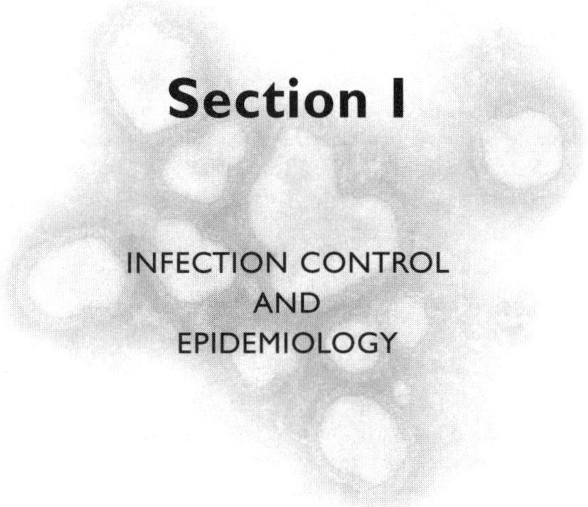

Program Requirements

Overview

- Each healthcare organization is unique and its specific needs should be considered when developing or reorganizing an IC program. Because of these differing needs, there may be various groups, individuals, and functions within the institution that are responsible for the IC program. This chapter outlines various persons and activities related to an effective IC program using three principal goals:
  - Protect the patient,
  - Protect the healthcare worker, visitors, and others in the healthcare environment, and
  - Accomplish the previous two goals in a cost-effective manner, whenever possible.
- Achieving these goals is the driving force behind every recommendation and action of an IC program. The goals are relevant to patient-care activities in any healthcare setting, not only in the acute-care hospital but also in skilled nursing facilities, nursing homes, rehabilitation units, urgent-care centers, same-day surgery facilities, ambulatory-care centers, and home-care programs.

Purpose

- The success or failure of the IC program is defined by its effectiveness in achieving its goals. It is imperative that every healthcare institution develops specific objectives and outcome measures to determine whether or not its IC program is effective. The recommendations listed fall into eight categories:
  - Managing critical data and information,

- Setting and recommending policies and procedures,
- Compliance with regulations, guidelines, and accreditation requirements,
- Employee health,
- Direct intervention to prevent transmission of infectious diseases,
- Education and training of healthcare workers,
- Personnel resources, and
- Non-personnel resources.

Risk Factors

➤ The preponderance of the risk of healthcare associated infections is found among the sickest patients; those who will continue to occupy acute-care hospitals. Despite shorter hospital stays and a decreasing census, there is an increased potential for infections due to the changing demographics of the population and new, increasingly invasive technology. Patients in hospitals will be sicker; there will be new antibiotic-resistant microorganisms; there will be new instruments and procedures; and there will be new infectious diseases. Thus, the need for IC as a specialty practice in the hospital will continue to increase. Infection control is a quality-improvement activity that focuses on improving the care of patients and protecting the health of staff.

Strategies for Prevention

➤ The following is a summary of recommendations from the Consensus Panel with members from the APIC, SHEA, AHA, JCAHO, IDSA, PIDS, HICPAC, NFID, and HIP-CDC. The panel used an evidence-based approach in developing recommendations. Although the recommendations address hospital-based IC programs, ICPs in other settings may adept them for their own settings.

RECOMMENDATION CLASSIFICATION

I Strongly recommended	Strongly recommended for implementation based on: • Evidence from at least one properly randomized, controlled trial, or • Evidence from at least one well-designed clinical trial without randomization, or • Evidence from cohort or case-control analytical studies (preferably from more than one center), or • Evidence from multiple time-series studies.
II Recommended	Recommended for implementation based on: • Published clinical experience or descriptive studies, or • Reports of expert committees, or • Opinions of respected authorities.
III Recommended	When required by government rules or regulations.

Managing critical data and information

➤ Surveillance of nosocomial infections should be performed.

➤ The surveillance process should incorporate at least the following elements:

- Identification and description of the problem or event to be studied,
- Definition of the population at risk,
- Selection of the appropriate methods of measurement, including statistical tools and risk stratification,
- Identification and description of data sources and data collection personnel and methods,
- Definition of numerators and denominators, or
- Preparation and distribution of reports to appropriate groups.

- Selection of specific events to be monitored, which should be guided by validated, nationally available benchmarks appropriately adjusted for patient risks, so that meaningful comparisons can be made.

Surveillance data should be analyzed appropriately and used to monitor and improve IC and healthcare outcomes. *(I)*

- Clinical performance and assessment indicators used to support external comparative measurements should meet the criteria delineated by SHEA and APIC. *(II)*
- Specifically, these indicators and their analyses should address the following parameters:
  - Relation to outcome or processes,
  - Ability to measure variation in quality,
  - Definition of numerators and denominators,
  - Reliability, completeness, and feasibility of data collection,
  - Appropriate risk adjustment,
  - Comparability of populations; severity and case-mix adjustments for external comparison,
  - Training required for indicator implementation, and
  - Applicable benchmarks of standards of care.

Setting and recommending policies and procedures

- Written infection prevention and control policies and procedures should be established, implemented, maintained, and updated periodically. *(II and III)*
- The policies and procedures should be scientifically valid.
- The policies and procedures should be reviewed for practicality and cost.

- The policies and procedures should lead to improved prevention or improved patient outcomes.
- Policies and procedures should be monitored periodically for performance. *(II and III)*

Compliance with regulations, guidelines, and accreditation requirements

- Healthcare facilities should use IC personnel to assist in maintaining compliance with relevant regulatory and accreditation requirements. *(II)*
- Infection control personnel should have appropriate access to medical or other relevant records and to staff members who can provide information on the adequacy of the institution's compliance with regard to regulations, standards, and guidelines. *(I)*
- The IC program should collaborate with, and provide liaison to, appropriate local and state health departments for reporting communicable diseases and related conditions, and to assist with control of infectious diseases. *(II and III)*

Employee health

- The IC program personnel should work collaboratively with the facility's employee health program personnel. *(II)*
  - The infection control program should review and approve all policies and procedures developed in the employee health program that relate to the transmission of infections in the hospital.
  - Infection control personnel should be available to the employee health program for consultation regarding infectious disease concerns.
- At the time of employment, all facility personnel should be evaluated for conditions relating to communicable diseases. *(II and III)*

- The evaluation should include the following:
  - Medical history, including immunization status and assessment for conditions that may predispose personnel to acquiring or transmitting communicable diseases,
  - Tuberculosis skin testing,
  - Serologic screening for vaccine-preventable diseases, if indicated, and
  - Such medical examinations as are indicated by the above.
- Appropriate employees or other healthcare workers should have periodic medical evaluations to assess for new conditions related to infectious diseases that may have an impact on patient care, the employee, or other healthcare workers, which should include review of immunization and tuberculosis skin-test status, if appropriate. *(II and III)*
  - All facilities should maintain confidential medical records on all healthcare workers.
  - The employee health program should have the capability to track employee immunization and tuberculosis skin-test status.
- Employees should be offered appropriate immunizations for communicable diseases. *(II and III)*
  - Immunizations should be based on regulatory requirements and Advisory Committee on Immunization Practices recommendations for healthcare workers.
- The employee health program should develop policies and procedures for the evaluation of ill employees, including assessment of disease communicability, indications for work restrictions, and management of employees who have been exposed to infectious diseases, including postexposure prophylaxis and work restrictions. *(I)*

Intervening directly to prevent transmission of infectious diseases

- All healthcare facilities should have the capacity to identify the occurrence of outbreaks or clusters of infectious diseases. *(I)*
  - Infection control personnel should review microbiology records regularly to identify unusual clusters or a greater than usual incidence of certain species or strains of microorganisms.
  - In patient areas of the healthcare facility in which active prospective surveillance is not conducted, IC programs should maintain regular contact with clinical, medical, and nursing staff to ascertain the occurrence of disease clusters or outbreaks, assist in maintenance and monitoring of IC procedures, and provide consultation as required.
- All healthcare facilities should have access to the services of personnel trained and experienced in conducting outbreak investigations. *(II)*
- When an outbreak occurs, the IC team should have adequate resources and authority to ensure a comprehensive and timely investigation of appropriate control measures. *(II)*

Education and training of healthcare workers

- Healthcare facilities should provide ongoing educational programs in infection prevention and control to healthcare workers. *(II and III)*
  - Infection control personnel with knowledge of epidemiology and infectious diseases should be active participants in the planning and implementation of the educational programs.
- Educational programs should be evaluated periodically for effectiveness, and attendance should be monitored. *(II and III)*

- Educational programs should meet the needs of the group or department for which they are given and should provide learning experiences for people with a wide range of educational backgrounds and work responsibilities.

Infection Control Resources

- The personnel and supporting resources, including secretarial services, available to the hospital epidemiology and IC program should be proportional to the size, complexity, and estimated risk of the population served by the institution. *(II)*
- All hospitals should have the continuing services of a trained hospital epidemiologist(s) and ICP(s). *(I)*
- ICPs should be encouraged to obtain Certification in Infection Control. *(II)*
- Healthcare facilities should provide or make available in a timely fashion sufficient office space and equipment, statistical and computer support, and clinical microbiology and pathology services to support the nosocomial infection surveillance, prevention, and control program of the institution. *(II)*
- Resources should be provided for continuing professional education of hospital epidemiologists and ICPs. *(II)*

EXAMPLE OF AN INFECTION CONTROL PROGRAM MODEL

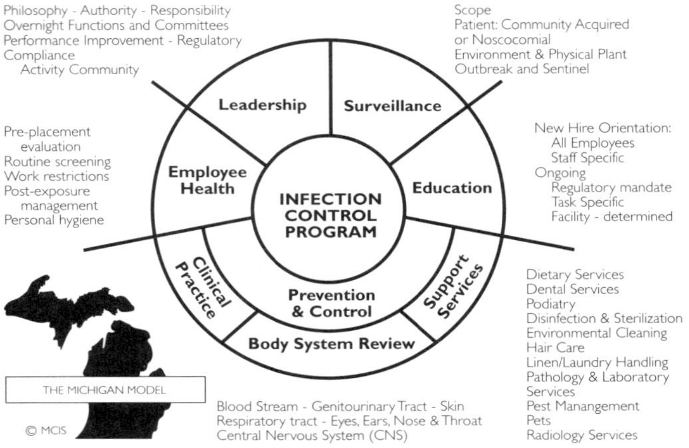

References/Resources

- Association for Professionals in Infection Control and Epidemiology. APIC Text of Infection Control and Epidemiology. 2000, chapters 2,5,6,7,8,9,10,11,12.
- APIC/CHICA Infection Control and Epidemiology: Professional and Practice Standards Am J Infect Control 1999; 27:47-51.
- APIC Consensus Panel Report: Requirements for Infrastructure and Essential Activities of ICE in Out-of-hospital Settings. Am J Infect Control 1999; 20:695-705.
- Michigan Society for Infection Control. www.msic-online.org
- Scheckler WE, Brimhall D, Buck AS, Farr BM, et al. Requirements for infrastructure and essential activities of infection control and epidemiology activities of infection control and epidemiology in hospitals: A Consensus Panel report. Am J Infect Control 1998; 26(1): 47–60.

Principles of Epidemiology

Overview

- Epidemiology is a combination of research methodology concerned with the distribution of health and disease in populations and a body of knowledge built upon evidence-based research and interventions to control disease and improve health. It is the scientific foundation for an effective IC program. In epidemiology as in surveillance, the unit of observation is individuals with like characteristics, similar risk factors, or similar exposures rather than individual cases. Comparisons to other similar populations and population trends are used to identify opportunities for intervention.
- Infection control epidemiology has as its core foundation the chain of infection.
- Each link in the chain provides opportunities for intervention and surveillance.

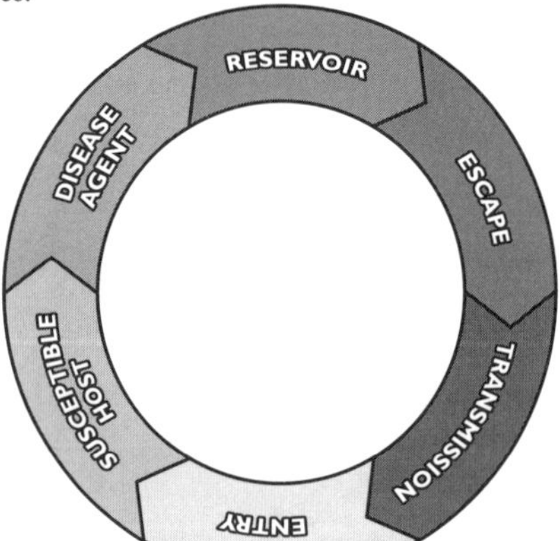

- Infection control surveillance categories:
  - Communicable Disease Surveillance
    (Refer to Section 1 - Communicable Disease Reporting)
  - Nosocomial Infection Surveillance
    (Refer to Section 1 - General Considerations for Surveillance, Acute, Long-Term Care and Home Care Surveillance)
  - Environmental Surveillance
    (Refer to Section 1 - Environmental Surveillance)

Definitions

- **Null hypothesis:** The claim that there is no difference between the population and the sample.
- **Type I (alpha) error:** The probability of rejecting a true null hypothesis. Indicates the significance level, or P value (usually set at <0.05). *Note: Statistical association based on small P values does NOT prove causation.*
- **Type II (beta) error:** The likelihood of not attributing statistical significance when it is there (i.e., failing to reject a null hypothesis that really is false).
- **Power:** The ability of a statistical test to detect a difference (one – Beta). Increasing samples size increases power and the ability to obtain meaningful results.
- **Mean:** Arithmetic average of a group of numbers.
- **Median:** The middle number in an ordered group of numbers.
- **Mode:** The most common value (number) in a group of numbers.
- **Range:** The largest value minus the smallest value in a data set.

- **Cohort study:** Performed prospectively (usually) to examine a population free of the disease being studied and looks for association between risk factors and appearance of disease.
- **Case-control study:** Performed retrospectively by comparing potential risk factors in those with a specific disease (cases) with those without disease (controls).
- **Experimental/clinical study:** Performed prospectively by intentionally exposing subjects to a factor (drug, infection, etc.) and measuring outcomes. Ideally performed by "double-blinding" (neither the subject nor the researcher knows which subjects were exposed to the factor being studied).
- **Standard deviation:** Square root of the sum of the difference between each individual value in a data set and the mean of the data set divided by the number of values in the data set minus one. Larger standard deviations are associated with more variability in the data set (i.e., more dispersion).
- **SIR:** Standardized infection rates with the mean infection rate set at 1.0.

Statistical Formulas:

Z ***test:*** *Test to compare two SIRs (x vs.y).*

DISEASE STATE		
Test Result	Present	Absent
Positive	True positive (TP)	False positive (FP)
Negative	False negative (FN)	True negative (TN)

Sensitivity = Percentage of cases with the disease that are detected by the test.

$$\frac{TP}{TP+FN} \times 100\%$$

Specificity = Percentage of people without the disease that were correctly labeled by the test as not diseased.

$$\frac{TN}{TN+FP} \times 100\%$$

Positive predictive value = Percentage of all test-positives that are truly positive (e.g., diseased).

$$\frac{TP}{TP+FP} \times 100\%$$

Negative predictive value = Percentage of all test-negatives that are truly negative (e.g., not diseased).

$$\frac{TN}{TN+FN} \times 100\%$$

$$\textit{Nosocomial infection rate by patient-discharge} = \frac{\textit{No. of nosocomial infections at all sites}}{\textit{No. of patients discharged}} \times 100$$

$$\textit{Nosocomial infection rate} = \frac{\textit{No. of nosocomial infections at all sites}}{\textit{No. of patient-days}} \times 1000$$

$$\textit{Device-day infection rate} = \frac{\textit{No. of device-associated infections for a site}}{\textit{No. of device-days}} \times 1000$$

$$\textit{Incidence rate} = \frac{\textit{No. of new cases of a disease for a specified time period}}{\textit{Population at risk for same time period}} \times k^{*}$$

$$\text{Device utilization ratio} = \frac{\text{No. of device-days}}{\text{No. of patient-days}}$$

$$\text{Prevalence rate} = \frac{\text{No. of existing cases of a disease at specified interval or point in time}}{\text{Population at risk for same time period}} \times k^{*}$$

*(e.g., 100 for discharges, 1000 for device-days)

$$\text{Risk} = \frac{\text{No. with disease}}{\text{Total no. exposed}}$$

$$\text{Relative Risk} = \frac{\text{Incidence rate among exposed}}{\text{Incidence rate among unexposed}}$$

$$\text{Attack rate} = \frac{\text{No. of new cases of diseases for a specified time period}}{\text{Population at risk for same time period}} \times 100$$

$$\text{Odds} = \frac{\text{No. of diseased persons exposed}}{\text{No. of well persons exposed}}$$

$$\text{Odds ratio} = \frac{\text{Odds of disease in those exposed}}{\text{Odds of disease in those not exposed}}$$

$$\text{SSI rate} = \frac{\text{No. of nosocomial SSIs}}{\text{No. of surgical procedures}} \times 100$$

$$\text{Standardized infection rate (SIR)} = \frac{\text{Observed no. of SSIs}}{\text{Expected no. of SSIs}}$$

$$Z \text{ (to compare to SIR)} = \frac{2(\sqrt{SIRy} - \sqrt{SIRx})}{\sqrt{1/Ey + 1/Ex}}$$

$$Z\ (\text{to compare Obs and Exp SSI}) = 2(\sqrt{\text{observed number of SSIs}} - \sqrt{\text{expected number of SSIs}})$$

$$Z\ (\text{to compare device assoc. rates}) = \frac{I - 0.5 - (i+I) \times p}{\sqrt{(i+I) \times p \times (1-p)}}$$

I = *No. of device-associated infections of the smaller rate*

I = *No. of device-associated infections of the larger rate*

d = *No. of device days of the smaller rate*

D = *No. of device days of the larger rate*

p = D/(D+d)

References/Resources

- Association for Professionals in Infection Control and Epidemiology. APIC Text of Infection Control and Epidemiology. 2000, chapters 9,10,12,17,18,19,20,21.
- Culver DH. Methods of comparing nosocomial infection rates. Preconference workshop, Sixth Annual Meeting of the Society for Healthcare Epidemiology of America. Washington, DC, April 20, 1996.
- Checko PJ. Use of statistics for epidemiology. In: Olmsted RN, editor. Infection control and applied epidemiology: principles and practice. St. Louis, MO: Mosby; 1996. P 2 - 1–2 - 24.
- Giesecke J. Modern infectious disease epidemiology. Boston: Edward Arnold; 1994.
- Mausner JS, Bahn AK. Epidemiology: an introductory text. Philadelphia: WB Saunders; 1974.

General Surveillance Principles

Overview

- Surveillance is an active process encompassing identification of opportunities for improvement, development of data collection and analytic procedures, development and implementation of quality improvement action plans, and evaluation of improvement efforts through measurement. Surveillance is best when the ICP engages the healthcare delivery team members in the process.

Purpose

- Improve nosocomial infection rates within a healthcare facility, and ultimately reduce morbidity, mortality, and cost.
- Establish endemic baseline infection rates with the aim of lowering these rates; endemic infections account for 90 – 95% of nosocomial infections.
- Identify outbreaks.
- Educate healthcare personnel concerning data relevant to their practice.
- Evaluate control measures designed to reduce infection rates.
- Defend malpractice claims through implementation of an active surveillance program.
- Research.
- Comply with accreditation requirements and standards.

Definitions

- **Denominator:** Represents the population at risk (e.g., persons, device days, patient days, etc.).

- **Nosocomial infection:** A localized or systemic condition resulting from an adverse reaction to the presence of an infectious agent(s) or its toxin(s) not present or incubating at the time of admission to the healthcare facility.
- **Numerator:** Each event (e.g., infection) that occurs during the study period. For surveillance purposes, the operational definitions of infection provide the description of numerators.
- **Prospective:** Patients with risk factors of interest (e.g., IV catheters, ventilators, etc.) are identified and concurrent surveillance is performed to monitor for infection.
- **Retrospective:** Infections are identified and research (e.g., medical record review) is performed to identify risk factors most often done in outbreak situations.
- **Surveillance:** Systematic method of collecting, consolidating, and analyzing data regarding the distribution and determinants of a given disease process or event, intended for dissemination of that information to those who can improve the outcomes.

Risk Factors

- Failure to implement effective IC programs in healthcare settings can lead to higher morbidity, mortality, costs, and decreased inpatient, provider, and staff satisfaction.
- Without active surveillance programs, infectious outbreaks are more likely to occur and go unnoticed for longer time periods.

Strategies for Prevention
(Steps in the Surveillance Process)

- Complete assessment.
  - Define patient/resident/client population profile.
    - Patient demographics (age, gender, ethnicity).

- Patient clinical characteristics (top diagnoses, top procedures, and special needs).
- Define staff profile.
  - Staff characteristics (knowledge, training, skills).
- Define facility profile.
  - Facility in general, unit/clinic characteristics (physical size, structure, traffic flow, air flow, geographic location).

➤ Collect baseline information based on assessment.

➤ Select the outcome(s) or process(es) to be surveyed.

- Ask the following questions:
  - What possibilities are there for improvement? (Quality, cost, utilization, satisfaction?)
  - What interventions can be developed to make improvements?
  - What measurements can be used to evaluate the impact of interventions?
  - Will measurements be focused or "whole-house"? (if "whole-house"—Why??)
- Include clinicians in the selection process.
- Seek administrative support/commitment.
- Rank surveillance priorities to align with available resources.
- Examples of Possible Measurements.
  - Outcomes
    - Nosocomial bloodstream infection.
    - Community acquired salmonella.
    - Patient satisfaction with operative care.
    - Staff satisfaction with sharps injury follow-up.
    - Noninfectious outcomes (e.g., fall, medication error).

    - Processes
        - Antibiotic appropriateness monitoring.
        - Environmental monitoring.
        - Disinfection/Sterilization practices.
        - Reporting of communicable diseases.
    - TB skin testing.
    - Compliance with precautions/isolation.
    - Sharps injuries follow up.

➤ Define methodology that will be used.

- Type of surveillance:
    - Prospective patient identification and concurrent surveillance are preferred.
    - Active data collection is preferred.
    - Design data collection tool.
- Surveillance definitions:
    - Adopt consistent definitions for surveillance (e.g., McGeer's, CDC). Note: These are not clinical definitions of infection.
    - If modifying or developing new definitions, address the limitations in the surveillance plan.
    - Use written definitions for both numerators and denominators.
- Data elements:
    - Demographics (name, ID, age, sex, location, admission date, discharge date).
    - Clinical and laboratory information to support case definition.
    - Risk factors for the infections being surveyed.
    - Optional data: clinician notes, interventions, costs.

- Data sources:
  - Patient records (e.g., history and physical examination, progress notes, vital signs, physician's orders, radiographic records, drugs).
  - Microbiology lab reports.
  - Pharmacy records.
  - Autopsy reports.
  - Admission records.
  - Interactions with caregivers.
  - Interactions with and observations of patients.
  - Post-discharge reports.
  - Activity records from operating room, labor and delivery, ICUs, respiratory care, emergency room, outpatient department.
  - Health information department (Medical Records).
  - Billing records.
- Analytic plan:
  - Selection of computer software.
  - Baseline and comparison information (e.g., NNIS data).

➤ Develop a Surveillance Plan.

- Written Plan components:
  - Assessment findings including baseline data.
  - Goals and objectives.
  - Roles and responsibilities.
  - Selected measurements and specifications.
  - Methods that will be used.
  - Success evaluation strategy.
  - Leadership approval.

- Examples of possible goals:
  - Improve procedure or treatment related infection rates to reduce morbidity, mortality, and costs by x% within X timeframe.
  - Identify clusters and outbreaks that may be related to practices.
  - Evaluate control measures designed and implemented to reduce procedure or treatment related infection rates.
  - Establish baseline prevalence rates of community-acquired infections.
  - Contribute to the scientific body of research.
- Comply with accreditation requirements and standards.
  - Develop a project plan.
  - Who will collect data?
  - What data sources will be used?
  - How often will data be collected?
  - How often will reports be generated?
  - Who will receive reports?

➤ Implement the measurement process.

- Conduct casefinding per measurement specifications.
- Collect additional data elements for verification.
- Record case specific results on worksheet (electronic or manual).
- Record time spent.
- Maintain consistency when identifying infections.
- Use systematic data collection methods.

➤ Create meaningful information from the data collected (electronic or manual).

- Record key information on line list to prepare monthly/quarterly report.

- Calculate rates, ratios, and proportions to summarize findings. A single number expressing a hospital's overall nosocomial infection rate is not a valid measure of the overall efficacy of the IC program, and therefore should not be used for inter-hospital comparison.
- Perform quality control on results.
- Prepare tables and graphs.

➤ Create actionable information to assist decision making.

- Be aware of the limitations of rate calculations with small numbers such as infrequent events or small sample sizes.
- Use statistical probability methods to determine whether observed differences in rates are meaningful.
- Analyze results to identify significant findings (identify trends, outliers, unusual patterns, comparisons to benchmarks, special vs. common cause variation).
- Apply risk stratification methods where appropriate.
  - Risk stratification means subdividing (stratifying) surveillance population into groups with similar risk of infection before performing any analyses or comparisons.
  - Evaluate surveillance cohort for obvious heterogeneity.
  - Ensure comparisons are valid.
- Solicit and welcome alternative interpretation of the data.
- Summarize issues and recommendations based on analysis and References/Resources.
- Prepare executive summary.
- Provide timely feedback to staff who can use the data to make improvements.

- Take action.
  - Convene interdisciplinary team to identify improvement strategies, actions.
  - Collaborate with clinical staff to develop action plans to address problems identified through surveillance.
  - Prepare action plans with defined tasks, responsibilities, and timelines.
  - Routinely prepare status reports including actions taken.
- Evaluate interventions and measurement strategies.
  - Routinely evaluate the efficiency and effectiveness of actions taken.
    - Document results of actions including identified changes in process or outcomes post intervention (quality, cost, utilization, satisfaction) and compare to targets or benchmarks).
    - For successful interventions, develop and implement ongoing measurement to ensure that benefits of the intervention are sustained.
    - For unsuccessful interventions, develop and implement new interventions.
  - Routinely evaluate the efficiency and effectiveness of measurement process.
    - Consider external validation of surveillance efforts.
- Tools used in the process.
  - Assessment Worksheet
  - Measurement Selection Grid
  - Measurement Definitions/Specifications
  - Project Plan
  - Data collection tools

- Computer
- Current literature and guidelines

COMPARISON OF SURVEILLANCE APPROACHES		
Approach	**Advantages**	**Disadvantages**
Comprehensive/ hospital-wide	Global view of all infections in all patients; may facilitate detection of outbreaks.	Labor intensive; may not be objective driven.
Priority directed (e.g., body site, patient ward, or procedure specific)	Offers flexibility and adaptability for specific needs and problems; more objective driven and resource efficient.	Limited information on endemic rates; may miss outbreaks.
Post discharge	Increases case finding.	Problems with timeliness and accuracy of data and patient follow up.

References/Resources

- Association for Professionals in Infection Control and Epidemiology. APIC Text of Infection Control and Epidemiology. 2000, chapters 1,13-16, 22 - 26,46,120,123,124.
- Gaynes RP, Horan TC. Surveillance of nosocomial infections. In Mayhall CG, editor. Infection control and hospital epidemiology. Baltimore: Williams and Wilkins; 1996. P 1017–1031.
- Lee TB, Baker OG, Lee JT, Scheckler WE, Steele L et al. Recommended practices for surveillance. Am J Infect Control 1998; 26:277–288.

Communicable Disease Surveillance

Overview

- Infectious/communicable diseases remain the leading cause of death worldwide and the third leading cause of death in the U.S. Since 1973, more than 30 new and reemerging diseases/syndromes have been recognized. Healthcare providers and organizations are an integral part of the community and play an important role in reporting, investigating outbreaks, preventing, and controlling these diseases. Public/community health authorities perform an essential role in promulgating regulations and requirements for reporting diseases and conditions of importance to the public on a variety of levels: local, regional, national, and worldwide.

Purpose

- Provide an informational summary of epidemiologically important communicable diseases in a table format. The reader should check the References/Resources for details.

Risk Factors

- Per the CDCs National Center for Infectious Diseases (NCID) *Preventing Emerging Infectious Diseases: A Strategy for the 21st Century*, plans to combat infectious diseases targets certain categories of emerging infectious disease problems and particular groups of people who are at special risk. They include:
  - Antimicrobial resistance.
  - Foodborne and water-borne diseases.
  - Vector-borne and zoonotic diseases.

- Diseases transmitted through blood transfusions or blood products.
- Chronic diseases caused by infectious agents.
- Vaccine development and use.
- Diseases of people with impaired host defenses.
- Diseases of pregnant women and newborns.
- Diseases of travelers, immigrants, and refugees.

Strategies for Prevention

- Preventing emerging and reemerging infection requires special strategies and partnerships between public health, the community, and healthcare providers.
- Each state and territorial health department classifies reportable diseases and prescribes the manner and time of reporting and the list in each state differs.
- All physicians, directors of medical care facilities, and directors of laboratories are required to report persons diagnosed with a notifiable disease to the local health department serving the jurisdiction in which the facility is located.

References/Resources

- Association for Professionals in Infection Control and Epidemiology. APIC Text of Infection Control and Epidemiology. 2000, chapters 93-120.
- Centers for Disease Control and Prevention. Case definitions for infectious conditions under public health surveillance. MMWR 1997; 46 (No. RR-10).
- Centers for Disease Control, www.cdc.gov
- Chin J. Control of communicable diseases manual, 17th edition. 2000, American Public Health Association, Washington, D.C.

NATIONALLY NOTIFIABLE INFECTIOUS DISEASES UNITED STATES, 2002

Acquired immunodeficiency syndrome (AIDS)
Anthrax
Botulism
Brucellosis
Chancroid
Chlamydia trachomatis, genital infection
Cholera
Coccidioidomycosis
Cryptosporidiosis
Cyclosporiasis
Diphtheria
Ehrlichiosis
Encephalitis, Arboviral
Enterohemorrhagic *Escherichia coli*
Giardiasis
Gonorrhea
Haemophilus influenzae, invasive disease
Hansen disease (leprosy)
Hantavirus pulmonary syndrome
Hepatitis, viral, acute (A, B, C)
HIV
Legionellosis
Lyme disease
Malaria
Measles
Meningococcal disease
Mumps
Pertussis
Plague
Poliomyelitis, paralytic
Psittacosis
Q fever
Rabies, animal
Rabies, human
Rocky Mountain spotted fever
Rubella
Salmonellosis
Shigellosis
Streptococcal disease, invasive, group A
Streptococcal toxic shock syndrome
Streptococcus pneumoniae, drug resistant
Streptococcus pneumoniae invasive in children <5 years
Syphilis
Tetanus
Toxic shock syndrome
Trichinosis
Tuberculosis
Tularemia
Typhoid fever
Varicella (deaths only)
Yellow fever

For updates: *www.cdc.gov/epo/dphsi/PHS/infdis.htm*

EPIDEMIOLOGICALLY IMPORTANT COMMUNICABLE DISEASES

IP = Incubation Period; **PC** = Period of Communicability; **E** = Means of Exposure
SP = Susceptible Persons; **PR** = Prophylaxis; **APT** = Asymptomatic Patient Precautions
PRS = Personnel Restrictions; **IPT** = Infected Patient Precautions (in addition to Standard Precautions)
PR = private room; **M** = mask; **GL** = gloves; **GW** = gown

ANTHRAX	**IP**	One to seven days, although periods up to 60 days are possible.
	PC	Transmission from person-to-person is very likely.
	E	1) Cutaneous contact with spores. 2) Inhalation of spores. 3) Ingestion of contaminated meat/food.
	PR	Tetracycline or Ciprofloxacin Immunization is indicated in certain instances.
	APT	None
	PRS	None
	IPT	None
CAMPYLOBACTER-ASSOCIATED DIARRHEA	**IP**	One to 10 days, usually three to five days.
	PC	Usually from several days to several weeks.
	E	1) Ingestion of contaminated food. 2) Handling of contaminated feces. 3) Transmission from pets.
	SP	Those having contact with infected feces.
	PR	None
	APT	None
	PRS	None
	IPT	PR if patient hygiene poor; GL for touching.

EPIDEMIOLOGICALLY IMPORTANT COMMUNICABLE DISEASES

IP = Incubation Period **PC** = Period of Communicability **E** = Means of Exposure
SP = Susceptible Persons **PR** = Prophylaxis **APT** = Asymptomatic Patient Precautions
PRS = Personnel Restrictions **IPT** = Infected Patient Precautions (in addition to Standard Precautions)
PR = private room; **M** = mask; **GL** = gloves; **GW** = gown

CHICKEN POX *(VARICELLA-ZOSTER)*	**IP**	10–21 days (usually 13–17 days).
	PC	From one to two days before appearance of rash until all lesions are crusted, which is usually five to seven days after appearance of rash.
	E	1) Physical contact with vesicles, or 2) Close proximity (three to six feet) to an infectious person for more than several minutes, or 3) Same-room proximity to an infectious person for one hour or more.
	SP	Those with no history of chicken pox and negative varicella antibody titers; all infants under six months of age.
	PR	Varicella-zoster immune globulin (VZIG) may attenuate infection. Postexposure VZIG (125 U/10 kg, maximum 625 U (5 vials), given within 96 hours is recommended for several categories of susceptible children and for susceptible immunosuppressed adults, provided there are no contraindications. Postexposure VZIG for other persons may be considered on an individual basis. No data exist regarding postexposure efficacy of current varicella virus vaccine or acyclovir in healthcare settings.
	APT	If VZIG is not taken: Isolate on days 10–21 after exposure. If VZIG is taken: Isolate on days 10–28 after exposure. *continues on next page*

EPIDEMIOLOGICALLY IMPORTANT COMMUNICABLE DISEASES

IP = Incubation Period
SP = Susceptible Persons
PRS = Personnel Restrictions
PC = Period of Communicability
PR = Prophylaxis
IPT = Infected Patient Precautions (in addition to Standard Precautions)
E = Means of Exposure
APT = Asymptomatic Patient Precautions

PR = private room; **M** = mask; **GL** = gloves; **GW** = gown

CHICKEN POX (*VARICELLA-ZOSTER*) *continued*	**PRS**	If VZIG is not taken: exclude from duty on days 10–21 after exposure.
	IPT	If VZIG is taken: Exclude from duty on days 10–28 after exposure. PR, with special ventilation, M, GL, GW, until all lesions are crusted. Non-immune personnel should avoid caring for infected patients whenever possible.
***CLOSTRIDIUM DIFFICILE*–ASSOCIATED DIARRHEA**	**IP**	May be days or weeks following antibiotic treatment.
	PC	Until diarrhea subsides.
	E	Handling of contaminated feces without gloves.
	SP	Those receiving antimicrobial therapy.
	PR	None
	APT	None
	PRS	None
	IPT	PR may be indicated; use GL and GW when providing care.

EPIDEMIOLOGICALLY IMPORTANT COMMUNICABLE DISEASES

IP = Incubation Period **PC** = Period of Communicability **E** = Means of Exposure
SP = Susceptible Persons **PR** = Prophylaxis **APT** = Asymptomatic Patient Precautions
PRS = Personnel Restrictions **IPT** = Infected Patient Precautions (in addition to Standard Precautions)
PR = private room; **M** = mask; **GL** = gloves; **GW** = gown

CONJUNCTIVITIS **Bacterial**	**IP**	24-72 hours
	PC	During the course of active infection.
	E	Direct contact with eye drainage or upper respiratory tract secretions, direct contact with contaminated equipment, cosmetics, or multi-dose solutions.
	SP	Universal susceptibility.
	PR	None
	APT	None
	PRS	Restrict personnel until signs and symptoms (e.g., purulent drainage) subside.
	IPT	GL for touching infective substances; contact precautions may be necessary during outbreaks.

EPIDEMIOLOGICALLY IMPORTANT COMMUNICABLE DISEASES

IP = Incubation Period | **PC** = Period of Communicability | **E** = Means of Exposure
SP = Susceptible Persons | **PR** = Prophylaxis | **APT** = Asymptomatic Patient Precautions
PRS = Personnel Restrictions | **IPT** = Infected Patient Precautions (in addition to Standard Precautions)

PR = private room; **M** = mask; **GL** = gloves; **GW** = gown

CONJUNCTIVITIS **Viral** [e.g., epidemic keratoconjuncitivis (EKC)]	**IP**	Four to 12 days
	PC	From the incubation period until 14 days after onset; persistent shedding can occur.
	E	Direct contact with eye drainage or upper respiratory tract secretions, direct contact with contaminated equipment, cosmetics, or multi-dose solutions.
	SP	Universal susceptibility.
	PR	None
	APT	None
	PRS	Restrict personnel until signs and symptoms subside.
	IPT	GL for touching infective substances; contact precautions may be necessary during outbreaks.

EPIDEMIOLOGICALLY IMPORTANT COMMUNICABLE DISEASES

IP = Incubation Period　**PC** = Period of Communicability　**E** = Means of Exposure
SP = Susceptible Persons　**PR** = Prophylaxis　**APT** = Asymptomatic Patient Precautions
PRS = Personnel Restrictions　**IPT** = Infected Patient Precautions (in addition to Standard Precautions)
PR = private room; **M** = mask; **GL** = gloves; **GW** = gown

COXSACKIE VIRUS (HAND, FOOT, AND MOUTH DISEASE)	**IP**	Three to five days.
	PC	During acute illness; shedding can persist for several weeks.
		Direct contact with upper respiratory secretions or feces.
	E	Universal susceptibility.
	SP	None
	PR	None
	APT	None
	PRS	None
	IPT	GL for handling infective substances; contact precautions for infants and children.

EPIDEMIOLOGICALLY IMPORTANT COMMUNICABLE DISEASES

IP = Incubation Period; PC = Period of Communicability; E = Means of Exposure
SP = Susceptible Persons; PR = Prophylaxis; APT = Asymptomatic Patient Precautions
PRS = Personnel Restrictions; IPT = Infected Patient Precautions (in addition to Standard Precautions)
PR = private room; M = mask; GL = gloves; GW = gown

DIPHTHERIA, PHARYNGEAL	**IP**	Two to five days, occasionally longer.
	PC	Treated persons who do not become carriers: usually from beginning of symptoms to ≥4 days after beginning effective therapy. Untreated persons who do not become carriers: from beginning of symptoms to two to four weeks. Persons who become carriers: from beginning of symptoms to six months or longer.
	E	1) Physical contact with respiratory secretions of an infectious person, or 2) Close proximity (three to six feet) to an infectious person for more than several minutes.
	SP	Primarily those with no history of diphtheria and incomplete vaccination; however, infection can occur even in immunized persons.

continues on next page

EPIDEMIOLOGICALLY IMPORTANT COMMUNICABLE DISEASES

IP = Incubation Period | **PC** = Period of Communicability | **E** = Means of Exposure
SP = Susceptible Persons | **PR** = Prophylaxis | **APT** = Asymptomatic Patient Precautions
PRS = Personnel Restrictions | **IPT** = Infected Patient Precautions (in addition to Standard Precautions)
PR = private room; **M** = mask; **GL** = gloves; **GW** = gown

DIPHTHERIA, PHARYNGEAL *continued*	**PR**	All exposed persons should be given a seven day course of oral erythromycin (40–50 mg/kg/d) or benzathine penicillin G (600,000 1,200,000U IM), provided there are no contraindications. Diphtheria toxoid vaccination: 1) *Exposed persons who have completed primary diphtheria series (>3 doses)*. If last dose was >5 years: Give booster, provided there are no contraindications; otherwise no vaccine is necessary. 2) *Exposed persons who have not completed primary diphtheria vaccination series (<3 doses)*. Give vaccine dose and complete primary series according to schedule, provided there are no contraindications.
	APT	Exposed patients should have nasal and pharyngeal cultures taken for *Corynebacterium diphtheriae*. If exposed patients develop symptoms of pharyngitis: contact precautions with mask, private room required until final culture results are negative. If exposed patients do not develop symptoms of pharyngitis: no isolation unless cultures are positive. Patients with positive cultures should be kept in isolation until two cultures from nose and pharynx taken at least 24 hours apart after cessation of antibiotics are negative.

continues on next page

EPIDEMIOLOGICALLY IMPORTANT COMMUNICABLE DISEASES

IP = Incubation Period | **PC** = Period of Communicability | **E** = Means of Exposure
SP = Susceptible Persons | **PR** = Prophylaxis | **APT** = Asymptomatic Patient Precautions
PRS = Personnel Restrictions | **IPT** = Infected Patient Precautions (in addition to Standard Precautions)
PR = private room; **M** = mask; **GL** = gloves; **GW** = gown

DIPHTHERIA, PHARYNGEAL *continued*	**PRS**	Exposed personnel should have nasal and pharyngeal cultures taken for *Corynebacterium diphtheria*. If exposed personnel develop symptoms of pharyngitis: Exclude from duty until final culture results are negative. If exposed personnel do not develop symptoms of pharyngitis: Do not exclude from duty unless cultures are positive. Personnel with positive cultures should be excluded from duty until two cultures from nose and pharynx, taken at least 24 hours apart after cessation of antibiotics, are negative.
	IPT	PR, M until two negative nose and throat cultures at least 24 hours apart after antimicrobial therapy stopped; GL for touching infective material; GW if soiling is likely.

IP = Incubation Period
SP = Susceptible Persons
PRS = Personnel Restrictions
PC = Period of Communicability
PR = Prophylaxis
IPT = Infected Patient Precautions (in addition to Standard Precautions)
E = Means of Exposure
APT = Asymptomatic Patient Precautions

PR = private room; **M** = mask; **GL** = gloves; **GW** = gown

E. COLI (0-157)–**ASSOCIATED DIARRHEA**	**IP**	Variable, usually three days.
	PC	During diarrhea and several days thereafter, until stool is culture negative.
	E	1) Ingestion of contaminated food. 2) Handling of contaminated feces.
	SP	Those having contact with infected feces or who have ingested contaminated food.
	PR	None
	APT	None
	PRS	None
	IPT	PR if patient hygiene poor; GL for handling feces; GW if soiling is likely.

EPIDEMIOLOGICALLY IMPORTANT COMMUNICABLE DISEASES

IP = Incubation Period | **PC** = Period of Communicability | **E** = Means of Exposure
SP = Susceptible Persons | **PR** = Prophylaxis | **APT** = Asymptomatic Patient Precautions
PRS = Personnel Restrictions | **IPT** = Infected Patient Precautions (in addition to Standard Precautions)
PR = private room; **M** = mask; **GL** = gloves; **GW** = gown

FIFTH'S DISEASE (HUNGARIAN MEASLES/ ERYTHEMA INFECTIOSUM/ HUMAN PARVOVIRUS)	**IP**	Variable; four to 20 days.
	CP	In rash illness—greatest before onset of rash; in aplastic crisis probably up to one week after onset of symptoms; in immunosuppressed persons with chronic disease—months to years.
	E	1) Direct contact with respiratory secretions. 2) From mother to fetus. 3) Rarely through transfusion of blood or blood products.
	SP	Universal susceptibility; protection appears to be conferred with development of B19 antibodies.
	PR	None
	APT	None; pregnant women should be advised of the potential for acquiring infection, the potential risks to the fetus; pregnant women with contact with sick children should wash hands frequently and avoid sharing eating utensils.
	PRS	None
	IPT	GL for handling contaminated items; droplet precautions.

EPIDEMIOLOGICALLY IMPORTANT COMMUNICABLE DISEASES

IP = Incubation Period · **PC** = Period of Communicability · **E** = Means of Exposure
SP = Susceptible Persons · **PR** = Prophylaxis · **APT** = Asymptomatic Patient Precautions
PRS = Personnel Restrictions · **IPT** = Infected Patient Precautions (in addition to Standard Precautions)
PR = private room; **M** = mask; **GL** = gloves; **GW** = gown

HEPATITIS A	**IP**	15–50 days (average 25–30 days).
	PC	Two weeks prior to onset of symptoms through the 10th day after onset.
	E	1) Intimate contact with infected person. 2) Ingestion of contaminated food. 3) Handling of contaminated feces.
	SP	Those who have had close person-to-person contact with infected persons or have ingested contaminated food. Persons without history of HAV infection.
	PR	IG prophylaxis (0.02 mL/kg) recommended within two weeks after exposure for: 1) Household members, 2) Residents/staff in institutions for mentally retarded, 3) Children/staff in day care setting, and 4) Food handlers.
	APT	None
	PRS	None
	IPT	PR if patient hygiene is poor; GL for touching infective material; GW if soiling is likely.

EPIDEMIOLOGICALLY IMPORTANT COMMUNICABLE DISEASES

IP = Incubation Period **PC** = Period of Communicability **E** = Means of Exposure
SP = Susceptible Persons **PR** = Prophylaxis **APT** = Asymptomatic Patient Precautions
PRS = Personnel Restrictions **IPT** = Infected Patient Precautions (in addition to Standard Precautions)
PR = private room; **M** = mask; **GL** = gloves; **GW** = gown

HEPATITIS B	**IP**	45–160 days (average of 120 days).
	PC	As long as blood tests positive for hepatitis B surface antigen.
	E	1) Percutaneous injury through contaminated needles or sharps. 2) Mucous membrane exposure to contaminated blood or body fluids. 3) Sexual exposure.
	SP	1) Persons who have a negative history for hepatitis B infection. 2) Persons who have not received hepatitis B vaccination. 3) Persons with negative hepatitis B surface antibody and core antibody.
	PR	Hepatitis B IG (HBIG 0.06 mL/kg) should be given within 24 hours of exposure plus initiation of hepatitis B vaccination. Pre-exposure vaccination recommended for persons at substantial risk for acquiring hepatitis B virus (HBV) infection.
	APT	None
	PRS	None
	IPT	Usually none; case-by-case decision in surgical setting. GL for touching infective material; GW if soiling is likely.

EPIDEMIOLOGICALLY IMPORTANT COMMUNICABLE DISEASES

IP = Incubation Period	**PC** = Period of Communicability	**E** = Means of Exposure
SP = Susceptible Persons	**PR** = Prophylaxis	**APT** = Asymptomatic Patient Precautions
PRS = Personnel Restrictions	**IPT** = Infected Patient Precautions (in addition to Standard Precautions)	

PR = private room; **M** = mask; **GL** = gloves; **GW** = gown

HEPATITIS C	**IP**	Two weeks to six months (most within six to nine weeks).
	PC	One or more weeks before onset of first symptoms through acute clinical course of the disease and indefinitely in chronic carriers.
	E	Percutaneous injury through contaminated needles or sharps.
	SP	Those persons who have percutaneous exposure to contaminated blood or plasma derivatives.
	PR	None
	APT	None
	PRS	None
	IPT	GL for touching infective material; GW if soiling is likely.

EPIDEMIOLOGICALLY IMPORTANT COMMUNICABLE DISEASES

IP = Incubation Period   **PC** = Period of Communicability   **E** = Means of Exposure
SP = Susceptible Persons   **PR** = Prophylaxis   **APT** = Asymptomatic Patient Precautions
PRS = Personnel Restrictions   **IPT** = Infected Patient Precautions (in addition to Standard Precautions)
PR = private room; **M** = mask; **GL** = gloves; **GW** = gown

HERPES SIMPLEX	**IP**	Two to 12 days.
	PC	Seven to 12 days.
	E	For HSV-1 direct contact with saliva, for HSV-2 usually sexual contact.
	SP	Universal susceptibility.
	PR	None
	APT	**C-section is advised before rupture of membranes when primary HSV infections occur late in pregnancy.**
	PRS	Genital infections—no restriction; hands (herpetic whitlow)-restrict from patient contact and contact with the patient's environment until lesions heal; orofacial—evaluate the need to restrict from care of high-risk patients.
	IPT	GL for touching infective material; GW if soiling is likely; contact precautions for neonatal patients and disseminated or primary severe lesions.

EPIDEMIOLOGICALLY IMPORTANT COMMUNICABLE DISEASES

IP = Incubation Period | **PC** = Period of Communicability | **E** = Means of Exposure
SP = Susceptible Persons | **PR** = Prophylaxis | **APT** = Asymptomatic Patient Precautions
PRS = Personnel Restrictions | **IPT** = Infected Patient Precautions (in addition to Standard Precautions)
PR = private room; **M** = mask; **GL** = gloves; **GW** = gown

HUMAN IMMUNODEFICIENCY VIRUS (HIV)	**IP**	Variable; time from infection to development of detectable antibodies generally one to three months. Time from HIV infection to diagnosis of AIDS <1 year to 10 years or longer (avg. 10 years).
	PC	Presumed to be indefinite; infectiousness increases with increased immunodeficiency and initial period after infection.
	E	1) Percutaneous injury through contaminated needles or sharps. 2) Mucous membrane exposure to contaminated blood or body fluids. 3) Sexual exposure.
	SP	Presumably all exposed persons.
	APT	None
	PRS	None
	IPT	GL for touching infective material; GW if soiling is likely.

EPIDEMIOLOGICALLY IMPORTANT COMMUNICABLE DISEASES

IP = Incubation Period | PC = Period of Communicability | E = Means of Exposure
SP = Susceptible Persons | PR = Prophylaxis | APT = Asymptomatic Patient Precautions
PRS = Personnel Restrictions | IPT = Infected Patient Precautions (in addition to Standard Precautions)
PR = private room; M = mask; GL = gloves; GW = gown

IMPETIGO	IP	Four to 10 days for *S. aureus;* One to three days for *S. pyogenes* (group A Strep).
	PC	As long as purulence continues for *S. aureus;* carrier states and autoreinfection can occur 10–21 days in uncomplicated cases due to *S. pyogenes*. (See *Streptococcus pyogenes* below.)
	E	Direct contact with drainage usually via unwashed hands.
	SP	Universal susceptibility.
	APT	None
	PRS	Restrict from patient care, contact with patient's environment, and food handling until 24 hours after initiation of appropriate antibiotic therapy.
	IPT	GL for touching infective material; GW if soiling is likely; contact precautions until 24 hours following appropriate antibiotic therapy; GL for touching infective material; GW if soiling is likely.

EPIDEMIOLOGICALLY IMPORTANT COMMUNICABLE DISEASES

IP = Incubation Period **PC** = Period of Communicability **E** = Means of Exposure
SP = Susceptible Persons **PR** = Prophylaxis **APT** = Asymptomatic Patient Precautions
PRS = Personnel Restrictions **IPT** = Infected Patient Precautions (in addition to Standard Precautions)
PR = private room; **M** = mask; **GL** = gloves; **GW** = gown

INFLUENZA	**IP**	Usually one to three days.
	PC	From 24 hours before onset of symptoms until three to five days after onset of symptoms in adults; in children, until seven or more days after onset of symptoms.
	E	1) Close proximity (three to six feet) to an infectious person for more than several minutes, or 2) Same-room proximity to an infectious person for 1 hour or more.
	SP	Those with no history of disease or vaccination of the specific vaccine protective against the current prevalent viral strain.
	PR	Amantadine or rimantadine hydrochloride is recommended after exposure to influenza A (not B), provided there are no contraindications, for susceptible elderly persons and persons with underlying health problems. Amantadine/rimantadine dosage: children >20 kg, adults 100 mg/day. Doses should be reduced for those >65 years or with decreased hepatic and renal function.
	APT	None
	PRS	None
	IPT	M; PR if possible.

EPIDEMIOLOGICALLY IMPORTANT COMMUNICABLE DISEASES

IP = Incubation Period **PC** = Period of Communicability **E** = Means of Exposure
SP = Susceptible Persons **PR** = Prophylaxis **APT** = Asymptomatic Patient Precautions
PRS = Personnel Restrictions **IPT** = Infected Patient Precautions (in addition to Standard Precautions)
PR = private room; **M** = mask; **GL** = gloves; **GW** = gown

LICE	**IP**	Seven to 10 days.
	PC	As long as lice or eggs remain viable on the infested person or fomites; may survive seven to 10 days away from host (eggs, 10 days); persons considered communicable until 24 hours after treatment with an effective insecticide.
	E	1) Direct contact with infested person. 2) Use of personal objects of an infested person (e.g., headgear, clothing, and combs).
	SP	Those who have person-to-person contact or have shared personal objects with the infested person.
	PR	None
	APT	None
	PRS	None
	IPT	GL for touching infective material.

EPIDEMIOLOGICALLY IMPORTANT COMMUNICABLE DISEASES		
IP = Incubation Period **SP** = Susceptible Persons **PRS** = Personnel Restrictions	**PC** = Period of Communicability **PR** = Prophylaxis **IPT** = Infected Patient Precautions (in addition to Standard Precautions)	**E** = Means of Exposure **APT** = Asymptomatic Patient Precautions
PR = private room; **M** = mask; **GL** = gloves; **GW** = gown		
LYME DISEASE *(Borrelia burgdorferi)*	**IP**	Seven to 14 days but can be as short as three days or as long as 30 days.
	PC	None
	E	Legged ticks *(Ixodes scapularis)* in the Northeastern and North-Central part of the US; western black legged ticks *(Ixodes pacificus)*.
	SP	All persons thought to be susceptible, however, persons who live or work in residential areas surrounded by woods or overgrown brush infested by vector ticks or persons who participate in outdoor activities in these areas.
	PR	Applying insect repellents containing DEET (n,n-diethyl-m-toluamide) to clothes and exposed skin and applying permethrin to clothes; also covering of all exposed body parts with light colored clothing; daily check for ticks and prompt removal.
	APT	None
	PRS	None
	IPT	None

EPIDEMIOLOGICALLY IMPORTANT COMMUNICABLE DISEASES

IP = Incubation Period **PC** = Period of Communicability **E** = Means of Exposure
SP = Susceptible Persons **PR** = Prophylaxis **APT** = Asymptomatic Patient Precautions
PRS = Personnel Restrictions **IPT** = Infected Patient Precautions (in addition to Standard Precautions)
PR = private room; **M** = mask; **GL** = gloves; **GW** = gown

MEASLES (RUBEOLA)	**IP**	Seven to 18 days.
	PC	From one to two days before onset of symptoms (three to five days before rash) until four days after onset of rash.
	E	1) Same-room proximity to an infectious person for any amount of time. 2) Presence in a room previously occupied by an infectious patient within the previous one to four hours, depending on room size and ventilation characteristics.
	SP	Those with negative measles antibody titers. When titers are not available, susceptible persons are presumed to be persons born after 1956 who do not have either documentation of physician-diagnosed measles or history of two doses of measles vaccine taken on and after the first birthday.
	PR	**Susceptible, immunocompetent, exposed persons >6 months of age:** Measles vaccine (0.5 mL SC), measles–rubella (MR), or measles–mumps–rubella (MMR) is recommended (provided there are no contraindications) and should be given as soon as possible within 72 hours of exposure.

EPIDEMIOLOGICALLY IMPORTANT COMMUNICABLE DISEASES

IP = Incubation Period | **PC** = Period of Communicability | **E** = Means of Exposure
SP = Susceptible Persons | **PR** = Prophylaxis | **APT** = Asymptomatic Patient Precautions
PRS = Personnel Restrictions | **IPT** = Infected Patient Precautions (in addition to Standard Precautions)
PR = private room; **M** = mask; **GL** = gloves; **GW** = gown

MEASLES (RUBEOLA) *continued*		**Susceptible, exposed persons <6 months of age and immunocompromised persons of any age:** Immune globulin 0.25 mL/kg body weight, IM. For immunocompromised persons 0.5 mL/kg IM (maximum 15 mL) is recommended (provided there are no contraindications) and should be given as soon as possible within six days of exposure.
	APT	If vaccine is taken <72 hours after exposure: no isolation. If vaccine is not taken or is taken >72 hours after exposure: isolation on days five to 21 after exposure.
	PRS	If vaccine is taken <72 hours after exposure: Do not exclude from duty. If vaccine is not taken or is taken >72 hours after exposure: exclude from duty on days five to 21 after exposure. In outstanding situations, susceptible exposed personnel should be relieved from direct patient contact on days five to 21 after exposure regardless of whether they received measles vaccine or IG or if they became ill, for four days after rash. The vaccine virus has not been shown to be communicable.
	IPT	PR with special ventilation; M; nonsusceptible persons do not need a mask. Susceptible persons should stay out of room if possible.

EPIDEMIOLOGICALLY IMPORTANT COMMUNICABLE DISEASES

IP = Incubation Period; **PC** = Period of Communicability; **E** = Means of Exposure
SP = Susceptible Persons; **PR** = Prophylaxis; **APT** = Asymptomatic Patient Precautions
PRS = Personnel Restrictions; **IPT** = Infected Patient Precautions (in addition to Standard Precautions)
PR = private room; **M** = mask; **GL** = gloves; **GW** = gown

MENINGOCOCCAL DISEASE, INVASIVE (e.g., respiratory tract infection, bacteremia, meningitis)	**IP**	One to 10 days (usually three to four days).
	PC	Until 24 hours after initiation of effective therapy.
	E	Face-to-face proximity to an infectious person while respiratory secretions are being handled (e.g., mouth-to-mouth resuscitation, intubation, suctioning) before initiation of appropriate treatment.
	SP	All persons are considered susceptible unless they have been recently infected by the same *N. meningitidis* strain as the source person.
	PR	Rifampin (10 mg/kg, maximum 600 mg) q12 h for two days (provided there are no contraindications). Alternative regimen: 18 years old: ciprofloxacin 500 mg × 1 dose. Pregnancy: ceftriaxone 250 mg, IM, × 1 dose
	APT	None
	PRS	None
	IPT	PR, M

EPIDEMIOLOGICALLY IMPORTANT COMMUNICABLE DISEASES

IP = Incubation Period **PC** = Period of Communicability **E** = Means of Exposure
SP = Susceptible Persons **PR** = Prophylaxis **APT** = Asymptomatic Patient Precautions
PRS = Personnel Restrictions **IPT** = Infected Patient Precautions (in addition to Standard Precautions)
PR = private room; **M** = mask; **GL** = gloves; **GW** = gown

MUMPS	**IP**	12–25 days (usually 16–18 days).
	PC	From seven days before onset of parotid swelling until nine days after onset.
	E	1) Contact with respiratory secretions of an infectious person; or 2) Close proximity (three to six feet) to an infectious person for more than several minutes; or 3) Same-room proximity to an infectious person for ≥1 hour.
	SP	Those with negative mumps antibody titers. When titers are not available, SP are presumed to be those born after 1956 who have no history of mumps or history of mumps vaccination on or after the first birthday.
	PR	None; vaccination may be considered for prevention of disease in susceptible persons following *future* exposure.
	APT	M, PR on days 10–25.
	PRS	Exclude from duty on days 10–25 after exposure.
	IPT	M, PR; Nonsusceptible persons need not wear a mask.

EPIDEMIOLOGICALLY IMPORTANT COMMUNICABLE DISEASES

IP = Incubation Period **PC** = Period of Communicability **E** = Means of Exposure
SP = Susceptible Persons **PR** = Prophylaxis **APT** = Asymptomatic Patient Precautions
PRS = Personnel Restrictions **IPT** = Infected Patient Precautions (in addition to Standard Precautions)
PR = private room; **M** = mask; **GL** = gloves; **GW** = gown

PERTUSSIS	IP	Five to 21 days (usually seven to 10 days).
	PC	From the beginning of the catarrhal stage until completion of seven days of effective antibiotic therapy. If effective antibiotic therapy is not taken, the period of communicability may last as long as three weeks.
	E	1) Contact with respiratory secretions of an infectious person; or 2) Close proximity (three to six feet) to an infectious person for more than several minutes.
	SP	Primarily those with no history of pertussis and incomplete vaccination; however, infection can occur even in immunized person.
	PR	**Persons ≥7 years of age;** erythromycin (40–50 mg/kg/d), maximum 2 g for 14 days (provided there are no contraindications) irrespective of vaccination status. **Persons <7 years of age;** erythromycin for 14 days (provided there are no contraindications) **and** pertussis vaccine, depending on age and vaccination history.

EPIDEMIOLOGICALLY IMPORTANT COMMUNICABLE DISEASES

IP = Incubation Period | **PC** = Period of Communicability | **E** = Means of Exposure
SP = Susceptible Persons | **PR** = Prophylaxis | **APT** = Asymptomatic Patient Precautions
PRS = Personnel Restrictions | **IPT** = Infected Patient Precautions (in addition to Standard Precautions)
PR = private room; **M** = mask; **GL** = gloves; **GW** = gown

PERTUSSIS *continued*	**APT**	If effective antibiotic therapy is not taken; precautions with mask, private room required on days five to 21 after exposure. If effective antibiotic therapy is taken, M, PR required until completion of five days of therapy.
	PRS	None
	IPT	PR, M
PINWORMS ***(Enterobius vermicularis)***	**IP**	Two to six weeks.
	PC	As long as eggs are being laid on perianal skin.
	E	Direct contact from anus to mouth usually via unwashed hands, contaminated food, clothing, or bedding.
	SP	Universal susceptibility.
	PR	Specific treatment with pyrantel pamoate (Antiminth®, Combantrin®), mebendazole (Vermox®), or albendazole (Zental®). Treatment should be repeated after two weeks. Concurrent treatment of all household and school contacts when there are several infected.
	APT	None
	PRS	None
	IPT	GL for touching infective material.

EPIDEMIOLOGICALLY IMPORTANT COMMUNICABLE DISEASES

IP = Incubation Period; PC = Period of Communicability; E = Means of Exposure
SP = Susceptible Persons; PR = Prophylaxis; APT = Asymptomatic Patient Precautions
PRS = Personnel Restrictions; IPT = Infected Patient Precautions (in addition to Standard Precautions)
PR = private room; M = mask; GL = gloves; GW = gown

RESPIRATORY SYNCYTIAL VIRUS (RSV)	**IP**	Two to eight days.
	PC	Shedding of virus occurs for several weeks following infection.
	E	Direct contact with infected respiratory secretions usually via unwashed hands.
	SP	Susceptibility is universal; illness is more severe in infants, children, and the elderly.
	PR	None
	APT	Exposed patients can be cohorted.
	PRS	Restrict personnel with URI symptoms from caring for high-risk infants/children; cohort exposed personnel with infected patients.
	IPT	Contact precautions in pediatric units; patients with laboratory-documented RSV infection can be cohorted; GL for touching infective material.

EPIDEMIOLOGICALLY IMPORTANT COMMUNICABLE DISEASES

IP = Incubation Period **PC** = Period of Communicability **E** = Means of Exposure
SP = Susceptible Persons **PR** = Prophylaxis **APT** = Asymptomatic Patient Precautions
PRS = Personnel Restrictions **IPT** = Infected Patient Precautions (in addition to Standard Precautions)
PR = private room; **M** = mask; **GL** = gloves; **GW** = gown

RINGWORM (FUNGUS)	**IP**	10–14 days.
	PC	As long as active lesions are present.
	E	1) Direct skin-to-skin contact with infected person or animal. 2) Contact with contaminated items such as barber clippers, combs, etc.
	SP	Children below the age of puberty are highly susceptible to *Microsporum canis*; all ages are susceptible to *Trichophytan* infections; reinfections are rare.
	PR	None
	APT	None
	PRS	None
	IPT	None; GL for touching infective material.

EPIDEMIOLOGICALLY IMPORTANT COMMUNICABLE DISEASES

IP = Incubation Period; **PC** = Period of Communicability; **E** = Means of Exposure
SP = Susceptible Persons; **PR** = Prophylaxis; **APT** = Asymptomatic Patient Precautions
PRS = Personnel Restrictions; **IPT** = Infected Patient Precautions (in addition to Standard Precautions)
PR = private room; **M** = mask; **GL** = gloves; **GW** = gown

ROTAVIRUS	**IP**	24–72 hours.
	PC	During the acute stages of the disease and later while virus shedding continues. Usually ≤ 8 days; can be prolonged in immunocompromised patients.
	E	Probably fecal–oral with possible contact and respiratory spread.
	SP	Susceptibility is greatest between six and 24 months of age.
	PR	None
	APT	None
	PRS	None
	IPT	GL for touching infective material; GW if soiling is likely. PR if cohort infected patients.

EPIDEMIOLOGICALLY IMPORTANT COMMUNICABLE DISEASES

IP = Incubation Period　**PC** = Period of Communicability　**E** = Means of Exposure
SP = Susceptible Persons　**PR** = Prophylaxis　**APT** = Asymptomatic Patient Precautions
PRS = Personnel Restrictions　**IPT** = Infected Patient Precautions (in addition to Standard Precautions)
PR = private room; **M** = mask; **GL** = gloves; **GW** = gown

RUBELLA	IP	14–23 days.
	PC	From seven days before and five days after onset of rash.
	E	1) Contact with respiratory secretions of an infectious person; or 2) Close proximity (three to six feet) to an infectious person for more than several minutes; or 3) Same-room proximity to an infectious person for ≥1 hour.
	SP	Those with negative rubella antibody titers. When titers are not available, SP are presumed to be those who have no history of rubella or history of rubella vaccination on or after the first birthday.
	PR	None, except that immune globulin (0.55 mL/kg) may be considered in certain situations during pregnancy.
	APT	PR, M on days seven to 23 after exposure.
	PRS	Exclude from duty on days seven to 23 after exposure.
	IPT	PR, M

EPIDEMIOLOGICALLY IMPORTANT COMMUNICABLE DISEASES

IP = Incubation Period; **PC** = Period of Communicability; **E** = Means of Exposure
SP = Susceptible Persons; **PR** = Prophylaxis; **APT** = Asymptomatic Patient Precautions
PRS = Personnel Restrictions; **IPT** = Infected Patient Precautions (in addition to Standard Precautions)

PR = private room; **M** = mask; **GL** = gloves; **GW** = gown

SALMONELLA DIARRHEA	**IP**	**six to 72 hours**
	PC	During acute illness and until organism no longer is present in the feces; usually several weeks, although some persons may be carriers for prolonged periods.
	E	1) Direct contact with feces usually via unwashed hands. 2) Ingestion of contaminated food (e.g., eggs, poultry) or water. 3) Direct contact with contaminated pets such as turtles or other reptiles.
	SP	Universal susceptibility increased by antacid therapy, immunosuppression, broad-spectrum antibiotic therapy, and GI surgery.
	PR	None
	APT	None
	PRS	None; may exclude infected personnel from food handling and care of high-risk patients.
	IPT	GL for touching infective material; GW if soiling is likely.

EPIDEMIOLOGICALLY IMPORTANT COMMUNICABLE DISEASES

IP = Incubation Period	**PC** = Period of Communicability	**E** = Means of Exposure
SP = Susceptible Persons	**PR** = Prophylaxis	**APT** = Asymptomatic Patient Precautions
PRS = Personnel Restrictions	**IPT** = Infected Patient Precautions (in addition to Standard Precautions)	

PR = private room; **M** = mask; **GL** = gloves; **GW** = gown

SCABIES	**IP**	Two to six weeks in those without previous exposure. One to four days in those with prior scabies infestation.
	PC	Transmission possible immediately after infestation. Persons considered communicable until 24 hours after treatment with an effective insecticide.
	E	1) Direct contact with infested person; or 2) Use of personal objects of an infested person: combs, bed linens, brushes, scarves, hats, pillows, towels, clothing, earphones.
	SP	Those who have person-to-person contact or have shared personal objects with the infested person.
	PR	Indicated for prolonged skin-to-skin contact or household contacts; 5% permethrin (Elimite®), 1% lindane (Kwell®) (avoid use for infants and pregnant women); or crotamiton (Eural®) lotion.
	APT	None
	PRS	None
	IPT	PR; GL, GW for touching infective material.

EPIDEMIOLOGICALLY IMPORTANT COMMUNICABLE DISEASES

IP = Incubation Period; PC = Period of Communicability; E = Means of Exposure
SP = Susceptible Persons; PR = Prophylaxis; APT = Asymptomatic Patient Precautions
PRS = Personnel Restrictions; IPT = Infected Patient Precautions (in addition to Standard Precautions)
PR = private room; M = mask; GL = gloves; GW = gown

SHIGELLA DIARRHEA (DYSENTERY)	IP	12–96 hours
	PC	During acute illness and while bacteria are being shed into the feces, usually within four weeks of infection.
	E	1) Direct contact with feces usually via unwashed hands, or 2) Ingestion of contaminated food or water.
	SP	Universal susceptibility after ingestion of a small number of organisms. Disease is more severe in young children, the elderly, and the debilitated.
	PR	None
	APT	None
	PRS	None; may exclude infected personnel from food handling and care of high-risk patients.
	IPT	GL for touching infective material; GW if soiling is likely.

EPIDEMIOLOGICALLY IMPORTANT COMMUNICABLE DISEASES

IP = Incubation Period PC = Period of Communicability E = Means of Exposure
SP = Susceptible Persons PR = Prophylaxis APT = Asymptomatic Patient Precautions
PRS = Personnel Restrictions IPT = Infected Patient Precautions (in addition to Standard Precautions)
PR = private room; M = mask; GL = gloves; GW = gown

SMALLPOX (VARIOLA)	IP	Seven to 19 days; commonly 10-14 days to onset of illness and two to four days more to onset of rash.
	PC	From the time of development of the earliest lesions to disappearance of all scabs; about three weeks. The most contagious period is before onset of rash by aerosol droplets from oropharyngeal lesions.
	E	By aerosol droplets from oropharyngeal lesions.
	SP	Unvaccinated or > 10 years since vaccination.
	PR	Immunization with vaccinia virus vaccine.
	APT/ PRS	IMMEDIATE TELEPHONIC COMMUNICATION WITH LOCAL AND STATE HEALTH AUTHORITIES AND THE CDC.
	IPT	PR, GL, GW; Respirator, Airborne isolation with negative pressure ventilation.

EPIDEMIOLOGICALLY IMPORTANT COMMUNICABLE DISEASES

IP = Incubation Period | **PC** = Period of Communicability | **E** = Means of Exposure
SP = Susceptible Persons | **PR** = Prophylaxis | **APT** = Asymptomatic Patient Precautions
PRS = Personnel Restrictions | **IPT** = Infected Patient Precautions (in addition to Standard Precautions)
PR = private room; **M** = mask; **GL** = gloves; **GW** = gown

STREPTOCOCCUS PYOGENES (Group A)	**IP**	Usually two to five days for pharyngitis; seven to 10 days for skin infection.
	PC	(**untreated**): 10–21 days. (**treated**): One to two days.
	E	Direct or intimate contact with patients or carriers.
	SP	Presumably all, but susceptibility may vary.
	PR	Not routinely recommended; may be considered in outbreak situations following culture documentation.
	APT	None
	PRS	None, except in outbreak situations with culture documentation of asymptomatic carriers.
	IPT	Respiratory tract infections in infants and young children: PR, M. Soft-tissue infections: PR; GL when touching infective material; GW if soiling is likely.

EPIDEMIOLOGICALLY IMPORTANT COMMUNICABLE DISEASES

IP = Incubation Period; **PC** = Period of Communicability; **E** = Means of Exposure
SP = Susceptible Persons; **PR** = Prophylaxis; **APT** = Asymptomatic Patient Precautions
PRS = Personnel Restrictions; **IPT** = Infected Patient Precautions (in addition to Standard Precautions)
PR = private room; **M** = mask; **GL** = gloves; **GW** = gown

TUBERCULOSIS (TB)	**IP**	From infection to positive PPD skin test or active TB disease, usually four to 12 weeks.
	PC	Depends on the number and virulence of bacilli discharged, adequacy of ventilation, coughing, sneezing, etc. Effective antimicrobial chemotherapy usually eliminates contagion within a few weeks.
	E	1) Same-room proximity to a person with AFB smear-positive, culture-positive respiratory tract TB for any amount of time; or 2) Same-room proximity to a person with AFB smear-negative, culture-positive respiratory tract TB during cough-inducing procedures or other procedures which aerosolize respiratory secretions; or 3) During autopsies, if precautionary measures are not taken, same-room proximity to the body of a patient with AFB smear-positive tuberculosis lesions in tissues.
	SP	All persons are presumed to be susceptible, although persons with preexisting latent TB infection or past BCG vaccination may be less susceptible to TB infection or active disease.
	PR	INH prophylaxis is used for persons whose PPD skin tests convert from negative to positive after exposure.

EPIDEMIOLOGICALLY IMPORTANT COMMUNICABLE DISEASES

IP = Incubation Period **PC** = Period of Communicability **E** = Means of Exposure
SP = Susceptible Persons **PR** = Prophylaxis **APT** = Asymptomatic Patient Precautions
PRS = Personnel Restrictions **IPT** = Infected Patient Precautions (in addition to Standard Precautions)
PR = private room; **M** = mask; **GL** = gloves; **GW** = gown

TUBERCULOSIS (TB) *continued*	**APT**	None, if no active disease.
	PRS	During active disease.
	IPT	PR, with negative pressure ventilation, use of respirator mask.
WEST NILE VIRUS	**E**	Mosquitoes become infected with West Nile virus when they feed on infected birds that carry the virus in their blood. After 10-14 days, mosquitoes can then transmit West Nile virus to humans and other animals while biting during blood feasting.
	SP	All persons are presumed to be susceptible; however, older adults are at higher risk.
	PR	None
	APT	None
	PRS	None
	IPT	None

* Durations apply to personnel who do not develop disease after exposure.
** Durations apply to patients who do not develop disease after exposure.
*** Exposure to an infectious source person who is not isolated.

Acute Care Nosocomial Surveillance

Overview

- Surveillance activities in acute-care facilities should include surveillance for nosocomial and community acquired infections in addition to quality of care surveillance and performance improvement. The Surveillance and Performance Improvement Process Steps should be followed (Refer to the chapter in this section).

Purpose

- Effective nosocomial surveillance in acute-care facilities can reduce morbidity, mortality, and costs associated with these infections and increase patient, provider, and staff satisfaction. Surveillance with associated performance improvement activities can be used to meet accreditation and regulatory requirements.

Risk Factors

- Use of invasive devices (e.g., indwelling urinary catheters, intravascular catheters).
- Invasive diagnostic and therapeutic procedures (surgery, diagnostic probes).
- Patient endogenous organisms.
- Exogenous organisms transmitted by staff, other patients, or contaminated equipment.

Strategies for Prevention

- Priority-based surveillance is preferred over comprehensive (total house) surveillance to focus on opportunities for improvement based on identified high-risk populations or activities, problem prone areas, or high-volume populations or activities.
- Definitions are not all inclusive but are focused on infections that are common and may be facility acquired.
- For the majority of bacterial nosocomial infections, the infection usually becomes evident 48 hours or more following admission; however, each infection must be assessed individually for evidence that links it to the healthcare facility.
  - All symptoms must be new or acutely worse.
  - Noninfectious causes of signs and symptoms should always be considered and ruled out before identifying as an infection.
- Data sources for identifying infections include clinical findings, microbiology results, other laboratory results, radiology findings, etc.
- Classification of infection as nosocomial usually is based on a combination of clinical and laboratory data; supportive data (e.g., X-rays, pathology reports) also may be used as appropriate.
- Physician/surgeon diagnosis of infection is an acceptable criterion, unless there is evidence to the contrary.
- Preventability of an infection is not a consideration when determining whether it is nosocomial.
- Surveillance definitions are not intended to be the reason for making treatment decisions.
- Conditions that are not infectious but may be misleading when doing surveillance:

- Colonization—presence of organisms in or on a body site, but not causing clinical signs or symptoms of infection.
- Inflammation—a condition that results from response to injury or stimulation by a noninfectious agent.

➤ Considered to be nosocomial:

- Infection acquired in the healthcare facility but not clinically evident until after discharge from the facility.
- Infection in neonates resulting from passage through the birth canal.

➤ Not considered to be nosocomial:

- Infection associated with a complication or extension of infection already present at the time of admission, unless a change in pathogen or symptoms strongly suggests the acquisition of a new infection.
- In infants, an infection known or proved to have been acquired transplacentally (e.g., cytomegalovirus, rubella), and becomes evident at or before 48 hours after birth.

➤ Analysis and interpretation are integral components of the surveillance process.

- Nosocomial infections should be analyzed as rates versus raw numbers. (Refer to Section 2 – General Surveillance Considerations for rate formulas.)
    - Numerators represent the number of infections in a specific category.
    - Denominators represent days or persons at risk for developing the infection in each category.
- Surveillance should be accompanied by analysis to identify improvement opportunities; action plans to address these opportunities, and evaluation of improvement efforts.

- National Nosocomial Infection Surveillance System (NNIS) can be used to compare facility rates to nationally reported rates provided that the NNIS methodology is used when collecting and analyzing data.
  - This system was established in 1970 when selected hospitals routinely began reporting their nosocomial infection surveillance data for aggregation into a national database. There are currently more than 300 hospitals participating in NNIS.
  - NNIS data are collected using standardized protocols called surveillance components for ICUs: adult, pediatric and high-risk nursery, and surgical cases.
  - Aggregated results are published annually in the *American Journal of Infection Control* providing:
    - Pooled means and percentiles of rates for each population and selected infection categories by risk factor (e.g., device type, birth weight, surgical site risk index).
    - Device utilization ratios by each ICU type.
    - Antimicrobial use and resistant rates by ICU versus non ICU populations.

➤ Interventions and action plans should be developed based on analysis. Refer to Sections 2 - 7 for topic specific prevention recommendations.

References/Resources

- Association for Professionals in Infection Control and Epidemiology. APIC Text of Infection Control and Epidemiology. 2000, chapter 13, appendices 13A and 13B.
- Association for Professionals in Infection Control and Epidemiology, Inc. APIC position statement on the release of nosocomial infections. Am J Infect Control 1998; 17(2).
- NNIS. National nosocomial infections surveillance (NNIS) system report, data summary from January 1992 - June 2001, issued August 2001. Am J Infect Control 2001; 29:404-21.

SELECTED ACUTE CARE DEFINITIONS OF INFECTIONS

Site/Infection	Criteria	Comments
Bloodstream Laboratory Confirmed Patient ≥ 12 months old	**One of:** ➤ Recognized pathogen isolated from one or more blood cultures. ➤ Common skin contaminant (e.g., Diphtheroids, Bacillus sp., Proprionobacterim sp., Coagulase-negative staphylococci) isolated from two blood culture drawn on separate occasions. ➤ Common skin contaminant isolated from at least one blood culture from person with intravascular access device and physician institutes appropriate antimicrobial therapy. ➤ Positive antigen test on blood (e.g., *H. influenzae*, *S. pneumoniae*, *N. meningitidis*, or group B streptococci).	Primary: Device related; no other source of infection identified. Secondary: Related to an infection at another site such as urinary tract, respiratory tract or wound site.
Clinical Sepsis ≥ 12 months old	**Two of:** ➤ At least one clinical sign/symptom: ▪ Fever (>38°C) ▪ Hypotension (systolic pressure ≤ 90 mm Hg ▪ Oliguria (> 20 mL/h output) *continued*	No other source of infection identified.

SELECTED ACUTE CARE DEFINITIONS OF INFECTIONS

Site/Infection	Criteria	Comments
	➤ And no blood culture performed or organisms isolated in culture or no antigen detected. ➤ Or physician institutes appropriate antimicrobial therapy for sepsis.	
Laboratory Confirmed Patient ≤ 12 months old	**Both:** ➤ At least one symptom: ▪ Fever ▪ Apnea ▪ Bradycardia ➤ And at least one of: ▪ Common skin contaminant isolated form two blood cultures drawn on separate occasions, ▪ Common skin contaminant isolated from patient with intravascular access device and physician institutes appropriate antimicrobial therapy, or ▪ Positive antigen test on blood (e.g., *H. influenzae*, *S. pneumoniae*, *N. meningitidis*, or group B streptococci).	Primary: Device related; no other source of infection identified. Secondary: Related to an infection at another site such as urinary tract, respiratory tract, or wound site.

SELECTED ACUTE CARE DEFINITIONS OF INFECTIONS		
Site/Infection	**Criteria**	**Comments**
Clinical Sepsis Patient ≤ 12 months old	**All of:** ➤ At least one clinical sign/symptom: ▪ Fever >38°C ▪ Hypothermia (<37°C) ▪ Apnea ▪ Bradycardia ➤ And no blood culture performed or organisms isolated in culture or no antigen detected. ➤ And physician institutes appropriate antimicrobial therapy for sepsis.	No other source of infection identified.
Respiratory Pneumonia Patients ≥ 12 months old	One of: ➤ Rales or dullness to percussion on physical examination of chest and at least one of: ▪ New onset of purulent sputum or change in character of sputum, ▪ Organism isolated from blood culture, or ▪ Isolation of pathogen from specimen obtained by transtracheal aspirate, bronchial brushing, or biopsy.	

SELECTED ACUTE CARE DEFINITIONS OF INFECTIONS

Site/Infection	Criteria	Comments
Respiratory Pneumonia Patients ≥ 12 months old *continued*	➤ Chest radiographic examination shows new or progressive infiltrate, consolidation, cavitation, or pleural effusion and at least one of: ▪ New onset of purulent sputum or change in character of sputum, ▪ Organism isolated from blood culture, ▪ Isolation of pathogen from specimen obtained by transtracheal aspirate, bronchial brushing, or biopsy, ▪ Isolation of virus or detection of viral antigen in respiratory secretions, ▪ Diagnostic single antibody titer (IgM) or fourfold increase in paired serum samples (IgG) for pathogens, or ▪ Histopathologic evidence of pneumonia. **Both:** ➤ Chest radiographic examination shows new or progressive infiltrate, consolidation, cavitation, or pleural effusion or at least two symptoms: ▪ Apnea ▪ Tachypnea	

SELECTED ACUTE CARE DEFINITIONS OF INFECTIONS

Site/Infection	Criteria	Comments
Respiratory Pneumonia Patients ≥ 12 months old *continued*	▪ Bradycardia ▪ Wheezing ▪ Rhonchi ▪ Cough ➤ And at least one of: ▪ Increased production of respiratory secretions, ▪ New onset of purulent sputum or change in character of sputum, ▪ Organism isolated from blood culture, ➤ Isolation of pathogen from specimen obtained by transtracheal aspirate, bronchial brushing, or biopsy, ➤ Isolation of virus or detection of viral antigen in respiratory secretions, ➤ Diagnostic single antibody titer (IgM) or fourfold increase in paired serum samples (IgG) for pathogens, or ➤ Histopathologic evidence of pneumonia.	

SELECTED ACUTE CARE DEFINITIONS OF INFECTIONS

Site/Infection	Criteria	Comments
Urinary Tract Symptomatic UTI ≥ 12 months old	**One of:** ➤ Urine culture obtained aseptically (e.g., by clean catch, bladder catheterization or suprapubic aspiration) and at least one of: ▪ Fever (>38°C) ▪ Urgency ▪ Frequency ▪ Dysuria ▪ Suprapubic tenderness	
	Both: ➤ At least two symptoms: ▪ Fever (>38°C) ▪ Urgency ▪ Frequency ▪ Dysuria ▪ Suprapubic tenderness ➤ With at least one of: ▪ Dipstick test positive for leukocyte esterase and/or nitrate ▪ Pyuria (≥ 10 white blood cells (WBC)/mL or 3 WBC/high power field of unspun urine), *continues on next page*	

SELECTED ACUTE CARE DEFINITIONS OF INFECTIONS

Site/Infection	Criteria	Comments
Urinary Tract Symptomatic UTI $\geq$ 12 months old *continued*	▪ Organisms seen on Gram stain of unspun urine, ▪ Two urine cultures with repeated isolation of the same uropathogen (Gram negative bacteria or *Staphylococcus saprophyticus*) with $\geq 10^2$ colonies/mL urine in nonvoided specimens, ▪ Urine culture with $\geq 10^5$ colonies/mL urine of single uropathogen in patient being treated with appropriate antimicrobial therapy, ▪ Physician's diagnosis, or ▪ Physician institutes appropriate antimicrobial therapy.	

SELECTED ACUTE CARE DEFINITIONS OF INFECTIONS

Site/Infection	Criteria	Comments
Urinary Tract Symptomatic UTI ≤ 12 months old	**One of:** ➤ Urine culture with ≥ 10^5 colonies/mL urine with no more than two species of organisms and at least one of: ▪ Fever (>38°C) ▪ Hypothermia (<37°C) ▪ Apnea ▪ Bradycardia ▪ Dysuria ▪ Lethargy ▪ Vomiting **Both:** ➤ At least two symptoms: ▪ Fever (>38°C) ▪ Hypothermia (<37°C) ▪ Apnea ▪ Bradycardia ▪ Dysuria ▪ Lethargy ▪ Vomiting	

SELECTED ACUTE CARE DEFINITIONS OF INFECTIONS

Site/Infection	Criteria	Comments
Urinary Tract Symptomatic UTI ≤ 12 months old *continued*	➤ **With at least one of:** ▪ Dipstick test positive for leukocyte esterase and/or nitrate, ▪ Pyuria (≥ 10 white blood cells (Wbc)/mL or 3 Wbc/high power field of unspun urine), ▪ Organisms seen on Gram stain of unspun urine, ▪ Two urine cultures with repeated isolation of the same uropathogen (Gram negative bacteria or *Staphylococcus saprophyticus*) with ≥ 10^2 colonies/mL urine in nonvoided specimens, ▪ Urine culture with ≥ 10^5 colonies/mL urine of single uropathogen in patient being treated with appropriate antimicrobial therapy, ▪ Physician's diagnosis, or ▪ Physician institutes appropriate antimicrobial therapy.	

SELECTED ACUTE CARE DEFINITIONS OF INFECTIONS

Site/Infection	Criteria	Comments
Asymptomatic Bacteriuria—Catheter related	**Both:** ➤ No symptoms: ▪ Fever ▪ Urgency ▪ Frequency ▪ Dysuria ▪ Suprapubic tenderness ➤ And urine culture with $\geq 10^5$ colonies/mL urine with no more than two species of organisms.	Catheter in place within seven days of culture.
Asymptomatic Bacteriuria—Not catheter related	**Both:** ➤ No symptoms: ▪ Fever ▪ Urgency ▪ Frequency ▪ Dysuria ▪ Suprapubic tenderness ➤ And two urine cultures with $\geq 10^5$ colonies/mL urine same organisms with no more than two species of organisms.	No catheter in place within seven days of culture.

SELECTED ACUTE CARE DEFINITIONS OF INFECTIONS

Site/Infection	Criteria	Comments
Surgical Site Superficial	**One of:** ➤ Purulent drainage from the superficial incision, ➤ Organisms isolated form an aseptically obtained culture of fluid or tissue form the superficial incision, or ➤ At least one sign or symptom of infection: ▪ Pain or tenderness at site ▪ Localized swelling ▪ Redness ▪ Heat and organisms cultured from site (pathogens, or if skin contaminants, pure culture) or organisms cultured from blood.	Infection within 30 days of surgical procedure (one year for implanted devices) involving skin and/or subcutaneous tissue. Data collection methods may include: ➤ Routine direct wound examination by trained professional. ➤ Outpatient chart review by trained professionals. ➤ Surgeon reporting (self/survey). ➤ Patient reporting (self/survey). ➤ Telephone survey of patient. ➤ Review of microbiology data.

SELECTED ACUTE CARE DEFINITIONS OF INFECTIONS		
Site/Infection	**Criteria**	**Comments**
Deep	**One of:** ➤ Purulent drainage from the deep incision but not from the organ/space component of the surgical site, ➤ Deep incision spontaneously dehisces or is deliberately opened by a surgeon and is culture positive or not cultured (a culture negative finding does not meet this criterion) when a patient has one of more of: ▪ Fever ▪ Localized pain or tenderness, ➤ An abscess or other evidence of infection involving the deep incision is found on direct examination during reoperation or by histopathologic or radiologic examination, or ➤ Diagnosis of a deep incisional SSI by a surgeon or attending physician.	Infection within 30 days of surgical procedure (one year for implanted devices) involving deep soft tissues (e.g., fascial and muscle layers). Data collection methods may include: ➤ Routine direct wound examination by trained professional. ➤ Outpatient chart review by trained professionals. ➤ Surgeon reporting (self/survey). ➤ Patient reporting (self/survey). ➤ Telephone survey of patient. ➤ Review of microbiology data.

SELECTED ACUTE CARE DEFINITIONS OF INFECTIONS		
Site/Infection	**Criteria**	**Comments**
Organ/Space	One of: ➤ Purulent drainage form a drain that is place through a stab wound into the organ/space, ➤ Organisms isolated form an aseptically obtained culture or fluid or tissue in the organ/space, ➤ Abscess or other evidence of infection that is found on direct examination of the organ/space during reoperation, or by histopathologic or radiologic examination, or ➤ Diagnosis of an organ/space SSI by a surgeon or attending physician.	Infection within 30 days of surgical procedure (one year for implanted devices) involving any part of the body; excluding skin incision, fascia, or muscle layers that is opened or manipulated during the operative procedure. Data collection methods may include: ➤ Routine direct wound examination by trained professional. ➤ Outpatient chart review by trained professionals. ➤ Surgeon reporting (self/survey). ➤ Patient reporting (self/survey).

SELECTED ACUTE CARE DEFINITIONS OF INFECTIONS

Site/Infection	Criteria	Comments
		➤ Telephone survey of patient. ➤ Review of microbiology. data
Surgical Site risk index	➤ One point if the surgical site is dirty or contaminated. ➤ One point if the patients ASA score is a three, four, or five prior to the procedures (American Society of Anesthesiology). ➤ One point if the procedure lasted longer than "T" hours where "T" is the approximate 75th percentile for the duration of surgery as published in the NNIS database (see reference).	Scores for surgical risk are zero, one, two, or three.
Additional sites		Refer to CDC Definitions of Infection—see references.

Long-Term Care Nosocomial Surveillance

Overview

- Surveillance activities in long-term care facilities should include identification of nosocomial and community acquired infections in addition to quality of care surveillance and performance improvement. Refer to Section 4-Long Term Care Facilities for more details. The Surveillance and Performance Improvement Process Steps should be followed (Refer to the chapter in this section). Because there is generally less laboratory and technological support in the long-term care facility, definitions of infection used in surveillance may be more symptoms based. Signs and symptoms of infection may be more difficult to identify in the elderly due to diminished immune status, mental status, etc.

Purpose

- Effective nosocomial surveillance in long-term care facilities can reduce morbidity, mortality, and costs associated with these infections and increase patient, provider, and staff satisfaction. Surveillance with associated performance improvement activities are required to meet state and federal (Centers for Medicaid and Medicare Studies or CMS previously known as HCFA) regulations.

Risk Factors

- Predominately populated by elderly and often debilitated, bedridden residents.
- Long stays.
- Use of invasive devices (e.g., indwelling catheters, intravascular devices) and procedures (e.g., respiratory suctioning, dialysis).

Strategies for Prevention

- Priority-based surveillance is preferred over comprehensive (total house) surveillance to focus on opportunities for improvement based on identified high-risk populations or activities, problem prone areas, or high-volume populations or activities.
- Definitions are not all inclusive but are focused on infections that are common and may be facility acquired.
- For the majority of bacterial nosocomial infections, the infection usually becomes evident 48 hours or more following admission; however, each infection must be assessed individually for evidence that links it to the healthcare facility.
  - All symptoms must be new or acutely worse.
  - Noninfectious causes of signs and symptoms should always be considered and ruled out before identifying as an infection.
- Data sources for identifying infections include clinical findings, microbiology results, other laboratory results, radiology findings, etc.
- Frequent indicators of infection in the elderly can be used as case finding events for possible infections and include:
  - The presence of delirium (acute confusional state).
  - A rise in body temperature.
  - Worsening mental or functional status.

- Loss of appetite.
- Decrease in blood pressure or pulse.
- Fall without previous history of falls.

➤ Conditions that are not infectious but may be misleading when doing surveillance:

- Colonization—presence of organisms in or on a body site, but not causing clinical signs or symptoms of infection.
- Inflammation—a condition that results from response to injury or stimulation by a noninfectious agent.

➤ Analysis and interpretation is an integral component of surveillance:

- Nosocomial infections should be analyzed as rates versus raw numbers (Refer to Section 2 – General Surveillance Considerations for rate formulas).
    - Numerators represent the number of infections in a specific category.
    - Denominators represent days or persons at risk for developing the infection in each category.
- Surveillance should be accompanied by analysis to identify improvement opportunities; action plans to address these opportunities, and evaluation of improvement efforts.

➤ Interventions and action plans should be developed based on analysis. Refer to Sections 2 - 7 for topic specific prevention recommendations.

References/Resources

- Association for Professionals in Infection Control and Epidemiology. APIC Text of Infection Control and Epidemiology. 2000, chapters 35,37,46.
- McGeer, A, Campbell B, Emori TG, et al. Commentary. Definitions of infections in long-term care facilities. Am. J Infect Control 1991; 19:1-7.
- Smith PW and Rushnak PG. Infection Prevention and Control in the Long-term care Facility. Infection Control and Hospital Epidemiology 1997; 18(12): 831-4.

LONG-TERM CARE DEFINITIONS OF INFECTIONS

Site/Infection	Criteria	Comments
Respiratory Tract Common cold	**Two or more:** ➤ Runny nose or sneezing, ➤ Stuffy nose, hoarseness, or difficulty swallowing, ➤ Dry cough, or ➤ Swollen or tender glands in the neck.	Symptoms must be acute and not allergy related. Fever not required, but does not exclude diagnosis.
Sinusitis	Diagnosis by a physician or practitioner.	
Influenza-like illness	**Fever and two or more:** ➤ Chills, ➤ Headache or eye pain, ➤ Myalgias (muscle aches), ➤ Sore throat, or ➤ Dry cough.	Symptoms must be acute. Usually during influenza season; generally November through March.
Pneumonia	**Both:** ➤ Interpretation by a radiologist of a chest X-ray as demonstrating pneumonia, probably pneumonia or the presence of new infiltrates with a compatible clinical syndrome, and ➤ At least two symptoms as described under lower respiratory tract infections.	Noninfectious causes must be ruled out (e.g., Congestive Heart Failure).

LONG-TERM CARE DEFINITIONS OF INFECTIONS

Site/Infection	Criteria	Comments
Other Lower Respiratory Tract Infection	**Three or more:** ➤ New or increased cough, ➤ New or increased sputum production, ➤ Fever, ➤ Pleuritic chest pain, or ➤ New physical findings on chest exam (rales, rhonchi, wheezing, bronchial breathing).	Symptoms must be acute. Either no chest X-ray done, or X-ray does not meet the definition for pneumonia above.
Urinary Tract Symptomatic UTI	**No catheter and three or more:** ➤ Fever or chills, ➤ New burning pain on urinating, or frequency or urgency, ➤ Flank or suprapubic pain or tenderness, ➤ Change in character of urine (visual, or by smell, or by lab testing), or ➤ Change in mental or functional status, including new or worse incontinence. **Catheter and two or more:** ➤ Fever or chills, ➤ Flank or suprapubic pain or tenderness, ➤ Change in character of urine, or ➤ Change in mental or functional status.	No other source of infection is identified.

LONG-TERM CARE DEFINITIONS OF INFECTIONS

Site/Infection	Criteria	Comments
Asymptomatic Bacteriuria	**Both:** ➤ Urinalysis showing >100,000 bacterial colonies, and ➤ No signs and symptoms of UTI above.	
GI Tract Gastroenteritis	**One of:** ➤ Two or more loose or watery stools above what is normal for the resident within a 24 hour period, ➤ Two or more episodes of vomiting within a 24 hour period, or ➤ Stool culture positive for a pathogen (Salmonella, Shigella, Campylobacter, *Clostridium difficile*, etc.) with at least one clinical symptom: ▪ Nausea ▪ Vomiting ▪ Abdominal pain/tenderness ▪ Diarrhea	For the first two criteria, there must be no evidence of a noninfectious cause (e.g., diarrhea due to laxative use, change in tube feeding or medication or vomiting due to change in medication, peptic ulcer).

LONG-TERM CARE DEFINITIONS OF INFECTIONS

Site/Infection	Criteria	Comments
Skin Cellulitis / Soft Tissue / Wound	**One of:** ➤ Pus is present at a wound, skin, or soft tissue site, or ➤ Four or more symptoms: ▪ Fever (>38°C) ▪ Worsening mental/functional status ▪ Worsening of status of wound site ▪ Heat ▪ Redness ▪ Swelling ▪ Tenderness ▪ Serous drainage	
Fungal skin infection	**Both:** ➤ Maculopapular rash (e.g., abnormally colored, usually red, flat, or slightly raised area of skin in varying sizes), and ➤ Physician or practitioner diagnosis or laboratory confirmation.	No evidence of a noninfectious cause (e.g., allergy to medication, lotions, etc.). Other diagnoses ruled out (e.g., Impetigo, Scabies).

LONG-TERM CARE DEFINITIONS OF INFECTIONS

Site/Infection	Criteria	Comments
Herpes Simplex (Cold Sores) or Varicella Zoster (Shingles)	**Both:** ➤ Vesicular rash (blister like skin lesions containing watery fluid), and ➤ Physician or practitioner diagnosis or laboratory confirmation.	Usually not a nosocomial infection.
Scabies	**One of:** ➤ Undiagnosed macular (flat) or popular (slightly raised) rash different in color or texture than skin, ➤ Dry thickened, scaling skin with documented tracks, or ➤ Itching rash and physician or practitioner diagnosis or laboratory confirmation.	Care must be taken to ensure that a rash is not allergic or secondary to a skin irritation.

LONG-TERM CARE DEFINITIONS OF INFECTIONS

Site/Infection	Criteria	Comments
Eye, Ear, Nose and Mouth Conjunctivitis (e.g., Pink Eye, Epidemic Keratoconjuncitivis)	**One of:** ➤ Pus appearing from one or both eyes for > 24 hours with or without redness, itching or pain, or ➤ Conjunctival redness often with itching and pain for > 24 hours.	No evidence of eye trauma (e.g., foreign body or allergy).
Ear	**One of:** ➤ Physician or practitioner diagnosis, or ➤ Drainage from one or both ears with or without pain.	
Mouth/Peri-Oral	Physician or practitioner or dentist diagnosis.	

LONG-TERM CARE DEFINITIONS OF INFECTIONS

Site/Infection	Criteria	Comments
Bloodstream (Primary)	**One of:** ➤ ≥ Two blood cultures positive for the same organism, ➤ One blood culture with a non contaminant organism (e.g., NOT Diphtheroids, Bacillus sp, Corynebacterium sp., or Coagulase-negative staphylococcus) and at least one of: ▪ Fever ≥ 38°C ▪ New hypothermia (≤ 34.5°C) or doesn't register on thermometer ▪ Drop in systolic blood pressure > 30 mm Hg from baseline ▪ Worsening of mental or functional status	Primary: Device related; no other source of infection identified.
Unexplained Febrile Episode	➤ Documentation in the medical record of fever on ≥ *two* or more occasions at least 12 hours apart in any three day period.	No other infectious or noninfectious (e.g., medication reaction) source identified.

Home Care Nosocomial Surveillance

Overview

- Surveillance activities in home care should be focused on identifying trends within the agency clientele over time and to provide staff and caregiver/patient education targeted at reducing risk of infection. Refer to Section 4-Home Care.
- The Surveillance and Performance Improvement Process Steps should be followed (Refer to the chapter in this section).

Purpose

- Describing infections as nosocomial or home health associated does not mean that they are caused by home care delivery, only that it they are identified by time, place, and definition as such so that appropriate interventions for infection prevention can be designed and implemented.

Risk Factors

- Various environmental factors may contribute to the development of infection including poor sanitation, inadequate utilities such as plumbing, electricity, or rodent infestation.
- Patient/family behaviors such as poor hygienic practices.
- Community exposures to disease.

Strategies for Prevention

- Home health associated infections refer to infections that develop in patients who are receiving home healthcare and that were neither present not incubating at the time the patient began receiving home healthcare (generally 48-72 hours after admission but may vary based on the incubation time of the infectious pathogen).
- An infection that develops in a patient who has been receiving home healthcare and is subsequently admitted to a healthcare facility may be considered a home health associated infection if it is determined to have been incubating at the time of discharge from home healthcare.
- Surgical site infection occurring within 30 days from the date of surgery (one year for surgically implanted devices) may be a nosocomial infection related to the surgical procedure performed in an acute or non-acute care facility. Surgical site infections should be reported to the facility where the surgery was performed.
- Conditions that are not infectious but may be misleading when doing surveillance:
  - Colonization—presence of organisms in or on a body site, but not causing clinical signs or symptoms of infection.
  - Inflammation—a condition that results from response to injury or stimulation by a noninfectious agent.
- Infections should be analyzed as rates versus raw numbers. Numerators represent the number of infections in a specific category and denominators represent days or persons at risk for developing the infection in each category.
- Surveillance should be accompanied by analysis to identify improvement opportunities; action plans to address these opportunities and evaluation of improvement efforts.

References/Resources

- Association for Professionals in Infection Control and Epidemiology. APIC Text of Infection Control and Epidemiology. 2000, chapter 13, appendices 13A and 13B,25,44,85-92,120.
- McGeer, A, Campbell B, Emori TG, et al. Commentary. Definitions of infections in long-term care facilities. *Am. J Infect Control* 1991; 19:1-7.
- Smith PW and Rushnak PG. Infection Prevention and Control in the Long-term care Facility. *Infection Control and Hospital Epidemiology* 1997; 18(12): 831-49.

HOME CARE DEFINITIONS OF INFECTIONS note: adults only

Site/Infection	Criteria	Comments
Respiratory Tract Common cold or pharyngitis	**Two or more:** ➤ Runny nose or sneezing, ➤ Stuffy nose, hoarseness, or difficulty swallowing, ➤ Dry cough, or ➤ New swollen or tender glands in the neck	Symptoms must be acute and not allergy related. Fever not required, but does not exclude diagnosis.
Sinusitis	Diagnosis by a physician or practitioner.	
Influenza-like illness	**Both:** ➤ Fever ➤ At lease three symptoms ▪ Chills ▪ Headache or eye pain ▪ Myalgias (muscle aches) or loss of appetite ▪ Sore throat ▪ New or increased dry cough	Symptoms must be acute. During influenza season (generally November through March) if both criteria for influenza-like illness and upper or lower respiratory tract infections are met, count only as influenza-like illness.

HOME CARE DEFINITIONS OF INFECTIONS note: adults only

Site/Infection	Criteria	Comments
Pneumonia	**One of:** ➤ Rales of dullness on physical examination of the chest and either one or both: ▪ New onset of purulent sputum or change in character of sputum, a/o ▪ Organisms cultured from the blood. ➤ Chest radiograph that shows new or progressive infiltrate, consolidation, cavitation, or pleural effusion and one or both: ▪ New onset of purulent sputum or change in character of sputum, a/o ▪ Organisms cultured from the blood.	Noninfectious causes such as congestive heart failure should be ruled out.

HOME CARE DEFINITIONS OF INFECTIONS note: adults only		
Site/Infection	**Criteria**	**Comments**
Other Lower Respiratory Tract Infection	**Three or more without chest film or the chest film did not confirm pneumonia:** ➤ New or increased cough ➤ New or increased sputum production ➤ New or increase purulence of sputum ➤ Fever ➤ Pleuritic chest pain ➤ New or increased physical findings on chest exam (rales, rhonchi, wheezing, bronchial breathing) ➤ Change in status (e.g., new or increased shortness of breath, increase respiratory rate, worsening mental or functional status)	Symptoms must be acute.

HOME CARE DEFINITIONS OF INFECTIONS note: adults only

Site/Infection	Criteria	Comments
Urinary Tract Symptomatic UTI	**Catheterized or noncatheterized** **Three or more:** ➤ Fever or chills (>100.4°F) ➤ Flank or suprapubic pain or tenderness ➤ Change in character of urine (e.g., new bloody urine, foul odor, increased or by lab testing) ➤ Change in mental or functional status, including new or worse incontinence **Two or more:** ➤ Urinalysis with pyuria (urine specimen with ≥ 3 WBC/high power field of unspun urine and positive nitrite and/or leukocyte esterase test	For urine specimens to be of value, they must be obtained aseptically using an appropriate technique or suprapubic aspiration.

HOME CARE DEFINITIONS OF INFECTIONS note: adults only		
Site/Infection	**Criteria**	**Comments**
GI Tract Gastroenteritis	**One of:** ➤ Two or more loose or watery stools above what is normal for the patient/client within a 24 hour period ➤ Two or more episodes of vomiting within a 24 hour period ➤ Stool culture positive for a pathogen (Salmonella, Shigella, Campylobacter, Clostridridium difficile, etc.) with at least one clinical symptom: ➤ Nausea ➤ Vomiting ➤ Abdominal pain/tenderness ➤ Diarrhea	For the first two criteria, there must be no evidence of a noninfectious cause (e.g., diarrhea due to laxative use, change in tube feeding or medication or vomiting due to change in medication, peptic ulcer).

HOME CARE DEFINITIONS OF INFECTIONS note: adults only		
Site/Infection	Criteria	Comments
Skin Cellulitis / Soft Tissue / Wound	**One of:** ➤ Pus is present at a wound, skin, or soft tissue site, or ➤ Two or more of: ▪ Worsening mental/functional status ▪ Pain or tenderness at sits ▪ Localized swelling ▪ Redness ▪ Swelling ▪ Heat and organisms cultured from site (pathogens, or if skin contaminants, pure culture) or organisms cultured from blood	

HOME CARE DEFINITIONS OF INFECTIONS note: adults only

Site/Infection	Criteria	Comments
Superficial surgical site infection	**One of:** ➤ Purulent drainage from the superficial incision ➤ Organisms isolated from an aseptically obtained culture of fluid or tissue form the superficial incision ➤ At least one sign or symptom of infection: ▪ Pain or tenderness at site ▪ Localized swelling ▪ Redness ▪ Heat and organisms cultured from site (pathogens, or if skin contaminants, pure culture) or organisms cultured from blood	Infection within 30 days of surgical procedure (one year for implanted devices) involving skin and/or subcutaneous tissue.

HOME CARE DEFINITIONS OF INFECTIONS note: adults only		
Site/Infection	**Criteria**	**Comments**
Deep surgical site infection	**One of:** ➤ Purulent drainage from the deep incision but not from the organ/space component of the surgical site ➤ Deep incision spontaneously dehisces or is deliberately opened by a surgeon and is culture positive or not cultured (a culture negative finding does not meet this criterion) when a patient has one of more of: ▪ Fever ▪ Localized pain or tenderness ➤ An abscess or other evidence of infection involving the deep incision is found on direct examination during reoperation or by histopathologic or radiologic examination ➤ Diagnosis of a deep incisional SSI by a surgeon or attending physician	Infection within 30 days of surgical procedure (one year for implanted devices) involving deep soft tissues (e.g., fascial and muscle layers) or the incision.

HOME CARE DEFINITIONS OF INFECTIONS note: adults only

Site/Infection	Criteria	Comments
Organ/space surgical site infection	**One of:** ➤ Purulent drainage from a drain that is place through a stab wound into the organ/space ➤ Organisms isolated form an aseptically obtained culture or fluid or tissue in the organ/space ➤ Abscess or other evidence of infection that is found on direct examination of the organ/space during reoperation, or by histopathologic or radiologic examination ➤ Diagnosis of an organ/space SSI by a surgeon or attending physician	Infection within 30 days of surgical procedure (one year for implanted devices) involving any part of the body; excluding skin incision, fascia, or muscle layers that is opened or manipulated during the operative procedure.
Fungal skin infection	**Two of:** ➤ Maculopapular rash (e.g., abnormally colored, usually red, flat or slightly raised area of skin in varying sizes) ➤ Physician or practitioner diagnosis or laboratory confirmation ➤ No evidence of a noninfectious cause (e.g., allergy to medication, lotions, etc.)	No evidence of a noninfectious cause (e.g., allergy to medication, lotions, etc.). Other diagnoses ruled out (e.g., Impetigo, Scabies).

HOME CARE DEFINITIONS OF INFECTIONS note: adults only		
Site/Infection	**Criteria**	**Comments**
Herpes Simplex (Cold Sores) or Varicella Zoster (Shingles)	**Two of:** ➤ Vesicular rash (blister like skin lesions containing watery fluid) ➤ Physician or practitioner diagnosis or laboratory confirmation	Usually not a healthcare associated infection.
IV site infection	**Two of:** ➤ Presence of purulent drainage at the entry site for a peripheral or centrally place intravascular line ➤ Blood culture no done or no organisms detected in blood cultures	
Eye, Ear, Nose and Mouth Conjunctivitis (e.g., Pink Eye, Epidemic Keratoconjuncitivis)	**One of:** ➤ Pus appearing from one or both eyes for > 24 hours with or without redness, itching or pain, or ➤ Conjunctival redness often with itching and pain for > 24 hours	No evidence of eye trauma (e.g., foreign body or allergy).

HOME CARE DEFINITIONS OF INFECTIONS note: adults only		
Site/Infection	**Criteria**	**Comments**
Ear	**One of:** ➤ Physician or practitioner diagnosis, or ➤ Purulent drainage fluid accumulated in the middle ear one or both ears with ear pain or tympanic redness	
Mouth/Peri-Oral	Physician or practitioner or dentist diagnosis.	
Bloodstream (Primary)	**One of:** ➤ ≥ Two blood cultures positive for the same organism ➤ One blood culture with a non contaminant organism (e.g., NOT Diphtheroids, Bacillus sp, Corynebacterium sp., or Coagulase-negative staphylococcus) and at least one of: ▪ Fever ≥ 38°C ▪ New hypothermia (≤ 34.5°C) or doesn't register on thermometer ▪ Drop in systolic blood pressure > 30 mm Hg from baseline ▪ Worsening of mental or functional status	

HOME CARE DEFINITIONS OF INFECTIONS note: adults only		
Site/Infection	**Criteria**	**Comments**
Clinical Sepsis	**Two of:** ➤ At least one clinical sign/symptom ▪ Fever $\geq$ 38°C ▪ Hypotension (systolic pressure $\leq$ 90 mm Hg) ▪ Oliguria (> 20 mL/h output) ➤ No blood culture performed or organisms isolated in culture or no antigen detected ➤ Physician institutes appropriate antimicrobial therapy for sepsis	No other source of infection identified

Environmental Surveillance

Overview

- The JCAHO mandates that "there is a safety management program that is designed to provide a physical environment free of hazards and to manage staff activities to reduce the risk of human injury."
- One method to accomplish the above, coupled with the opportunity to capture information related to risk assessment and management, is to perform environmental surveillance.

Purpose

- Provide a collection tool for environmental surveillance that may be adapted to the healthcare organization.

Risk Factors

- Processes, worker knowledge, competencies, and the physical environment may contribute to increased risk of infectious agent transmission.

Strategies for Prevention

- Combine a routine visit (e.g., education and training program) to a healthcare delivery setting with an opportunity to evaluate risks related to healthcare associated infection. Include interviews with management and employee(s), review of resources and records (e.g., policy/procedure manuals, training competencies), observation of procedure, and walk-through evaluation of the physical environment.
- Data collected and actions taken may be used for quality/process improvement activities.

References and Resources

- Association for Professionals in Infection Control and Epidemiology. APIC Text of Infection Control and Epidemiology. 2000, chapters 4, 24, 72-78.
- Centers for Disease Control and Prevention, Healthcare Infection Control Practices Advisory Committee (HICPAC). Draft guideline for environmental infection control in healthcare facilities, 2001. 2001, Federal Register
- Ibid. Draft guidelines for hand hygiene in healthcare settings. November 2001, Federal Register.
- Henry Ford Health Systems, Detroit, MI, Site visit tool, adapted with permission.

QUESTION/POLICY REFERENCE	YES	NO	N/A	COMMENTS	F/U DATE
A. ADMINISTRATOR/MGR INTERVIEW					
A1. Do you notify IC of reportable communicable diseases? (Pol #___)					
A2. Do you have a current IC manual available to all personnel? (Pol#___)					
A3. Have personnel (full time, part time, agency, volunteer) received IC training within the past 12 months? (Pol #___)					
A4. Do you documentation of personnel training/competency for cleaning, disinfection, and sterilzation? (Pol #___)					
A5. Do you have a triage process in place to identify and separate patients with contagious borne diseases? (Pol#___)					
A6. Do you have a screening process for latex allergic patients?					

QUESTION/POLICY REFERENCE	YES	NO	N/A	COMMENTS	F/U DATE
A7. Do you have latex free supplies available? (Pol#___)					
B. EMPLOYEE INTERVIEW (sample)					
B.1. Do you know what to do if you have an exposure? (Pol#___)					
B.1.a. Needlestick/sharp?					
B.1.b. Other blood/body fluid exposure?					
B.1.c. Tuberculosis?					
B.1.d. Scabies/lice?					
B.2. Do you know the process for triaging patients with communicable diseases? (Pol#___)					

QUESTION/POLICY REFERENCE	YES	NO	N/A	COMMENTS	F/U DATE
C. PROCESS OBSERVATION					
C.1. CLEANING, DISINFECTION, STERILIZATION (IF PERFORMED)					
C.1.a. Appropriate PPE used? (Pol#___) Nitrile gloves for chemical handling, gown, facial protection.					
C.1.b. Enzymatic solution used? (Pol#___)					
C.1.c. Space and ventilation adequate? (Pol#___)					
C.1.d. Workflow acceptable? (Pol#___)					
C.1.e. Approved disinfectant used? (Pol#___)					
C.1.f. Are disinfectant containers covered? (Pol#___)					

QUESTION/POLICY REFERENCE	YES	NO	N/A	COMMENTS	F/U DATE
C.1.g. Are containers labeled with chemical name? (Pol#___)					
C.1.h. Are containers labeled with expiration date? (Pol#___)					
C.1.i. Is the solution tested for dilution? (Pol#___)					
C.1.j. Is an automatic reprocessor used? If yes,					
Is reprocessor maintained appropriately? (Pol#___)					
C.1.k. Are reprocessing procedures posted? (Pol#___)					
C.1.l. Do employees follow established procedures? (Pol#___)					

QUESTION/POLICY REFERENCE	YES	NO	N/A	COMMENTS	F/U DATE
C.1.m. Is a sterilizer used? C.1.m.1 Are BIs used per policy? (Pol#___) C.1.m.2 Are chemical indicators used per policy? (Pol#___)					
C.1.n. Is appropriate packaging used?					
C.1.o. Is event related sterility policy followed? (Pol#___)					
C.2. ASEPTIC TECHNIQUES					
C.2.a. Do employees wash hands when appropriate? (Pol#___) # observed:					
C.2.b. Do employees follow aseptic technique? (Pol#___)					
C.1.p. Are safety showers and eyewash stations available and are they tested per policy? (Pol#___)					

QUESTION/POLICY REFERENCE	YES	NO	N/A	COMMENTS	F/U DATE
D.1. UTILITY ROOM ASSESSMENT					
D.1.a. Are clean and soiled utility areas separated? (Pol#___)					
D.1.b Is space and ventilation adequate? (Pol#___)					
D.1.c. Are external shipping cartons removed? (Pol#___)					
D.1.d. Does storage meet fire regulations? (Pol#___)					
D.1.e. Is stock rotated? (Pol#___)					
D.1.f. Is clean linen stored appropriately? (Pol#___)					

QUESTION/POLICY REFERENCE	YES	NO	N/A	COMMENTS	F/U DATE
E.1. EXAM ROOM ASSESSMENT					
E.1.a. Are appropriate PPE available? (Pol#___)					
E.1.b. Are handwashing facilities adequate? (Pol#___)					
E.1.c. Are handwashing sinks clean? (Pol#___)					
E.1.d. Are only appropriate items stored under sink? (Pol#__)					
E.1.e.Are sharps containers < 3/4 full? (Pol#___)					
E.1.f. Are multi use opened solutions dated and disposed of per policy? (Pol#___)					
E.1.g.Are appropriate waste receptacles (regular, red, Chemotherapy) used? (Pol#___)					

QUESTION/POLICY REFERENCE	YES	NO	N/A	COMMENTS	F/U DATE
E.1.h. Is equipment clean (exam tables, IV poles, monitors, etc.)? (Pol#____)					
F.1.MEDICATION REFRIGERATORS					
F.1.a. Appropriately labeled? (Pol#___)					
F.1.b.Thermometer present? (Pol#___)					
F.1.c.Temperature logged daily? (Pol#___)					
F.1.d.Appropriate items stored? (Pol#___)					
F.1.e.Appropriate action when temperature not adequate? (Pol#___)					
F.1.f.Alarms on when appropriate? (Pol#___)					

QUESTION/POLICY REFERENCE	YES	NO	N/A	COMMENTS	F/U DATE
G.1.FOOD REFRIGERATORS					
G.1.a.Appropriately labeled? (Pol#___)					
G.1.b.Thermometer present? (Pol#___)					
G.1.c.Temperature logged daily? (Pol#___)					
G.1.d.Appropriate items stored? (Pol#___)					
G .1.e. Appropriate action when temperature not adequate? (Pol#___)					
H.1.SPECIMEN REFRIGERATORS					
H.1.a.Appropriately labeled? (Pol#___)					
H.1.b.Thermometer present? (Pol#___)					
H.1.c.Temperature logged daily? (Pol#___)					

QUESTION/POLICY REFERENCE	YES	NO	N/A	COMMENTS	F/U DATE
H.1.d.Appropriate items stored? (Pol#___)					
H.1.e.Appropriate action when temperature not adequate? (Pol#___)					
I.1 TISSUE/BLOOD REFRIGERATORS					
I.1.a.Appropriately labeled? (Pol#___)					
I.1.b.Thermometer present? (Pol#___)					
I.1.c.Temperature logged daily? (Pol#___)					
I.1.d.Appropriate items stored? (Pol#___)					
I.1.e.Appropriate action when temperature not adequate? (Pol#___)					
I.1.f.Alarms on when appropriate? (Pol#___)					

QUESTION/POLICY REFERENCE	YES	NO	N/A	COMMENTS	F/U DATE
J.1.PROCEDURE/TREATMENT ROOMS					
J.1.a Are adequate sterile supplies available? (Pol#___)					
J.1.b. Are appropriate hand scrubs available? (Pol#___)					
J.1.c. Is room size and ventilation appropriate? (Pol#___)					
J.1.d.Is there an adequate method for transporting soiled instruments/equipment to reprocessing area? (Pol#___)					
J.1.e.Is all reprocessing done in appropriate reprocessing area? (Pol#___)					

QUESTION/POLICY REFERENCE	YES	NO	N/A	COMMENTS	F/U DATE
K.1.FACILITY MAINTENANCE					
K.1.a.Are appropriate environmental cleaning agents used? (Pol#___)					
K.1.b.Are cleaning chemicals appropriately diluted? (Pol/Proc#___)					
K.1.c.Are mop heads and cleaning rags changed and Laundered per established procedure? (Pol#___)					
K.1.d. Are cleaning supplies appropriately stored?					
K.1.e.Are horizontal surfaces free of dust? (Pol#___)					
K.1.f. Are ventilation grills dust free? (Pol#___)					

QUESTION/POLICY REFERENCE	YES	NO	N/A	COMMENTS	F/U DATE
K.1.g.Are floors clean? (Pol#___)					
K.1.h. Are surfaces in good repair (e.g., walls, floors, ceiling, grout, caulking)?					
K.1.i. Is there a pest management plan in place? (Pol#____)					
K.1.j.Are ceiling tiles in place and good condition? (Pol#___)					
K.1.k.Is caulking clean and in place where appropriate? (Pol#___)					

QUESTION/POLICY REFERENCE	YES	NO	N/A	COMMENTS	F/U DATE
L.1.CONSTRUCTION/ RENOVATION (if applicable)					
L.1.a.Is there an infection control review of plans? (Pol#___)					
L.1.b.Are dust barriers present and intact? (Pol#___)					
L.1.c.Is signage in place? (Pol#___)					
L.1.d.Is traffic rerouted? (Pol#___)					
L.1.e.Is interim life-safety plan in place? (Pol#___)					

Outbreak Investigation

Overview

- An outbreak (epidemic) of disease can occur at any level of care as well as in the community.
- Outbreaks may be identified by one case of an unusual disease or an increase over the expected number of cases of a disease within a facility or geographic area.
- Outbreaks can cause significant morbidity and in some cases mortality, making expedient identification and prevention strategies a primary goal.
- Surveillance data can often detect outbreaks of diseases but many are detected through clinicians, laboratory workers, or reports to public health officials.

Purpose

- Once an outbreak is recognized, the goal of an investigation is to identify and eliminate the source of infection to prevent additional cases. The results of the investigation in many cases will lead to recommendations or strategies for preventing similar future outbreaks.

Risk Factors

- Late identification of clusters and outbreaks can lead to serious morbidity and mortality outcomes.

- Risks for outbreaks include:
  - Lack of adherence to infection control preventive practices (e.g., aseptic technique, handwashing, immunization, disinfection and sterilization, safe food handling, etc.-refer to Sections 4 and 5 of this handbook for guidelines and recommended practices).
  - Deliberate acts exposing susceptible persons to known pathogens (e.g., bioterrorism).
- Populations at higher risk:
  - Neonates
  - Immunocompromised persons
  - Elderly persons

Strategies for Prevention

- Establish methods and communication practices to assist in early identification of potential clusters and outbreaks.
- Follow basic steps when a suspected or known cluster or outbreak has been identified.
  - Begin preliminary evaluation. Develop a case definition, identify site(s), pathogen(s), and affected host population.
  - Verify the diagnosis. Review each case to meet the definition.
  - Confirm that an outbreak exists. Compare rate of potential outbreak to the usual rate of this infection in the facility.
  - Notify and involve appropriate departments and personnel (e.g., administration, nursing, occupational health) as necessary.
  - Search for additional cases. Identify missed cases using medical and microbiology records. Frequently, records are searched back two to three months prior to the identified initial case.
  - Develop line listings (e.g., person, place, time).

- Develop an epidemic curve. Analyze the data.
- Formulate tentative hypothesis. Perform a literature search and make educated guesses as to what the cause(s) may be of the outbreak.
- Test the hypothesis. Consider morbidity, why the outbreak crosses several services, etc. Remember, hypotheses can be proven false. The hypothesis may be consistent and support the data collected. If the hypothesis is not supported by data, consider another with the additional data and analysis.
- Implement control measures appropriate to the findings in your data and analysis.
- Continue to monitor for further cases and the effectiveness of the control measures. Add or delete new measures to bring the outbreak under control.
- Write up the results and make a report. Summarize the information from the previous steps to show the outcome of the investigation and control measures used. Distribute to appropriate persons and committees.

References/Resources

- Checko P. Outbreak Investigation. APIC Text of Infection Control and Epidemiology, 2000: 15; 1-9.
- Reingold A. Outbreak Investigations – A Perspective. Emerging Infectious Diseases, 1998. 4(1).
- www.cdc.gov/ncidod/eid/vol4no1/reingold.htm

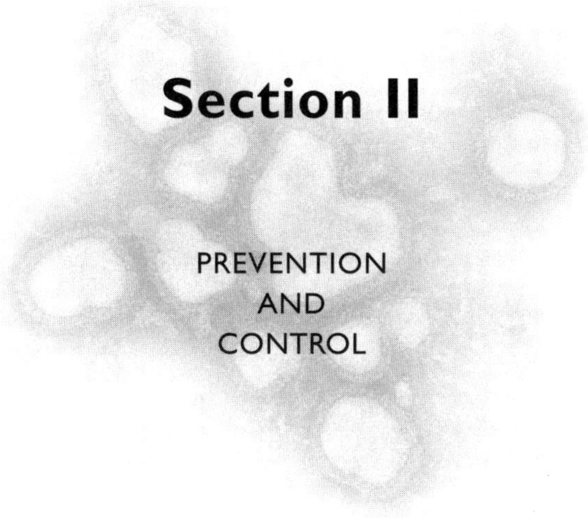

Section II

PREVENTION AND CONTROL

Asepsis

Overview

- Antiseptics, handwashing agents, skin cleansers, and medications should be used in an aseptic and safe manner to prevent harm to patients, clients, or personnel. Safe handling of these items is necessary to prevent contamination.

Purpose

- Aseptic principles and practices are fundamental in reducing infection and related safety risks in the healthcare settings, and success is dependent on effective education and surveillance.

Risk Factors

- Contamination, improper handling, incorrect storage, and/or inappropriate use of antiseptics, handwashing agents, skin cleansers, and medications could increase the risk of infection or adversely affect patient safety.
- Contamination may occur from extrinsic or intrinsic sources, however, some preparations more readily promote microbial growth than others.

Strategies for Prevention

- Personnel should follow basic IC principles, including aseptic technique, to protect themselves, clients, visitors, and others from infectious agents and to maximize safety.

- Only categories and brands of antiseptics, handwashing agents, and skin cleansers approved by the appropriate committee(s) should be used (e.g., Infection Control, Products, and/or the Pharmacy/Therapeutics).
- Only Pharmacy/Therapeutics approved medications should be used.
- Nursing personnel, physicians, physician extenders, medical assistants, therapists, pharmacists, and pharmacy technical who have been trained are responsible for the appropriate use and/or storage of medications and antiseptics.
- Personnel are responsible for the appropriate use of handwashing agents.
- Antiseptics, handwashing agents, and wound cleansers should be used only for the purposes indicated by the manufacturer and as approved by the appropriate committee.
- These items should not be used as equipment or environmental cleansers or disinfectants.
- Single-use unit dose packaging is recommended.
- Multi-use patient care agents and medications should be used in a manner that prevents cross-contamination.
- Multi-use patient items should be patient-specific, whenever possible.
- Agents should be drawn up or dispensed as close as possible to the time of administration to decrease the risk of microorganism proliferation and/or related endotoxin formation.
- Medications from a single syringe should not be given to several patients even if the needle on the syringe is changed.
- Syringes and needles are sterile, single-use items.
- Agents should be handled using a "no-touch" technique. (e.g., do not touch rim, tip or dropper with gauze, applicator, glove, finger, etc.)

- Agents should be discarded if contamination occurs (e.g., bottle lip/rim, tip, or dropper touches a contaminated surface or hand).
- Agents should be discarded if contamination is suspected (e.g., change in color, clarity, odor) or known contaminating event.
- Containers should be labeled with the date and time first entered; unlabeled containers should be discarded.
- Multi-use agents should be aliquoted from their containers in a manner that prevents contamination (e.g., diaphragms on vials and necks of glass ampoules should be swabbed with alcohol and friction and be allowed to dry before entering/opening).
- Agents should be used and disposed of as stated and in the Formulary/Policy/Procedures.
- Consider policy/procedure/protocol for multiple-dose vials without a preservative - discard 24 hours after opening or by the manufacturer's expiration date (whichever occurs first).
- Multiple-dose vials containing a preservative should be discarded by the manufacturer's expiration date.
- Containers should not be reused (e.g., rinsed and refilled).
- Agents should never be transferred from one container to another. (DO NOT "Top Off" - fill a partially used container from another partially used container).
- Agents should be discarded if containers are left open after use; agent containers should be closed.
- Medications used externally or internally should be stored separately in designated and labeled areas.
- Medication refrigerators should be maintained according to manufacturer's recommendations.
- Medications refrigerators should be dedicated for use whenever feasible; segregate/separate when refrigerator should be shared for other purposes.

- Temperatures should be checked and recorded daily; action should be taken and documented if temperature is out of expected range.

References/Resources

- American Society of Anesthesiologists, Recommendations for infection control for the practice of anesthesiology. 1999.
- American Society of Anesthesiologists www.asahq.org
- Association of Operating Room Nurses, Inc., Standards and Recommended Practices, 2000.
- Association for Professionals in Infection Control and Epidemiology. APIC Text of Infection Control and Epidemiology. 2000, chapter 27, 28, 42.
- Association For Professionals on Infection Control and Applied Epidemiology, Inc. Handwashing and skin preparation for invasive procedures. Infection Control and Applied Epidemiology - Principles and Practice. Mosby. 1996.
- Bischoff W., Franchi D., Wenzel R., and Edmond M. Use of multidose-vials in a tertiary care center: cost analysis of 30-day expiration policy versus manufacturer's date policy. Poster Presentation, Infectious Disease Society of America. 1997.
- Bischoff, W., Franchi,D., Wenzel, R., Edmond, M. Multiple dose vial (MDV) policies: Survey of U.S. hospitals. Poster Presentation, Infectious Disease Society of America. 1997.
- Centers for Disease Control and Prevention, Healthcare Infection Control Practices Advisory Committee (HICPAC). Draft guideline for environmental infection control in healthcare facilities, 2001. 2001, Federal Register.
- Ibid. Draft guidelines for hand hygiene in healthcare settings. November 2001, Federal Register.

- Kretzer E., Larson E. Do antiseptic agents reduce surgical wound infections: preoperative bathing, operative site preparation, and surgical hand scrub? Chemical Germicides in Healthcare, International Symposium, May 1994.
- Larson, E. APIC Guidelines for infection control practice-guideline for use of topical antimicrobial agents. Am J of Infect Control 1988; 16:253-266.
- Larson, E. A causal link between handwashing and risk of infection? Examination of the evidence. Infection Control and Hospital Epidemiology 1988; 9: 28-36.
- Loeb M., Wilcox L., Smail F., Walters S. and Duff Z. A randomized trial of surgical scrubbing with brush compared to antiseptic soap alone. American Journal of Infection Control. 1997; 25:11-15.
- Organization for Safety and Asepsis Procedures http://www.osap.org

Bioterrorism and Disaster Preparedness

Overview

- Bioterrorism may occur as covert events, in which persons are unknowingly exposed and an outbreak is suspected only upon recognition of unusual disease clusters or symptoms.
- Hospitals, emergency rooms, and clinics may have the first opportunity to recognize and initiate a response to a bioterrorism-related outbreak of infectious disease or biological toxins.
- Bioterrorism may also occur as announced events, in which warnings of an exposure are provided.

Purpose

- Facilities should be prepared to recognize, identify, and manage patients, visitors, personnel, and the environment following suspected or confirmed bioterrorism events.

Risk Factors

- Four agents are recognized as having the most bioterrorism potential —anthrax, botulism, plague, and smallpox.
- Additional agents with bioterrorism potential include those that cause tularemia, brucellosis, Q fever, viral hemorrhagic fevers, viral encephalitis, and disease associated with staphylococcal enterotoxin B.
- Most agents are not spread person-to-person.

- Aspects of dose size, route of exposure, time exposed to agent, and personal factors can influence time to symptoms and extent of illness.

Strategies for Prevention and Control

- **Policy/procedure**
  - Bioterrorism Readiness Plan (BRP) should be reviewed on a regular basis.
  - Notification/communication protocol in BRP should include contact information for: ICP, administration, local and state health departments, FBI, local police, CDC, and medical emergency services.
  - The BRP should include protocol for communication with local emergency planning and health department.
  - The BRP should be included when scheduling internal and external emergency preparedness drills.
  - Include BRP in education/training for new and existing HCWs.
  - The BRP should include procedures, equipment, training, and locations for decontamination of patients prior to entry into facility.
  - The BRP should designate in advance internal and external care sites for potentially large numbers of patients, including practical alternatives for isolation and possible cohorting, if required; base plan on patterns of airflow and ventilation, availability of adequate plumbing, waste disposal, and capacity to safely handle many patients.
- **Current resources**

    Should be available onsite, and

    Should be accessible if power and/or information systems were disrupted.

- **Syndrome-based criteria**
  - Due to the rapid progression to illness and potential for dissemination of some of these agents, it may not be practical to await diagnostic laboratory confirmation.
  - It may be necessary to initiate a response based on the recognition of high-risk syndromes.
  - Agent-specific information in Table includes clinical syndrome description (i.e., typical combination of clinical features of the illness at presentation), which should alert healthcare practitioners to the possibility of a bioterrorism-related outbreak.
- **Epidemiologic features**
  - Epidemiologic principles should be used to assess whether a patient's presentation is typical of an endemic disease (e.g., "flu") or is an unusual event that should raise concern.
  - Features that should alert healthcare providers to the possibility of a bioterrorism-related outbreak include:

    A rapidly increasing disease incidence (e.g., within hours or days) in a normally healthy population,

    An epidemic curve that rises and falls during a short period of time,

    An unusual increase in the number of people seeking care, especially with fever, respiratory, or gastrointestinal complaints,

    An endemic disease rapidly emerging at an uncharacteristic time or in an unusual pattern,

    Lower attack rates among people who had been indoors, especially in areas with filtered air or closed ventilation systems, compared with people who had been outdoors,

    Clusters of patients arriving from a single locale,

Large numbers of rapidly fatal cases, and

Any patient presenting with a disease that is relatively uncommon and has bioterrorism potential (e.g., pulmonary anthrax, tularemia, or plague).

- **IC practices for patient management**
  - **Isolation precautions**

    Agents of bioterrorism are generally not transmitted from person-to-person; re-aerosolization of these agents is unlikely; certain diseases or syndromes (e.g., smallpox and pneumonic plague) require additional precautions to reduce risk of transmission.

    Patients should be managed with Standard Precautions, which includes handwashing and PPE (Refer to Section 2 - Handwashing and Hand Hygiene).
  - **Patient placement**

    In small-scale events, routine facility patient placement and IC practices should be followed.

    If the number of patients presenting to a facility is too large to allow routine triage and isolation strategies (if required), it will be necessary to apply practical alternatives such as cohorting.
  - **Patient transport**

    Most infections are not transmitted from patient-to-patient, however there are exceptions that should be planned for (e.g., smallpox).

    The transport and movement of patients with bioterrorism-related infections, as for patients with any epidemiologically important infections (e.g., pulmonary tuberculosis, chickenpox, measles), should be limited to essential movement.
  - **Cleaning, disinfection, and sterilization of equipment and environment.**

Standard Precautions should be used for the management of patient-care equipment and environmental control.

Procedures for the routine care, cleaning, and disinfection of environmental surfaces, beds, bedrails, bedside equipment, and frequently touched surfaces and equipment should be followed.

EPA-approved germicidal cleaning agents available inpatient care areas for cleaning spills of contaminated material and disinfecting non-critical equipment should be readily available.

Used patient-care equipment that is soiled or potentially contaminated with blood, body fluids, secretions, or excretions should be handled in a manner that prevents exposures to skin and mucous membranes, avoids contamination of clothing, and minimizes the likelihood of transfer of microbes to other patients and environments.

Policies should be in place to ensure that reusable equipment is not used for the care of another patient until it has been appropriately cleaned and reprocessed, and to ensure that single-use patient items are appropriately discarded (Refer to Section 2 - Disinfection and Sterilization, SUDS).

Patient linen should be handled in accordance with Standard Precautions; facility policy, and local/state regulations should determine the methods for handling, transporting, and laundering soiled linen (Refer to Section 2 - Laundry Handling).

Contaminated waste should be sorted and discarded in accordance with federal, state, and local regulations (Refer to Section 2 - Environmental Maintenance).

- **Discharge management**

  Ideally, patients with bioterrorism-related infections will not be discharged from the facility until they are deemed noninfectious.

Consideration should be given to developing home care instructions in the event that large numbers of persons exposed may preclude admission of all infected patients.

Depending on the exposure and illness, home care instructions may include recommendations for the use of appropriate barrier precautions, handwashing, waste management, and cleaning and disinfection of the environment and patient-care items.

Home care instructions should be coordinated with health department/CDC information.

- **Post-mortem care**

  Pathology departments and clinical laboratories should be informed of a potentially infectious outbreak prior to submitting any specimens for examination or disposal.

  All autopsies should be performed carefully using Standard Precautions.

  Instructions for funeral directors should be developed and incorporated into the BRP for communication.

- **Postexposure management**

  Decontamination of patients and environment.

  The need for decontamination depends on the suspected exposure and in most cases will not be necessary.

  The goal of decontamination after a potential exposure to a bioterrorism agent is to reduce the extent of external contamination of the patient and contain contamination to prevent further spread.

  Decontamination should only be considered in instances of gross contamination.

  Decisions regarding the need for decontamination should be made in consultation with state and local health departments.

Decontamination of exposed individuals prior to receiving them in the healthcare facility may be necessary to ensure the safety of patients/staff.

Depending on agent, the likelihood for re-aerosolization associated with cutaneous exposure may exists, and clothing of exposed persons may need to be removed.

After removal of contaminated clothing, patients should be instructed (or assisted if necessary) to immediately shower with soap and water.

Potentially harmful practices, such as bathing patients with bleach solutions, are unnecessary and should be avoided.

Clean water, saline solution, or commercial ophthalmic solutions are recommended for rinsing eyes.

If indicated, after removal at the decontamination site, patient clothing should be handled only by personnel wearing appropriate personal protective equipment and placed in an impervious bag to prevent further environmental contamination.

Prophylaxis/postexposure immunization

Recommendations for prophylaxis are subject to change; up-to-date recommendations should be obtained in consultation with local and state health departments and CDC.

Policies should be in place to identify and manage healthcare workers exposed to infectious patients.

Accurate occupational health records will facilitate identification, contact, assessment, and delivery of postexposure care to potentially exposed HCWs.

- **Triage and management of large scale exposures and suspected exposures.**

  Each healthcare facility, with input from IC committee, administration, building engineering staff, emergency department, laboratory, and nursing directors, should plan in advance how best be able to deliver care in the event of a large-scale exposure.

Facilities should incorporate into their BRP processes for triage, safe housing, and care for potentially large numbers of affected individuals.

Facility needs will vary with the size of the regional population served and proximity to other healthcare facilities and external assistance.

Triage and management planning for large-scale events may include:

Establishing networks of communication and lines of authority required to coordinate onsite care.

Planning for cancellation of non-emergency services and procedures.

Identifying sources able to supply available vaccines, immune globulin, antibiotics, and botulinum anti-toxin (with assistance from local and state health departments).

Planning for the efficient evaluation and discharge of patients.

Developing discharge instructions for patients determined to be non-contagious or in need of additional onsite care, including details regarding if and when they should return for care or if they should seek medical follow up.

Determining availability and sources for additional medical equipment and supplies (e.g., ventilators) that may be needed for urgent large-scale care.

Planning for the allocation or re-allocation of scarce equipment in the event of a large-scale event (e.g., duration of ventilator support of terminally afflicted individuals).

With assistance from the Pathology service, identifying the institution's ability to manage a sudden increase in the number of cadavers onsite.

- **Psychological aspects of bioterrorism.**
  - Following a bioterrorism-related event, fear, and panic can be expected from both patients and healthcare providers.

    Psychological responses following a bioterrorism event may include horror, anger, panic, unrealistic concerns about infection, fear of contagion, paranoia, social isolation, or demoralization.

    ICPs should assist in developing prior working relationships with mental health support personnel (e.g., psychiatrists, psychologists, social workers, clergy, and volunteer groups) and assist in their collaboration with emergency response agencies and the media.

    Local, state, and federal media experts can provide assistance with communications needs.

    In the BRP, consider the following to address patient/general public fears:

      Minimize panic by clearly explaining risks, offering careful but rapid medical evaluation/treatment, and avoiding unnecessary isolation or quarantine, and

      Treat anxiety in unexposed persons who are experiencing somatic symptoms (e.g., with reassurance, or diazepam-like anxiolytics as indicated for acute relief of those who do not respond to reassurance).

    Consider the following for HCW fears:

      Provide bioterrorism readiness education, including frank discussions of potential risks and plans for protecting healthcare providers.

      Invite active, voluntary involvement in the BRP process.

Encourage participation in disaster drills.

Fearful or anxious HCWs may benefit from their usual sources of social support, or by being asked to fulfill a useful role (e.g., volunteer at triage site).

➤ **Laboratory Support and Confirmation**

- Subject to updates - current work is underway to improve the diagnostic capacity of labs to isolate and identify these agents rapidly.
- Facilities should work with local, state, and federal public health services to tailor diagnostic strategies to specific events.
- Obtaining diagnostic samples.

See specific recommendations for diagnostic testing for each agent.

Use Standard Precautions and Good Laboratory Practice.

Collect acute phase serum sample to be aliquoted and saved for later testing with a convalescent sample.

Laboratory proposed criteria for processing potential bioterrorism agents is based upon a Bio Safety level according to ability to support diagnostic needs and type of agent.

Level A: Clinical laboratories – minimal identification of agents.

Level B: County/ State/other laboratories – identification, confirmation, susceptibility testing.

Level C: State and other large facility laboratories with advanced capacity for testing – some molecular technologies.

Level D: CDC or select Department of Defense laboratories, such as U.S. Army Medical Research Institute of Infectious Diseases (USAMRIID) – Bio Safety Level (BSL) 3 and 4 labs with special surge capacity and advanced molecular typing techniques.

Specimen transport requirements:

Specimen packaging and transport should be coordinated with local and state health departments and FBI; should meet DOT regulations for packaging.

A chain of custody document should accompany the specimen from the moment of collection.

Advance planning may include identification of appropriate packaging materials/transport media in collaboration with the clinical laboratory and health departments.

➤ **Patient, Visitor, and Public Information**

- Clear, consistent, understandable information should be provided (e.g., fact sheets) to patients, visitors, and the general public.
- During bioterrorism-related outbreaks, visitors may be strictly limited.
- A well-designed BRP should clarify the lines of authority and communication flow.
- To minimize the anticipated responses of fear, confusion, and anger, healthcare facilities should plan in advance the methods and channels of communications to be used to inform the public.
- ICPs working with the IC committee and administration should coordinate in advance with state and local health agencies, local emergency services, and local broadcast media systems to decide how communication and action across agencies will occur.
- Failure to provide a public forum for information exchange may increase anxiety and misunderstanding, increasing fear among individuals who attribute non-specific symptoms to exposure to the bioterrorism agent.

Agent and Incubation	Clinical Syndrome	Diagnostic Testing
Anthrax Two to 60 days	Nonspecific viral syndrome followed in two to five days by severe respiratory distress, mediastinitis, shock, and death.	Widened mediastinum on CXR, Gram stain, culture (blood).
Botulinum One to five days	Blurred vision; diplopia; dry mouth; ptosis; symmetrical, descending, flaccid paralysis.	Largely clinical, serum and stool for detection of toxin by mouse bioassay if oral route of exposure.
Brucella Five to 60 days	Irregular fever, headache, fatigue, osteoarticular involvement.	Blood and bone marrow culture (hold six weeks); serum agglutination test.
Plague Two to three days	Acute onset of fever, cough with bloody sputum, may develop respiratory failure.	Gram stain and culture of blood, Sputum.
Q fever 10-40 days	Nonspecific, fever, cough, pleuritic chest pain.	ELISA or IFA on serum.
Ricin 18-24 hours	Weakness, fever, cough, pulmonary edema, respiratory failure, and death.	Clinical, serology on acute and Convalescent serum can confirm.

Agent and Incubation	Clinical Syndrome	Diagnostic Testing
Smallpox Seven to 17 days	Acute fever, followed in two to three days by macules progressing to pustules, most on extremities and face, synchronous.	Pharyngeal swab, scab material for PCR (reference laboratory only).
Staph. enterotoxin B Three to 12 hours	Fever, headache, nonproductive cough.	Clinical.
Tularemia Three to five days	Acute febrile illness, often pneumonia, may develop respiratory failure.	Culture of blood, sputum; difficult to isolate, largely a clinical diagnosis.
Viral encephalitis VEE: two to six days EEE,WEE: seven to 14 days	Systemic febrile illness, encephalitis.	Leukopenia, lymphopenia, serology: ELISA.

References/Resources

- American Psychiatric Association, Disaster Psychiatry Page www.psych.org/pract_of_psych/disaster_psych.cfm
- Association for Professionals in Infection Control and Epidemiology. APIC Text of Infection Control and Epidemiology. 2000, chapter 27, 1-11
- Bioterrorism alleging use of anthrax and interim Guidelines for management -United States, 1998. MMWR Morb Mortal Wkly Rep 1999; 48:69-74.
- Bioterrorism Readiness Plan, A Template for Healthcare Facilities. Association for Professionals in Infection Control and Epidemiology (APIC) and Centers for Disease Control (CDC). 1999 www.apic.org/educ/readinow.html
- Canadian Center for Emergency Preparedness www.ccep.ca/
- Chin J, ed., Control of communicable diseases manual, 17th edition. Washington DC: American Public Health Association; 2000
- CDC, Bioterrorism Preparedness and Response www.bt.cdc.gov
- CDC, National Center for Infectious Diseases www.cdc.gov/ncidod/diseases/index.htm
- Federal Emergency Management Agency (FEMA), The Federal Response Plan (FRP) 9230.1-PL, April 1999. www.fema.gov/r-n-r/frp/
- Flu Pandemic. Pandemic Influenza, A Planning Guide for State and Local Officials www.cdc.gov/od/nvpo/pandemicflu.htm#State
- Franz D, Jahrling PB, Friedlander AM, McClain DJ, Hoover DL, Bryne WR, et al. Clinical recognition and management of patients exposed to biological warfare agents. JAMA 1997; 278:399-411.

- Pile JC, Malone JD, and Eitzen et al. Anthrax as a potential biological warfare agent. Arch Intern Med 1998; 158:429-34.
- Simon JD. Biological terrorism. JAMA 1997; 278: 428-30
- Tucker JB. National health and medical services response to incidents of chemical and biological terrorism. JAMA 1997; 278:362 - 8.

Construction and Renovation

Overview

- Infection control risks, interventions, and management should be included in planning construction and renovation in the healthcare setting.
- The institutional philosophy, infection control policies, and relationship of the planned structural design to expected practice should be considered in this process.
- Preventing transmission of infectious agents to patients, healthcare workers, and visitors related to construction/renovation is fundamental to the provision of a safe environment of care in all healthcare venues.

Purpose

- Construction and renovation activities can pose infection transmission risks in the healthcare environment. Strategies to reduce these risks include early involvement in the conceptual phase to ascertain risks in patient populations, proactive design to address potential environmental sources of microorganisms during and following the construction/renovation activities, and architectural design to augment infection control practices.

Definitions

- **AII** – Airborne infection isolation room; single occupancy room for patient care where environmental factors are controlled to minimize transmission of infectious agents (e.g., TB, varicella).

- **CRP** – Construction and renovation policy. A comprehensive protocol that operationalizes the facility's ICRA and specifies essential participants. It supports IC involvement from conception through completion. The committee(s) and the board of trustees with periodic review/revision, as appropriate, should approve the CRP.
- **Environment of Care** – Those aspects within a healthcare facility/organization that are created, structured, and maintained to support quality healthcare; a section within the JCAHO standards.
- **ICRA** – Infection Control Risk Assessment that is conducted by facility owner during the programming phase of construction/renovation. Determination of potential risk of transmission of various agents in the facility; by multidisciplinary team with expertise in: IC, risk management, facility design, construction, ventilation, safety, and epidemiology. Constant process that is initiated in design/planning and continues through construction and renovation.
- **Handwashing station** – an area providing a sink with hot and cold water and a faucet that facilitates easy on/off/mixing. The station includes provision of cleansing agents and drying capability.
- **HEPA filtration** – High efficiency particulate air filtration filters out 99.97% of 0.3-micron particles.
- **PE** – Protective or protected environment; patient room or unit that provides care to severely immunosuppressed patients, such as bone marrow transplant units.

Risk Factors

- Construction/renovation activities may enhance the dispersal of microorganisms into the environment thus increasing the risk of transmission. There are numerous descriptions in the literature that provide scientific-based evidence to support construction/renovation as a cause of infections that have resulted in significant morbidity and mortality.

Strategies for Prevention and Control

- A Construction and Renovation Policy (CRP) policy should be developed. Elements should include:
  - Inclusion of an ICRA in all renovation and construction activities,
  - Planning, designing, and monitoring that defines authority and responsibility; communication; air handling and water systems, as appropriate; expectations for contractor accountability when breaches in IC practices occur; patient area risk assessment; criteria for emergency work interruptions including a start and stop process; education that indicates content, audience, and by whom; occupational health expectations for subcontractors (e.g., TB skin test, bloodborne pathogen training); traffic patterns for patients, healthcare workers, and visitors; transport of and approval for disposal of waste materials (e.g., asbestos, lead); emergency preparedness plans for major utility failures, including locations and responsibilities,
  - Establish processes that includes continuous input from IC into the structural design process that requires: routine submission of scheduled project lists to allow proactive anticipation by ICP; submission of an "IC permit" or "project approval signature block" before and during phases, as appropriate; review of risks and prevention strategies based upon changes in project once underway,

- Develop and utilize a matrix that provides assessment of type of construction/renovation project activity vs. patient risk groups affected (e.g., Construction Group 1 through 4 with 1 having the least disruption or dust production and 4 having the most and Patient Risk Group A through D with A the least susceptible through D as the most susceptible),
- Assemble and review pertinent resources including, but not limited to: The AIA Guidelines for Design and Construction of Hospital and HealthCare Facilities; state and local standards; and the APIC State-of-the-Art Report: The role of infection control during construction in healthcare facilities, and
- Be prepared to support the ICP position and recommendations with published citations whenever possible (e.g., APIC Toolkit has numerous References/Resources including scientific resources, online access listings, standards, guidelines).

➤ Other ICP and related safety/risk concerns:

- Carpeting, although not generally associated with infection, has a higher potential risk of contamination than hard-surfaced floors.
- Carpeting should be considered as a potential harbor for fungal infection during demolition and after events such as fires.
- A procedure should be developed for routine maintenance of carpeting; use disinfectants recommended by manufacturer for microbial contamination.
- Hard-surfaced floors are recommended for spillage, heavy soiling, and odor control areas.
- An educational program should be for internal and external workers presented related to construction/renovation on the risks of infection transmitted via dust, vermin, contaminated materials, etc. and expectations with corrective measures to prevent; educate healthcare staff to look for dust, footprints, open doors, flies, and wet ceiling tiles.

- Monitoring should be done to ensure infection control practices during and after construction; ensure accountability corresponding to the facility's RCP.
- Airtight barriers and exhaust airflow to maintain negative air pressure in construction zones should be used.
- Immunocompromised patients should be relocated to areas away from construction.
- Pedestrian traffic should be directed away from construction.
- Construction/renovation areas should be thoroughly cleaned prior to patients reentering the area; disinfect nonporous surfaces with appropriate disinfectant.
- Water lines in construction/renovation areas should be flushed prior to reuse as appropriate.
- Patients should be monitored for possible construction related infections (e.g., Aspergillus); investigate any clusters of fungal infection potentially caused by air contamination.

References/Resources

- American Institute of Architects (AIA) www.e-architect.com
- American Institute of Architects, Guidelines for design and construction of hospital and healthcare facilities, 2001 edition, The American Institute of Architects, Washington, D.C.; 2001.
- Association for Professionals in Infection Control and Epidemiology. APIC infection control tool kit series construction and renovation. Bartley J, editor. 1999.
- Association for Professionals in Infection Control and Epidemiology. www.apic.org

- Association for Professionals in Infection Control and Epidemiology. APIC Text of Infection Control and Epidemiology. 2000, chapters 72, 76,77,78,98.
- Bartley, JM. APIC State-of-the-art report: the role of infection control during construction in healthcare facilities. Am J of Infect Control 2000; 156-169.
- Centers for Disease Control and Prevention, Healthcare Infection Control Practices Advisory Committee (HICPAC). Draft guideline for environmental infection control in healthcare facilities, 2001. 2001, Federal Register.
- Jensen PA, Schafer MP. In : The NIOSH Manual of Analytical Methods. Sampling and characterization of bioaerosols. January 1998, pp. 82 - 112.
- Joint Commission on Accreditation of Healthcare Organizations, Environment of Care Standards – http://www.JCAHO.org.
- Michigan Department of Consumer and Industry Services (MDCIS), Division of Health Facilities and Services, Health Facility Evaluation Section. http://www.cis.state.mi.us/bhs/hfs/hfes/hfeshome.htm
- MDCIS – Healthcare facility projects: Project planning to opening survey recommendations. January 2000.
- MDCIS - Recommendations for developing an operational narrative for healthcare facilities. January 1998.
- MDCIS - Recommendations for the submission of plans and specifications for healthcare facilities. January 1998.
- MDCIS - Ventilation primer for healthcare facilities. July 2000.
- Society of Critical Care Medicine. ACCM Guidelines for Intensive Care Unit Design. http://www.sccm.org/accm/guidelines.

- U.S. Department of Health and Human services, Public Health Service. TB respiratory protection program respiratory protection program in healthcare facilities in healthcare facilities. Administrator's guide DHHS (NIOSH) Publication No. 99-143, September 1999.
- U.S. Department of Labor. OSHA technical manual, section III: chapter 7 Legionnaires' disease, pp. 1-46. www.osha.slc.gov/Tech_Man_data/III_7.html

Disinfection and Sterilization

Overview

- Reusable medical devices, patient-care equipment, and environmental surfaces require different approaches to remove soil and bioburden, decrease the risk of microorganism transmission, and maximize safety for patients and healthcare workers. The approach for reprocessing is based upon intended use of the item/device as established in Spaulding's hallmark classification system. Revised assessment methods and scientific-based evidence coupled with innovative technology have changed many methodologies to achieve best practice; nonetheless, the fundamental principles remain.

Purpose

- Numerous factors are essential in destroying microorganisms and achieving safe medical device for use on patients. Understanding these issues will assist the ICP in selecting/recommending the correct processes to follow when cleaning and disinfecting/sterilizing reusable patient items and environmental surfaces.

Definitions

- **Cleaning** – removal of all foreign material (e.g., dirt, body fluids, lubricants) from objects by using water and detergents/soaps/ enzymes and washing or scrubbing the object. Thorough cleaning should be done before any disinfection or sterilization process so the foreign material will not prevent the process from working.

- **Creutzfeldt-Jakob Disease (CJD)** – A transmissible spongiform encephalopathy allegedly caused by a prion (proteinaceous infectious particle), CJD is a degenerative, always fatal brain disorder that typically occurs in older people. A new variant of CJD (vCJD), caused by "mad cow disease", can occur in younger people; most reported cases are in Great Britain. Classic CJD is insidious, taking up to 20 or more years for symptoms to appear, with death taking place within five to 14 months after onset of symptoms.
- **Disinfection** – elimination of many or all microorganisms except bacterial spores; accomplished with liquid chemicals or by wet pasteurization.
- **High-level disinfection** - process expected to destroy all microorganisms, with the exception of high numbers of bacterial spores. Whenever high-level disinfection is used, the disinfectant solution should be routinely tested with an indicator to ensure efficacy.
- **Intermediate disinfection** – inactivation of *M. tuberculosis,* vegetative bacteria, most viruses, and most fungi, but not necessarily killing of bacterial spores.
- **Low-level disinfection** - can kill most bacteria, some viruses, and some fungi; cannot be relied on to kill resistant microorganisms (e.g., *M. tuberculosis* or bacterial spores).
- **Sterilization** - a process that completely eliminates or kills all microorganisms by using sterilizers that provide steam under pressure, dry heat, and/or ethylene oxide (EtO) and/or other gases, or liquid chemical for prolonged contact time. Whenever sterilants are used, they should be routinely tested with biological indicators (e.g., spore challenge) to ensure that they are working properly. Items that are sterilized should remain sterile until the package is torn, wet, or damaged (event related); sterility is a function of intact packaging, not time (e.g., expiration date).

Risk Factors

- The use of medical devices can increase the risk of infection in patients.
- The chemical and/or physical features of agents used to disinfect/ sterilize may pose a safety hazard to those in contact with and/or exposed to these agents.
- Microorganisms vary in how easily they are destroyed or inactivated; some are difficult to kill, others are not. The following microorganisms are arranged in order from most difficult to easy to destroy: Bacterial spores (e.g., *B. subtilis*), mycobacteria (e.g., *M. tuberculosis*), nonlipid or small viruses (e.g., poliovirus, hepatitis A virus), fungi (e.g., *Trichophyton spp.*), vegetative bacteria (e.g., *Ps. aeruginosa; S. aureus*), lipid or medium-sized viruses (e.g., herpes simplex virus, hepatitis B virus, HIV).

Strategies for Prevention and Control General

- The method of disinfection or sterilization selected should be based on the type of device, how it is used, related safety factors, current guidelines, and manufacturer's recommendations.
- Policies and procedures should be developed and regularly reviewed related to cleaning, disinfection, sterilization, quality control/verification of process, packaging, storage, recall due to process failure, borrowed/loaner instruments, and implants.
- Training programs should be presented that include competencies and return demonstration.
- Appropriate PPE, hazard communication, emergency equipment/procedures, monitoring, and documentation/tracking should be provided.

Products and processes

- When selecting an agent, consideration should be given for how it is to be used, chemical composition (where applicable) and manufacturer recommendations.
    - Agents may cause damage due to corrosive structure or incompatibility with components.
- Disinfection/sterilization processes cannot be accomplished unless the proper concentration is used and the time of exposure (time and contact) to the agent is adequate; agent can't contact surfaces if cleaning is inadequate.
- Workflow should proceed from dirty to clean in the soiled item reprocessing area.
- When a new disinfection/sterilization technology is implemented, a thorough review of factors and analysis of the agent/process should be completed; policy/procedure, validation, education, and training should be completed prior to use.
- Directions on the label should be followed; ***caution***—certain types of devices and some microorganisms require special handling, and the labels may not provide information on every subject.
- **The following agents have been shown to inactivate HBV:** glutaraldehyde (2%), glutaraldehydephenate (0.13% glutaraldehyde/0.44% phenol), iodophor (80 ppm), isopropyl alcohol (70%), ethyl alcohol (80%), hydrogen peroxide (0.3%), and sodium hypochlorite (500 ppm).
- **The following disinfectants have been shown to inactivate HIV:** glutaraldehyde (2%), hydrogen peroxide (0.3%), ethyl alcohol (50%), isopropyl alcohol (70%), phenolics, and sodium hypochlorite (50 ppm).

- Note: Environmental surfaces in rooms of patients with HBV or HIV infection can be cleaned with any Environmental Protection Agency (EPA)-approved hospital disinfectant, including quaternary ammonium germicidal disinfectants, provided instructions are followed (e.g., for wet time).
- **CJD agent** requires special process owing to extreme resistance of prions to normal inactivation methods. The following sterilization/ disinfection techniques are recommended:
  - Steam sterilization for at least 30 min at a temperature of 132°C (269°F) in a gravity displacement sterilizer is the preferred method for treatment of contaminated material; when a prevacuum sterilizer is used, 18 min at 134–138°C (273–280°F) is also effective.
  - Alternatively, immersion in 1 N sodium hydroxide (a caustic solution) for 1 hour at room temperature followed by steam sterilization at 121°C (249°F) for 30 min may be used for critical and semicritical items.
  - After initial sterilization process, items should be washed, scrubbed, and resterilized.
  - Noncritical patient care items or surfaces (e.g., autopsy table, floors) may be disinfected with either undiluted or up to 1:10 dilution of bleach, or 1 N sodium hydroxide at room temperature for 15 min.

General points to remember

- Never use quaternary ammonium germicides or other low-level disinfectants to disinfect critical devices that will enter sterile tissue or the vascular system or semicritical devices that touch mucous membranes or broken skin.
- Do not use glutaraldehyde or other high-level disinfectants to clean environmental surfaces or other noncritical devices.

- Always use the right dilution of disinfectants; stronger concentrations of disinfectants do not work better and can be toxic to the user and/or damage the item.
- Endoscopes and other semicritical devices should be managed the same way regardless of whether the patient is infected with *M. tuberculosis,* HIV, or HBV.
- Glutaraldehyde (2%) reliably kills C. *difficile* spores with short exposure times (20 min).
- Phenolics should not be used to clean infant bassinets and incubators during an infant's stay; when used for terminal cleaning in this setting, all surfaces should be thoroughly rinsed with water and dried.

Endoscopy (APIC Guidelines)

- *Note:* These guidelines represent minimum standards of care. Facilities may wish to adopt more stringent criteria. These recommendations should be followed for all patients, regardless of whether they are suspected or known to be infected.
- Meticulous cleaning of the endoscope with an enzymatic detergent recommended by the endoscope manufacturer should be performed immediately after use. All of the channels should be irrigated and brushed, if accessible, to remove particulate matter. Irrigation adapters should be used to facilitate cleaning of all channels. All immersible parts of the endoscope should then be rinsed with water. Detergent solutions should be discarded after each use. Cleaning brushes should be disposable or thoroughly cleaned and receive high-level disinfection or sterilization after each use.
- Leak testing is recommended for flexible endoscopes before immersion.

- Endoscopes that pass through normally sterile tissue should be subjected to a sterilization procedure before each use; if this is not feasible, they should receive at least high-level disinfection. Disinfection should be followed by a rinse with sterile water.
- Endoscopes that come in contact with mucous membranes are classified as semicritical items and should receive at least high-level disinfection.
- An FDA-cleared sterilant/disinfectant should be used for sterilization or high-level disinfection.
- Products and methods for cleaning and disinfection/sterilization should be compatible with the endoscopic equipment and design. Contact instrument manufacturer(s) to confirm compatibility.
- If glutaraldehyde is used, all immersible internal and external surfaces should be in contact with the disinfectant for not less than 20 minutes to achieve high-level disinfection.
- Personnel assigned to reprocess endoscopes should receive device-specific reprocessing instructions to ensure proper cleaning and disinfection or sterilization.
- Nonimmersible endoscopes should be phased out immediately.
- After chemical disinfection, endoscopes should be rinsed with sterile water or with tap water followed by a 70% ethyl or isopropyl alcohol rinse.
- The instrument and its channels should be thoroughly air-dried. A final drying step that includes flushing all channels with alcohol followed by purging the channels with air greatly reduces the possibility of recontamination of the endoscope by waterborne microorganisms.

- Endoscopes should be stored in a manner that will protect the endoscope and minimize the potential for accumulation of residual moisture. They should not be coil-stored in cases that cannot be properly cleaned. Endoscopes should be hung in a vertical position to facilitate drying.
- Reusable accessories that penetrate mucosal barriers (e.g., biopsy forceps, cytology brushes) should be mechanically cleaned (i.e., by ultrasonics) and then steam sterilized between each patient or used once and discarded.
- Sterile water should be used to fill the water bottle. The water bottle and its connecting tube should be sterilized or receive high-level disinfection at least daily.
- Flexible endoscopes that cannot withstand the processes described in these guidelines because of age, design, or damage should not be used.
- A log should be maintained for each procedure indicating the patient's name and medical record number, the procedure, the endoscopist, and the serial number or other identifier of the endoscope used.
- In the event of an outbreak caused by a suspected infectious or chemical etiology, the investigation should be performed according to standard methods of outbreak investigation.
- Endoscopy related infection or pseudoinfection should be reported to: (1) persons responsible for institutional infection control and risk management, (2) FDA, (3) state health department, (4) CDC, and (5) manufacturer(s).

- Facilities where endoscopes are used and disinfected should be designed to provide a safe environment for healthcare workers as well as patients. Air-exchange equipment (ventilation system, exhaust hoods, etc) should be used to minimize the exposure of all persons to potentially toxic vapors. The concentration of glutaraldehyde, if it is used, in the air should never exceed allowable limits. There should be adequate space for drying and storage of endoscopes and endoscopic accessories.
- Personal protective equipment (gloves, eyewear, respiratory protective devices, etc) should be readily available and should be used to protect workers from exposure to infectious agents (HIV, hepatitis B virus, *M tuberculosis,* etc.) and toxic chemicals.
- All endoscopy personnel should be educated about the biologic and chemical hazards present while performing or assisting at endoscopic procedures and during the reprocessing of endoscopic equipment.
- Endoscopy personnel should be trained according to the Occupational Safety and Health Administration's Hazardous Communications Standard. There should be a spill containment plan specific for the liquid chemical sterilant/disinfectant available whenever and wherever endoscope reprocessing occurs.
- Personnel should be vaccinated against preventable diseases such as hepatitis B. Those at risk for exposure to tuberculosis should be screened for infection by Mantoux skin testing with purified protein derivative.
- Routine testing of liquid sterilants/high-level disinfectants should be performed to ensure minimal effective concentration of the active ingredient.

TABLES OF CRITICAL, SEMICRITICAL, AND NONCRITICAL ITEMS

Device Classification	Device Examples	Type of Process	Process Examples
Critical Enters sterile tissue of vascular system (includes dental instruments)	Implants, scalpels, needles, or other surgical instruments; endoscopic accessories including biopsy forceps	Sterilization (cycle time per manufacturer) Liquid sterilants (exposure time in hours per manufacturer)	Steam under pressure Dry heat EtO gas Chemical gas sterilizers Glutaraldehyde based formulations (2%) Stabilized hydrogen peroxide (6%) Peracetic acid (variable conc.)
Semicritical Touches mucous membranes or broken skin	Flexible endoscopes, laryngoscopes, Endotracheal tubes, respiratory therapy and anesthesia equipment, diaphragm fitting rings, and other similar devices	High-level disinfection (exposure time ≥ 20 min)	Glutaraldehyde based formulations (2%) OPA 0.55% Stabilized H_2O2 (6%) Peracetic acid (variable conc.) Wet pasteurization (70°C - 30 min) Sodium hypochlorite (1:50 dilute)

TABLES OF CRITICAL, SEMICRITICAL, AND NONCRITICAL ITEMS

Device Classification	Device Examples	Type of Process	Process Examples
Semicritical Touches mucous membranes or broken skin	Other smooth, hard objects that are semicritical (e.g., hydrotherapy tanks) Thermometers (oral and rectal)	Intermediate-level disinfection (exposure time ≤10 min)	Sodium hypochlorite (dilute) Ethyl or isopropyl alcohol (70–90%) Phenolic germicidal detergent (dilute per label) Iodophor germicidal detergent (per label)
Noncritical Touches intact skin	Stethoscopes, tabletops, floors, bedpans, furniture, crutches, some food utensils, bedside tables, etc.	Low-level disinfection (exposure time ≤10 min)	Ethyl or isopropyl alcohol (70–90%) Sodium hypochlorite (1:100) Phenolic germicidal detergent (dilute per label) Iodophor germicidal detergent (per label) Quaternary ammonium germicidal detergent (per label)

References/Resources

- Alvarado CJ, Reichelderfer M. APIC guideline for infection prevention and control in flexible endoscopy. Am J Infect Control 2000; 28:138-55.
- AAMI standards and recommended practices, sterilization, Part 1: sterilization in healthcare facilities, 1(1). Arlington, VA, Association for the Advancement of Medical Instrumentation. 2000.
- American Society of Healthcare Central Service Professions www.ashcsp.org
- Association for the Advancement of Medical Instrumentation www.aami.org
- Association for Professionals in Infection Control and Epidemiology, Inc. www.apic.org
- Association for Professionals in Infection Control and Epidemiology. APIC Text of Infection Control and Epidemiology. 2000, chapters 53, 54, 55, 56, 58, 64, 65, 108.
- Rutala WA. APIC guideline for selection and use of disinfectants. Am J Infect Control 1996; 24:313–342.
- Rutala, WA. Disinfection, sterilization, and antisepsis: principles and practices in healthcare facilities. Washington, DC: Association for Professionals in Infection Control and Epidemiology, Inc. 2000.

Environmental Maintenance

Overview

- Issues related to infection control in the healthcare environment are numerous and diverse; they should be approached with consideration of scientific literature. Major attention is focused on engineering and infection control concerns during construction, demolition, renovation, and repairs of healthcare facilities (Refer to Section 2 - Construction and Renovation). However, IC measures used to recover from catastrophic events (e.g., flooding, sewage spills, loss of electricity and ventilation, disruption of the water supply) should be addressed. Additionally, the effect of environmental surfaces, laundry, plants, animals, medical wastes, cloth furnishings, and carpeting on disease transmission in healthcare facilities merit review.

Purpose

- Facility IC programs should address the fundamentals and control measures for preventing infections associated with air, water, or other environmental concerns within healthcare facilities. The scope of this subject is vast and it is recommended that the reader review the References/Resources listed at the end of this section for more details.

Definitions

- **AII** - Airborne Infection Isolation; single occupancy room for patient care where environmental factors are controlled to minimize transmission of infectious agents (e.g., TB, varicella).

- **Air changes per hour (ACH)** - the ratio of the volume of air flowing through a space in a certain period of time (i.e., the airflow rate) to the volume of that space (i.e., the room volume).
- **Air conditioning** - process of treating air to meet the requirements of a conditioned space by controlling its temperature, humidity, cleanliness, and distribution.
- **Biosafety level** - a combination of microbiological practices, laboratory facilities, and safety equipment determined to be sufficient to reduce or prevent occupational exposures of laboratory personnel to the microbiological agents; there are four biosafety levels based on the hazards associated with the various microbiological agents.
- **Cooling tower** - a structure engineered to receive accumulated heat from ventilation systems and equipment and transfer this heat to water, which then releases the stored heat to the atmosphere through evaporative cooling.
- **HEPA filter** - High Efficiency Particulate Air filters capable of removing 99.97% of particles > 0.3 µm in diameter; may assist in controlling the transmission of airborne disease agents. These filters may be used in ventilation systems to remove particles from the air or in personal respirators to filter air before the person wearing the respirator inhales it.
- **High efficiency filter** - a filter with a particle-removal efficiency of 90% - 95%.
- **HVAC** - Heating, Ventilation, Air Conditioning.
- **Laminar flow** - HEPA filtered air that is blown into a room at a rate of 90 ± 10 feet/min in a unidirectional pattern with 100 - 400 ACH.
- **Laser plume** - the transfer of electromagnetic energy into tissues that results in a release of particles, gases, and tissue debris.

- **PE** – Protective/protected environment; patient room or unit that provides care to severely immunosuppressed patients (e.g., bone marrow transplant).
- **Potable (drinking) water** - water that is fit to drink. The quality of this water is defined by EPA microbiological standards.
- **Reservoir** - a non-clinical source of infection.
- **Ventilation** - the process of supplying and removing air by natural or mechanical means to and from any space; air may or may not be conditioned.

Risk Factors

- Air
  - A variety of airborne infections in susceptible hosts can result from exposures to clinically significant microorganisms.
  - Reservoirs include individuals and/or environmental sources (i.e., soil, water, dust, and decaying matter); outdoor or indoor origins.
  - Aerosolized oral/nasal secretions represent an important source of pathogens that can be dispersed into the air, either as droplets (e.g., influenza virus, rhinoviruses, adenoviruses, and respiratory syncytial virus [RSV]) or droplet nuclei (e.g., TB, VZV, and measles virus).
  - Spores of *Aspergillus* spp. are ubiquitous and survive in air, dust, and moisture present in healthcare facilities; their presence is an important extrinsic risk factor for opportunistic invasive aspergillosis.
  - Other opportunistic fungi have been linked with healthcare-associated infections; they proliferate in moist environments, such as water-damaged wood/building materials and are easily spread though the air.
  - Airborne bacteria, viruses, and fungi are particularly dangerous if a host has underlying disease or immunosuppressive therapy.

➤ Water

- Moist environments and aqueous solutions in healthcare settings have the potential to serve as reservoirs for waterborne microorganisms.
- Under favorable environmental circumstances (e.g., temperature, nutrition source), microorganisms can proliferate and linger in highly-stable, environmentally resistant, and infectious forms.
- Modes of transmission for waterborne infections include: 1) direct contact, 2) ingestion, 3) indirect contact, 4) aerosol inhalation, and 5) aspiration of contaminated water.
- The first three modes of transmission are commonly associated with infections due to gram-negative bacteria and non-tuberculous mycobacteria (NTM).
- *Legionella* spp. may be spread as an aerosol from water sources.
- Gram-negative bacteria in tap or potable water can cause opportunistic infections including: *Pseudomonas aeruginosa* and *Ps. spp., Burkholderia cepacia, Ralstonia pickettii, Stenotrophomonas maltophilia,* and *Sphingomonas spp.*
- Tap water used for medical care (e.g., diluent for solutions, water source for medical instruments/equipment, for instrument rinsing) impart a potential risk.
- *Pseudomonas* spp. and other gram-negative, non-fermentative bacteria have minimal nutritional requirements (i.e., can grow in distilled water) and tolerate varying conditions (e.g., temperature fluctuations); contributing persistence and dispersion in moist environments.
- *Acinetobacter spp.* and *Enterobacter spp.* can proliferate in moist environments and may be responsible for episodes of colonization, BSIs, pneumonia, and UTIs among medically-compromised patients, especially in ICUs and burn units.

- NTM, found in potable water, are of low pathogenicity, and opportunistic; the most common forms of human disease associated with NTM are: 1) pulmonary disease in adults; 2) cervical lymph node disease in children; 3) skin, soft tissue, and bone infections; and 4) disseminated disease in immunocompromised patients.
- NTM occur in natural and manmade environments and have been reported in pseudo-outbreaks (e.g., *M. chelonae, M. gordonae,* and *M. xenopi*) associated with both bronchoscopy and endoscopy.
- *Cryptosporidium parvum*, a protozoan parasite, causes self-limiting gastroenteritis in normal hosts but can cause severe, life-threatening disease in the immunocompromised; oocysts are highly resistant to chlorine and may be present in natural and community water after fecal contamination from human or animal sources.
- Microorganisms may be found in ice, ice-storage chests, and ice-making machines; a variety of opportunistic microorganisms, mainly gram-negative bacilli, originate from the water source used to make ice or from contaminated hands.
- Therapy pools/tubs/tanks and water containing equipment (e.g., hydrotherapy pools, whirlpools, hot tubs, physiotherapy tanks, birthing tanks, dialysis equipment, automated endoscopic reprocessors, dental unit lines) may become contaminated with microorganisms.
- Flooding from external or internal sources may result in water- or sewer-related damage can initiate microorganism proliferation.

➤ **Environmental services**

- Environmental surfaces include medical equipment surfaces (e.g., monitor knobs, controls on hemodialysis machines, X-ray machines, instrument carts, dental units) and housekeeping surfaces (e.g., floors, walls, tabletops); the later carries a lesser risk of microbial transmission.

- Improper/inadequate cleaning and disinfection of these surfaces can increase risk of infection.
- Item composition (material, porosity, agent compatibility), type of soiling (touch contamination vs. gross blood/body fluid; fresh vs. dried), work flow (clean to dirty), supplies (agents, cloths and mops, contaminated solution), worker competencies, and preventative maintenance (carpets, caulking, grout) contribute to the effectiveness of cleaning and disinfection in reducing the risk of microbial spread from environmental surfaces.
- Pests (ants, cockroaches, flies/maggots, mosquitoes, spiders, mites, midges, rats, and mice) may carry a variety of microorganisms.

➤ **Environmental sampling**

- Routine, random, and/or undirected sampling without purpose may yield confusing and difficult to interpret results; conclusions may misdirect resources without reducing risk of infection to patients or HCWs.

➤ **Laundry and Bedding**

- Soiled laundry (e.g., sheets, blankets, towels, cloths, clothing, uniforms, scrub suits, gowns, and drapes for surgical procedures) can contain large numbers of pathogenic microorganisms.
- Reports of healthcare-associated diseases linked to soiled fabrics are few in number thus the overall risk of disease transmission during the laundry process appears to be negligible.

➤ **Animals in healthcare facilities**

- Pets/animals may be a reservoir for microorganisms, parasites, and allergens.

➤ **Regulated medical waste**

- The quantity and type of etiologic agents present in waste from healthcare facilities varies, thereby imparting a variety of risks (infection or injury) from generation point to ultimate disposal.

- Risk reduction for handling, storage, treatment, transportation, and disposal is incorporated into a range of regulations and guidelines.

Strategies for Prevention

- **Selected excerpts from the *CDC/HICPAC Guideline for Environmental Infection Control in Healthcare Facilities,*** 2001 (***Draft*** 3/2001). Each recommendation is categorized on basis of existing scientific data, theoretical rationale, applicability, and economic impact. The system for categorizing recommendations is as follows:
  - **Category IA** *(IA)*. Strongly recommended for implementation and strongly supported by well-designed experimental, clinical, or epidemiological studies.
  - **Category IB** *(IB)*. Strongly recommended for implementation and supported by some experimental, clinical, or epidemiological studies and a strong theoretical rationale.
  - **Category IC** *(IC)*. Required by state or federal regulations, rules, or standards.
  - **Category II** *(II)*. Suggested for implementation and supported by suggestive clinical or epidemiological studies or a theoretical rationale.
  - **No recommendation; unresolved issue** *(UI)*. Practices for which evidence is insufficient or no consensus regarding efficacy exists.
- **Air-handling systems in healthcare facilities**
  - Monitor ventilation systems in accordance with engineering and manufacturers' recommendations to ensure process management through preventive engineering, optimal performance for removal of particulates, and elimination of excess moisture. *(IC)*

    Ensure that HVAC filters are properly installed and maintained to prevent air leakages and dust. *(IC)*

Monitor areas with special ventilation requirements (e.g., AII, PE) for ACH, and pressure differentials; document pressure differentials. *(IB)*

Engineer humidity controls into the HVAC system and monitor these to ensure proper moisture removal. *(IC)*

Maintain the air intakes and inspect filters periodically to ensure proper operation. *(IC)*

Remove bird roosts and nests near air intakes and prevent birds from gaining access to these structures. *(IB)*

Prevent dust accumulation by regularly cleaning air-duct grilles when patients do not occupy rooms. *(IC)*

- Conduct a risk assessment and provide an adequate number of AII and PE rooms or areas to meet the needs of the patient population. *(IC)*

HVAC systems should not be shut down except for maintenance, repair, testing of emergency back-up capacity, or for new construction.

If the HVAC system should be shut down, do not inactivate entire system at one time. *(IC)*

Provide backup emergency power and redundant air handling and pressurization systems to maintain filtration, constant ACH and pressure differentials in PE units, AII, operating rooms, and critical care areas. *(IC)*

Coordinate HVAC system maintenance with infection control staff to allow for relocation of immunocompromised patients if necessary. *(II)*

Develop a contingency plan for a general power failure, with emphasis on restoration of proper air-quality and ventilation conditions in AII, PE, operating rooms, emergency departments, and intensive-care units. *(IC)*

Coordinate system start-ups with infection control staff to protect patients in PE units from bursts of mold spores. *(IC)*

- Clean ventilation ducts as per the manufacturer's recommendations for maintaining HVAC performance. *(IC)*

➤ **Construction, renovation, remediation, repair, and demolition**

- Establish a multidisciplinary team that includes an ICP to coordinate demolition, construction, and renovation projects (Refer to Section 3 - Construction and Renovation). *(IC)*

➤ **Environmental infection control measures in special healthcare settings** (Refer to Sections 2, 3, and 4)

- Maintain redundant ventilation equipment for emergency replacement in PE, AII, and operating rooms. *(IC)*
- Implement infection control measures in care areas for high-risk patients (i.e., patients who require PE rooms, solid organ transplant patients, non-allogeneic, and neutropenic patients):

  Minimize exposures of these immunocompromised patients to activities that might cause aerosolization of fungal spores (e.g., vacuuming, disruption of ceiling tiles). *(IB)*

  Install central or point-of-use HEPA filters for incoming air. *(IB)*

  Ensure that rooms are well sealed by: 1) properly constructing windows, doors, and intake and exhaust ports; 2) ensuring that ceilings are smooth and free of fissures, open joints, and crevices; and 3) sealing walls above and below the ceiling. *(IC)*

  Incorporate ... [recommended] ventilation engineering specifications into the planning and construction of new PE units. *(IC)*

- When immunocompromised patients who normally would be in PE require isolation for airborne diseases (e.g., VZV infection, tuberculosis), place these patients in an AII room with an anteroom having an independent exhaust. *(IC)*

- Implement infection control measures for AII [as recommended].
- Implement infection control measures for operating rooms [as recommended].
- Other aerosol hazards in special settings:

  In settings where surgical lasers are used, wear appropriate personal protective equipment, including high-filtration surgical masks. *(IC)*

➤ **Controlling the spread of waterborne microorganisms**

- Practice consistent handwashing/hand hygiene to prevent the spread of waterborne pathogens; use barrier precautions (e.g., gloves) in accordance with current guidelines. *(IA)* (Refer to Section 2 - Handwashing and Hand Hygiene, Isolation and Precautions.
- Eliminate contaminated environmental reservoirs (e.g., equipment, solutions) whenever possible. *(IB)*
- **Water systems in healthcare facilities**

  Maintain hot water temperature at the outlet at the highest temperature allowable by state regulations or codes, preferably >51°C (>124°F), and maintain cold water temperature at <20°C (<68°F). *(IC)*

  If the hot water temperature can be maintained at >51°C (>124°F), install preset thermostatic valves in point-of-use fixtures to help minimize the risk of scalding. *(II)*

  When state regulations or codes do not allow hot water temperatures >43°C (>110°F), follow alternative preventive measures to minimize the growth of *Legionella* spp. in water systems. *(II)*

  When water disruptions occur, use the following infection control measures:

Prepare a contingency plan to estimate water demands for entire facility. *(IC)*

Post signs advising patients, families, staff, and visitors not to drink tap water until the system is cleared for use by the facility engineer. *(IC)*

When the system function is restored: 1) Thoroughly flush the system with water at ambient temperatures, or 2) Use high-temperature water flushing or chlorination; 3) Flush and restart equipment and fixtures according to manufacturers' instructions. *(IC)*

- When corrective decontamination of the hot water system is necessary after a disruption in service or a cross-connection with sewer lines has occurred:

  Decontaminate the system when the fewest occupants are present in the building (e.g., nights, weekends). *(II)*

  If using high-temperature decontamination, raise the hot-water temperature to 71°C -77°C (160°F -170°F), progressively flushing each outlet; flush system for a minimum of five min. *(IC)*

  If using chlorination, add enough chlorine, preferably overnight, to achieve a free chlorine residual of >2 mg/L (>2 ppm) throughout system. *(IC)*

- Adhere to any "boil water" advisory issued by the municipal water utility. *(IC)*

  After the advisory is lifted, run faucets and drinking fountains at full flow for several minutes; maintain a high level of surveillance for waterborne disease in patients. *(IC)*

- Implement procedures to manage a sewage system failure or flooding:

  Develop a contingency plan in accordance with JCAHO requirements. *(IC)*

Relocate patients and clean/sterile supplies from affected areas, and close off these areas during clean-up procedures. *(IC)*

Ensure that the sewage system is fully functional before beginning remediation so that contaminated solids and standing water can be removed. *(IC)*

If hard-surface equipment, floors, and walls remain in good repair, allow them to dry out and clean with detergent according to standard cleaning procedures. *(IC)*

Remove absorbent structural items (e.g., carpeting, wallboard, wallpaper) and cloth furnishings if they cannot be easily and thoroughly cleaned and dried within 72 hours; replace with new materials as soon as the underlying structure is declared thoroughly dry by the hospital engineer. *(IC)*

Clean wood furniture and materials (if still in good repair); allow them to dry thoroughly before restoring varnish or other surface coatings. *(IC)*

- **Strategies for preventing healthcare-associated Legionellosis**

Use proper decontamination strategies as needed to eliminate legionellae from the healthcare facility's hot water supply. *(IB)*

No recommendation for treating water with ozone, UV light, heavy-metal ions, or monochloramines. *(UI)*

Implement strategies for preventing Legionnaires' disease. *(IB and II)*

No recommendation on routine culturing of water systems in healthcare facilities that do not have patient-care areas (i.e., transplant units) for persons at high risk for Legionella infection. *(UI)*

If one case of laboratory-confirmed, definite healthcare-associated Legionnaires' disease is identified, OR if two or more cases of laboratory-confirmed, possible healthcare-associated Legionnaires' disease occur during a six month period, report the cases to the state and local health departments, and conduct an epidemiologic investigation. *(II)*

Clean hot-water storage tanks and water heaters to remove accumulated scale and sediment. *(II)*

No recommendation for the removal of faucet aerators in areas for immunocompetent patients. *(UI)*

Do not use large-volume room air humidifiers that create aerosols (e.g., by Venturi principle, ultrasound, or spinning disk) unless are subjected to high-level disinfection and filled only with sterile water. *(II)*

- **Cooling towers and evaporative condensers**

When planning construction of new healthcare facilities, locate cooling towers so that the drift is directed away from the air-intake system, and design the towers to minimize the volume of aerosol drift. *(IC)*

Implement infection control procedures for operational cooling towers. *(IB and IC)*

- **Dialysis water quality and dialysate (Refer to Section 4-Dialysis)**

Adhere to current AAMI standards for quality assurance performance of devices and equipment used to treat, store, and distribute water in hemodialysis centers (both acute and maintenance settings) and for the preparation of concentrates and dialysate. *(IA)*

No recommendation on whether more stringent requirements for water quality should be imposed in hemofiltration and hemodiafiltration. *(UI)*

Conduct microbiological testing specific to water in dialysis settings. *(IA)*

In conjunction with microbiological testing, perform endotoxin testing, especially on samples from water used to reprocess hemodialyzers. *(IA)*

Disinfect water distribution systems in dialysis settings at least weekly. *(IA)*

Design and engineer water systems in dialysis settings so that they are free of joints, dead-end pipes, and unused branches and taps that can harbor bacteria. *(IC)*

Do not use storage tanks in dialysis systems unless they are routinely drained, disinfected, and have an ultrafilter (membrane filter with a pore size sufficient to remove small particles and molecules >1 kilodalton in size) installed in the water line distal to the storage tank. *(IC)*

- **Ice machines and ice**

Do not handle ice directly by hand, and wash hands before obtaining ice. *(II)*

Use a smooth-surface ice scoop to dispense ice; keep the ice scoop on a chain short enough so the scoop cannot touch the floor, or keep the scoop on a clean, hard surface when not in use. *(II)*

Do not store pharmaceuticals or medical solutions on ice intended for consumption; use sterile ice to keep medical solutions cold, or use equipment specifically manufactured for this purpose. *(IB)*

Limit access to ice-storage chests, and keep the container doors closed except when removing ice. *(II)*

Clean and disinfect ice-storage chests on a regular basis. *(II)*

To ensure performance and maintain infection control, perform regular maintenance of ice machines according to manufacturers' instructions or, in the absence of manufacturers' instructions, clean, disinfect, and maintain ice machines on a regular basis. *(II)*

Conduct microbiologic sampling of ice, ice chests, and ice-making machines if indicated for an epidemiologic investigation. *(IB)*

- **Hydrotherapy tanks and pools**
  (Refer to Section 4-Rehabilitation Services)

  Drain and clean hydrotherapy equipment (e.g., Hubbard tanks, tubs, whirlpools, Jacuzzis, birthing tanks) after each patient, and disinfect equipment surfaces and components in accordance with manufacturers' instructions and relevant scientific literature. *(IC)*

- **Miscellaneous medical equipment connected to water systems**

  Clean, disinfect, and maintain automated endoscope reprocessor (AER) equipment according to manufacturers' instructions and relevant scientific literature. *(IB)*
  (Refer to Section 3-Disinfection and Sterilization)

  Take precautions to prevent waterborne contamination of dental unit water lines and instruments. *(IC and II)*
  (Refer to Section 4-Dentistry)

➤ **Environmental services**

- **Use appropriate cleaning and disinfecting strategies for environmental surfaces in patient-care areas.**

  Do not use high-level disinfectants/liquid chemical sterilants on non-critical surfaces for disinfection. *(IC)*

  Follow manufacturers' instructions for cleaning and maintaining non-critical medical equipment. *(II)*

  In the absence of manufacturers' cleaning instructions, follow [recommended] procedures. *(II)*

Keep housekeeping surfaces (e.g., floors, walls, tabletops) visibly clean on a regular basis and as spills occur. *(II)*

Use a one-step process and water/detergent or an EPA-registered hospital-grade disinfectant/detergent designed for general housekeeping purposes. *(II)*

Follow manufacturers' instructions for proper use of cleaning/disinfecting products, paying close attention to specified use dilutions and stated contact times. *(II)*

Clean and disinfect high-touch surfaces (e.g., doorknobs, bedrails, light switches, surfaces in and around toilets in patients' rooms) on a more frequent schedule compared to that for minimal touch housekeeping surfaces. *(II)*

Clean walls, blinds, and window curtains in patient-care areas when they are visibly dusty or soiled. *(II)*

Avoid large-surface cleaning methods that produce mists or aerosols or disperse dust in patient-care areas. *(IB)*

Follow proper procedures for effective use of mops, cloths, and solutions [as recommended]. *(II)*

Take precautions when using phenolic disinfectants in neonatal units. *(IB)*

- **Dusting and Vacuuming**

Use proper dusting and vacuuming methods for patient-care areas. *(IB)*

Wet dust horizontal surfaces daily using cloths moistened with an EPA-registered hospital disinfectant. *(IB)*

Avoid dusting methods that disperse dust (i.e., feather dusting). *(IB)*

Keep vacuums in good repair, and equip vacuums with HEPA filters for use in high-risk patient-care areas. *(IB)*

Close the doors of immunocompromised patients' rooms when vacuuming corridor floors to minimize exposure to airborne dust. *(IB)*

- **Spills of blood and body substances**

  Promptly clean and decontaminate spills of blood or OPIM. *(IC)*

  Follow proper procedures for site decontamination of spills of blood or blood-containing body fluids. *(IC)*

  Use intermediate-level germicides (germicides registered by the EPA for use as hospital disinfectants and labeled tuberculocidal) at recommended dilution and full-contact time to decontaminate spills of blood and other body fluids. *(IC)*

  Use a one-step cleaning/disinfecting procedure for small spills. *(II)*

  If sodium hypochlorite solutions (e.g., household chlorine bleach) are selected for use:

    Use a 1:100 dilution (500 ppm available chlorine) to decontaminate nonporous surfaces after cleaning a spill of either blood or body fluids in patient-care settings. *(IB)*

    If a spill involves large amounts of blood or body fluids, or if a blood or culture spill occurs in the laboratory, use a 1:10 dilution (5,000 ppm available chlorine) for the first application of germicide before cleaning. *(IB)*

- **Carpeting and cloth furnishings**

  Vacuum carpeting in public areas of healthcare facilities and in general patient-care areas regularly with well-maintained equipment designed to minimize dust dispersion. *(II)*

  Perform a thorough, deep cleaning of carpeting periodically as determined by facility policy using a method that minimizes the production of aerosols and leaves little or no residue. *(II)*

Avoid the use of carpeting in high-traffic zones in patient-care areas or where spills are likely (e.g., burn therapy units, operating rooms, labs, intensive care units). *(II)*

Follow proper procedures for managing spills on carpeting. *(II)*

No recommendation on the routine use of fungicidal or bactericidal treatments for carpeting in public areas of a healthcare facility or in general patient-care areas. *(UI)*

Avoid the use of carpeting in hallways and patient rooms in areas housing immunosuppressed patients (i.e., PE areas). *(IB)*

Avoid the use of upholstered furniture and furnishings in high-risk patient-care areas and in areas with increased potential for body substance contamination (e.g., pediatrics units). *(II)*

No recommendation on the use of upholstered furniture and furnishings in general patient-care areas. *(UI)*

- **Flowers and plants in patient-care areas**

Flowers and potted plants need not be restricted from areas for immunocompetent patients. *(II)*

Designate the care and maintenance of flowers and potted plants to staff not directly involved with patient care. *(II)*

Do not allow flowers (fresh or dried) or potted plants in patient-care areas for immunosuppressed patients. *(II)*

- **Pest control**

Develop pest control strategies, with emphasis on kitchens, cafeterias, laundries, central sterile supply areas, operating rooms, loading docks, and other areas prone to infestations. *(II)*

Install screens on all windows that open to the outside; keep screens in good repair. *(II)*

Contract for routine pest control service by a credentialed pest control specialist who will tailor the application to the needs of a healthcare facility. *(II)*

- **Special pathogens**

  Develop and maintain cleaning and disinfection procedures to control environmental contamination with antibiotic-resistant gram-positive cocci (e.g., MRSA, and VRE). *(IB)*

  Develop and maintain cleaning and disinfection procedures to control environmental contamination with *Clostridium difficile*. *(IB)*

  Develop and maintain cleaning and disinfection procedures to control environmental contamination with respiratory and enteric viruses in pediatric-care units. *(II)*

  Develop and maintain cleaning and disinfection procedures to control environmental contamination with Creutzfeldt Jakob disease (CJD) agent in patient-care areas. *(II)*

➤ **Environmental Sampling**

- Do not conduct random, undirected microbiologic sampling of air, water, and environmental surfaces in healthcare facilities. *(IB)*
- When indicated, conduct microbiologic sampling as part of an epidemiologic investigation. *(IB)*
- Limit microbiologic sampling for quality assurance purposes to: 1) biological monitoring of sterilization processes; 2) monthly cultures of water and dialysate in hemodialysis units; and 3) short-term evaluation of the impact of infection control measures or changes in infection control protocols. *(IB)*

➤ **Air, water, environmental surface sampling**

- Select a high-volume air-sampling device if anticipated levels of microbial airborne contamination are expected to be low. *(II)*
- Do not use settle plates to quantify the concentration of airborne fungal spores. *(II)*

- When sampling water, choose growth media and incubation conditions that will facilitate the recovery of waterborne organisms. *(II)*
- When using a sample/rinse method for sampling an environmental surface, develop and document a procedure for manipulating the swab, gauze, or sponge in a reproducible manner so that results are comparable. *(II)*
- When environmental samples and patient specimens are available for comparison, perform the laboratory analysis on the recovered microorganisms down to the species level at a minimum and beyond the species level if possible. *(II)*
- When conducting any form of environmental sampling, fully document departures from standard methods. *(II)*

➤ **Laundry and Bedding**

- Employers should launder workers' personal protective garments or uniforms that are contaminated with blood or other potentially infectious materials. *(IC)*
- No recommendation on home laundering of uniforms or apparel not considered personal protective equipment if these garments are not soiled with blood or other potentially infectious material. *(UI)*
- **Laundry facilities and equipment**
  (Refer to Section 2 - Laundry Handling)

  Maintain the receiving area for soiled linens at negative pressure compared to the clean areas of the laundry. *(IC)*

  Ensure that laundry areas have handwashing facilities and products and appropriate personal protective equipment available for workers. *(IC)*

  Use and maintain laundry equipment according to manufacturers' instructions. *(II)*

  Handle soiled textiles and fabrics with minimum agitation to avoid contamination of air, surfaces, and persons. *(IC)*

Bag or otherwise contain soiled textiles and fabrics at the point of use. *(IC)*

If laundry chutes are used, ensure that they are properly designed and maintained; toss bagged laundry into chutes as opposed to loose items. *(IC)*

Package, transport, and store clean textiles and fabrics by methods that will ensure their cleanliness and protect them from dust and soil during interfacility loading, transport, and unloading. *(IC)*

Do not conduct routine microbiological sampling of clean linens. *(IB)*

- **Mattresses and pillows**

  Keep mattresses dry; discard them if they become and remain wet or stained, particularly in burn units. *(IB)*

  Maintain mattress cover integrity. *(IB)*

    Clean and disinfect mattress covers using disinfectants that are compatible with the cover materials to prevent the development of tears, cracks, or holes in the cover. *(IB)*

    Replace mattress covers if they become torn or otherwise in need of repair. *(II)*

    Do not stick needles into the mattress through the cover. *(II)*

  Change mattress covers between patients. *(IB)*

  Launder pillow covers and washable pillows in the hot-water cycle. *(IB)*

- **Air-fluidized beds**

  Follow manufacturers' instructions for bed maintenance and decontamination. *(II)*

  Change the polyester filter sheet at least weekly or as indicated by the manufacturer. *(II)*

Clean and disinfect the polyester filter sheet thoroughly, especially between patients. *(IB)*

Consult the facility engineer to determine the proper location of air-fluidized beds in negative-pressure rooms. *(IC)*

- **Animals in healthcare facilities**
  (Refer to Section 2 - Service and Companion Animals)

- **Research animals in healthcare facilities**
  (see References/Resources)

- **Regulated medical waste**
  - Designate the following as major categories of medical waste that require special handling and disposal precautions: 1) microbiology laboratory wastes [e.g., cultures and stocks of microorganisms]; 2) bulk blood, blood products, blood and body fluid specimens; 3) pathology and anatomy waste; and 4) sharps [e.g., needles, scalpels]. *(II)*
  - Consult federal, state, and local regulations to determine if other waste items are considered regulated medical wastes. *(IC)*
  - Disposal plan for regulated medical wastes.

    Develop a plan for the collection, handling, pre-disposal treatment, and terminal disposal of regulated medical wastes. *(IC)*

    Designate a person or persons to be responsible for establishing, monitoring, reviewing, and administering the plan. *(II)*
  - Handling, transport, and storage of regulated medical wastes.

    Inform personnel involved in the handling and disposal of potentially infective waste of the possible health and safety hazards; ensure that they are trained in appropriate handling and disposal methods. *(IC)*

Manage the handling and disposal of regulated medical wastes generated in isolation areas using the same methods as for similar wastes from other patient-care areas. *(II)*

Use proper sharps disposal strategies. *(IC)*

Store regulated medical wastes awaiting treatment in a properly ventilated area that is inaccessible to vertebrate pests; use waste containers that prevent the development of noxious odors. *(IC)*

If treatment options are not available at the site where the medical waste is generated, transport regulated medical wastes in closed, impervious containers to the onsite treatment location or to another facility for treatment as appropriate. *(IC)*

- **Treatment and disposal of regulated medical wastes**

Treat regulated medical wastes using a method approved by the state (e.g., steam sterilization, incineration, interment, or an alternative treatment technology) before disposal in a sanitary landfill. *(IC)*

Follow precautions for treating microbiological wastes (e.g., amplified cultures and stocks of microorganisms). *(II)*

Biosafety level three laboratories should autoclave microbiological wastes in the laboratory or incinerate them at the facility before transport to and disposal in a sanitary landfill. *(II)*

Biosafety levels one and two laboratories should develop strategies to reinstate the capacity of autoclaving amplified microbial cultures and stocks onsite instead of packaging and shipping untreated wastes to an offsite facility for treatment and disposal. *(II)*

Sanitary sewers may be used for the safe disposal of blood, suctioned fluids, ground tissues, excretions, and secretions, provided that local sewage discharge requirements are met and that the state has declared this to be an acceptable method of disposal. *(II)*

Special precautions for wastes generated during care of patients with rare diseases.

When discarding items contaminated with blood and body fluids from viral hemorrhagic fever patients, use methods that minimize the production of aerosols. *(II)*

Manage properly contained wastes from areas providing care to viral hemorrhagic fever patients in accordance with recommendations for other isolation areas. *(II)*

Decontaminate bulk blood and body fluids from viral hemorrhagic fever patients using either autoclaving or chemical treatment before disposal. *(II)*

Follow the recommendation for managing isolation room medical wastes when disposing waste from clinical areas providing care for CJD patients. *(II)*

References/Resources

- American Institute of Architects, Guidelines for design and construction of hospital and healthcare facilities, 2001 edition, The American Institute of Architects, Washington, D.C.; 2001.
- American Society of Heating, Refrigerating, and Air-Conditioning Engineers. 1999 ASHRAE Handbook: Heating, Ventilating, and Air-Conditioning Applications. Chapter 7: Healthcare Facilities. Atlanta GA; 1999:p 7.1-7.13.
- American Society of Heating, Refrigerating and Air-conditioning Engineers, Inc. Ventilation for Indoor Air Quality. ASHRAE Standard 62 - 1999; Atlanta GA; 1999: p. 1-27.
- Association for Professionals in Infection Control and Epidemiology. APIC Text of Infection Control and Epidemiology. 2000, chapters 74, 76, 77, 78, 123.

- Centers for Disease Control and Prevention, Healthcare Infection Control Practices Advisory Committee (HICPAC). Draft guideline for environmental infection control in healthcare facilities, 2001. March 6, 2001, Federal Register.
- Centers for Disease Control and Prevention (CDC), National Institutes of Health (NIH). Biosafety in Microbiological and Biomedical Laboratories, 4th Ed. Washington DC; U.S. Government Printing Office; 1999.

Food Handling

Overview

➤ The safety of the food supply in the United States is of concern to all consumers. Even though in recent years public health efforts have focused on educating consumers on proper food handling techniques, food-related illness remains a serious public health problem. Each year up to 33 million cases of foodborne illness occurs in the U.S. and more than 9,000 die from foodborne illness. Economically, the costs of foodborne illness can be into the billions of dollars related to treatment, medications, and missed work time. Symptoms (cramps, diarrhea, vomiting, fever) can be mild to serious, with illness occurring from 30 minutes to two weeks after eating food containing harmful bacteria. Healthcare facilities should follow the U.S. Food and Drug Administration Food Code, establishing policies and procedures and training employees on the food laws. Strict adherence to food handling guidelines with foods that are consumed orally, enterally, or via the parental route can prevent most cases of foodborne illness.

Purpose

➤ Provide an overview to assist with evaluation and/or revision of IC practices related to food handling to decrease the incidence and prevent foodborne illness.

Definitions:

➤ **Hazard Analysis and Critical Control Point** (HACCP) is a prevention-based food safety system designed to stop the occurrence of potential problems by identifying and monitoring specific hazards—biological, chemical, or physical properties that can adversely affect the safety of the food product.

- **Potentially Hazardous Foods** (PHF) is a natural or synthetic food that requires temperature control because it is capable of supporting:
  - The rapid and progressive growth of infectious or toxigenic microorganisms.
  - The growth and toxin production of *Clostridium botulinum*.
  - In raw egg shells, the growth of *Salmonella enteritidis*.
  - Examples of PHFs: milk and milk products, meats, shell eggs, fish, poultry, shellfish, onions, cooked rice, soy protein products (tofu), potatoes, cut melons, raw seed sprouts.

Risk Factors

- Five leading causes of foodborne illness are:
  - Inadequate cooling of foods,
  - Improper holding temperatures,
  - Poor personal hygiene of food workers,
  - Contaminated equipment, and
  - Obtaining food from unsafe sources, e.g., oysters from contaminated oyster beds.
- Enteral/Parenteral Nutrition risks:
  - Contamination of formulas, solutions:

    During preparation,

    Addition of formula, additives to feeding bag, and

    Manipulation of tubing.
  - Initial contamination or long hang or delivery times.
  - Risk of *Clostridium difficile* diarrhea due to contamination of formulas or delivery set (enteral).

- Foodborne Pathogens
  - *E. coli, Salmonella enteritidis, Listeria monocytogenes, Campylobacter jejuni, Shigella, Vibro vulnificus, Yersinia enterocolitica, Clostridium perfringens, Staphylococcus aureus.*
  - Viral Pathogens transmitted by infected food handlers or through contact with sewage:

    Hepatitis A, Norwalk Virus
  - Parasites:

    Trichinella spiralis (causes trichinosis)

    Cryptosporidium
- Chemical contamination risks:
  - Cleaning agents
  - Additives
  - Pesticides
  - Non-organism Toxins:

    Scombroid toxin in tuna

    Mushrooms
- Physical agent contamination risks:
  - Glass chips
  - Insulation
  - Radioactive materials
- Populations at higher risk for foodborne illness include:
  - Infants, young children
  - Elderly
  - Immunocompromised
  - Critically ill and trauma patients

Strategies for Prevention and Control

➤ **Five key food safety tools:**

- Preventing sick employees from working with foods.
- Demonstrating food facility manager knowledge.
- Ensuring proper time and temperature food controls.
- Preventing contamination of foods by employee hands.
- Advising consumers of the risks of eating raw or undercooked foods of animal origin.

➤ **General food handling practices:**

- Wash hands after using the restroom, after handling raw meat, after removing gloves, and when soiled.
- Use liquid soap; antimicrobial soap is not required.
- A foot operated or uncovered receptacle for disposable towels.
- Use gloves for contact with ready to eat unwrapped food, raw meats, and vegetables.

➤ **Food considerations for highly susceptible populations (e.g., immunocompromised persons)**

- Unpasteurized, prepackaged juice or beverage containing juice; raw or partially cooked animal foods (includes meringue made from unpasteurized eggs); and raw seed sprouts should not be served.
- Food in unopened original containers should not be re-served (includes condiments).
- Pasteurized eggs and egg products should be substituted for raw shell eggs in the preparation of ready to eat or partially cooked foods (e.g., Caesar salad, hollandaise sauce, eggnog), or in recipes in which more than one egg is broken and combined. This is the case except when eggs are combined immediately before cooking for one consumer's serving, such as scrambled eggs (no holding

time permitted); before baking and the eggs are thoroughly cooked, such as cakes or muffins; or if food preparation is conducted under an HACCP plan.

- **Cleaning/Sanitizing**
  - All food contact surfaces should be washed, rinsed, and sanitized. Sanitizer should be at the proper concentration, and/or temperature to effectively eliminate pathogenic bacteria.
  - Food contact surfaces should be maintained in good repair without cracks or crevices and made of material that can be effectively sanitized.
  - Dishes should be allowed to air dry; do not stack dishes together until water is dried.
  - Wiping cloths should be stored in an approved sanitizing solution.
  - Thermometers should be sanitized between each measurement.
- **Thawing of frozen foods**
  - Food should be properly thawed to ensure that pathogenic bacteria do not grow on the portion of food that is not frozen.
  - Proper thawing is done in a refrigerator, under cold running water, in a microwave (cook immediately following thawing), or during the cooking process.
- **Cooking**
  - Potentially hazardous foods should have carefully controlled times and temperatures to ensure safety. Proper internal temperature varies with different cuts and types of meats and poultry when cooking or reheating.
  - Temperatures should be measured with an approved, appropriate calibrated food thermometer. Test temperatures at the center of the food product furthest from the heat source.

- Pasteurized shell eggs, pasteurized frozen liquid, or dry eggs or egg products should be substituted for raw shell eggs unless raw eggs are combined as an ingredient in a food item to be baked immediately. Raw shell eggs cooked at 145°F or above for 15 seconds may be used for an immediate consumption, single serving such as an omelet, soufflé, or scrambled eggs.

➤ **Cooling of heated foods**

- All potentially hazardous foods should be cooled within two hours from 140°F to 70°F, then an additional four hours to cool from 70°F to 41°F. If this time cannot be met, food should be cooled from 140°F to 41°F in four hours.

➤ **Holding of heated foods**

- Potentially hazardous foods, which are being held prior to serving: Hot food should be maintained at or above 140°F and cold foods maintained at or below 41°F.
- If a refrigerator is maintained at or below 41°F at all times, potentially hazardous leftover foods may be kept for seven days, which includes the day the product is prepared. If the refrigerator reaches above 41°F at any time, the shelf life of the leftover food is limited to four days.

➤ **Refrigeration of foods**

- Refrigerators should be able to maintain potentially hazardous foods at or below 41°F, and should be set at approximately 37°F or below to accomplish this.
- Freezers should be set at or below 0°F at all times.
- Thermometers should be provided in units to ensure that proper temperatures are maintained.
- All foods should be properly covered.
- Potentially hazardous foods, ready-to-eat foods, and foods held in refrigeration for more than a cumulative total of 24 hours should be clearly marked with the date they should be discarded.

- Meats, poultry, shellfish, and eggs may not be stored over food products that will not be cooked prior to being served.

➤ **Storage of foods**

- Dented or bulging cans should not be used and should be immediately discarded.
- Foods should not be stored under overhead sewer pipes.
- Chemicals should be stored separately from food to prevent contamination.
- Light bulbs should be shielded from breakage in food storage areas.

➤ **Enteral Nutrition**

- Enteral tube feedings are preferred over parenteral.
- Minimal mixing/diluting of formulas is preferred to reduce contamination risks.
- Strict handwashing with any manipulation of formula or equipment should be enforced.
- In most cases, clean technique is adequate for preparations. However, for high-risk neonates and immune deficient persons, sterile technique should be used.
- Undiluted/canned formula or prefilled containers should be used when possible.
- The use of additives should be minimized.
- Hang times should not exceed times stated in the facility policy.
- Tubing and bags should be changed at established times.

- Parenteral (TPN) Nutrition
  - Protocols for aseptic care and maintenance of the access site (catheter) should be maintained.
  - Bacterial filters should be used.
  - Lipids should not be allowed to infuse for longer than 12 hours.
- **HACCP system**
  - Monitoring and verification steps are included to ensure that potential risks are controlled.
  - The hazard analysis, critical control points, critical limits, and monitoring and verification steps are documented in a HACCP plan.
  - Seven principles are in an effective HACCP plan (see resources for details):

    Identify potential food safety hazards,

    Identify the critical control points (CCP) in food preparation,

    Establish critical limits/control procedures for preventive measures,

    Establish monitoring procedures,

    Establish corrective actions,

    Establish effective record-keeping systems to document the HACCP system, and

    Establish procedures to verify that the HACCP system is working.
  - Local regulations should also be addressed and followed.

References/Resources

- American Society for Parenteral and Enteral Nutrition: www.aspen@nutr.org
- Association for Professionals in Infection Control and Epidemiology. APIC Text of Infection Control and Epidemiology. 2000, chapters 37,57,121.
- Association for Professionals in Infection Control and Epidemiology (APIC), Food Safety Pamphlet www.apic.org
- Food Code, 1999. Recommendations of the United States Public Health Service, Food and Drug Administration. National Technical Information Service Publication PB99115917. Washington, DC: US Government Printing Office; 1999
- Guidelines for the Use of Parenteral and Enteral Nutrition in Adult and Pediatric Patients, Routes to Deliver Nutrition Support in Adults, 2001 www.nutritioncare.org
- Schmeichel P., Michigan Department of Consumer and Industry Services, Prescription for Safe Food Handling Practices, 2000.
- U. S. Department of Health and Human Services, Public Health Service, Food and Drug Administration, 2001 Food Code Available online in both HTML and PDF versions at www.fda.gov

Handwashing and Hand Hygiene

Overview

- Handwashing is considered one of the most important measures for reducing transmission of infectious agents in healthcare settings. Evidence has shown that adherence of HCWs to recommended handwashing practices is poor.

Purpose

- Provide ICPs with specific recommendations to promote improved hand hygiene practices and reduce transmission of pathogenic microorganisms to patients and personnel in healthcare settings.
- Explore References/Resources listed for a thorough review of evidence and further information related to handwashing and hand antisepsis in healthcare settings.

Risk Factors

- Failure of healthcare workers to wash hands has been associated with the transmission of infections.
- Poor skin integrity may enhance the risk of infection.

Strategies for Prevention and Control

- **CDC/HICPAC Guidelines for Hand Hygiene in Healthcare Settings** ***(Draft 11/9/01)*** recommendations are designed to improve hand hygiene practices of HCWs and to reduce transmission of pathogenic microorganisms to patients and personnel in healthcare settings. Each recommendation is categorized on the basis of existing scientific data, theoretical rationale, applicability, and economic impact. The system for categorizing recommendations is as follows:

- **Category IA** *(IA)*. Strongly recommended for implementation and strongly supported by well-designed experimental, clinical, or epidemiological studies.
- **Category IB** *(IB)*. Strongly recommended for implementation and supported by some experimental, clinical, or epidemiological studies and a strong theoretical rationale.
- **Category IC** *(IC)*. Required by state or federal regulations, rules, or standards.
- **Category II** *(II)*. Suggested for implementation and supported by suggestive clinical or epidemiological studies or a theoretical rationale.
- **No recommendation; unresolved issue** *(UI)*. Practices for which evidence is insufficient or no consensus regarding efficacy exist.

Strategies for Prevention

➤ Handwashing and decontamination

- Wash hands with a non-antimicrobial soap and water or an antimicrobial soap and water when hands are visibly dirty or contaminated with proteinaceous material. *(IA)*
- If hands are not visibly soiled, use an alcohol-based waterless antiseptic agent for routinely decontaminating hands in all other clinical situations described below. *(IA)*
- On nursing units where an alcohol-based waterless antiseptic agent is available, provide personnel with a non-antimicrobial soap for use when hands are visibly dirty or contaminated with proteinaceous material. It is not necessary and may be confusing to personnel to have both an alcohol-based waterless antiseptic agent and an antimicrobial soap available on the same nursing unit. *(II)*
- Although waterless antiseptic agents are highly preferable, hand antisepsis using an antimicrobial soap may be considered in

settings where time constraints are not an issue and easy access to hand hygiene facilities can be ensured or in rare instances when a caregiver is intolerant of the waterless antiseptic product used in the institution. *(IB)*

- Decontaminate hands after contact with a patient's intact skin (as in taking a pulse or blood pressure, or lifting a patient). *(IB)*
- Decontaminate hands after contact with body fluids or excretions, mucous membranes, non-intact skin, or wound dressings, as long as hands are not visibly soiled. *(IA)*
- Decontaminate hands if moving from a contaminated body site to a clean body site during patient care. *(II)*
- Decontaminate hands after contact with inanimate objects (including medical equipment) in the immediate vicinity of the patient. *(II)*
- Decontaminate hands before caring for patients with severe neutropenia or other forms of severe immune suppression. *(II)*
- Decontaminate hands before donning sterile gloves when inserting a central intravascular catheter. *(IB)*
- Decontaminate hands before inserting indwelling urinary catheters or other invasive devices that do not require a surgical procedure. *(IB)*
- Decontaminate hands after removing gloves. *(IB)*
- To improve hand hygiene adherence among personnel in units or instances where high workloads and high intensity of patient care are anticipated, make an alcohol-based waterless antiseptic agent available at the entrance to the patient's room, at the bedside, in other convenient locations, and in individual pocket-sized containers to be carried by HCWs. *(IA)*

➤ **Hand hygiene technique**

- When decontaminating hands with a waterless antiseptic agent such as an alcohol-based handrub, apply product to palm of one hand and rub hands together, covering all surfaces of hands and fingers until hands are dry. *(IB)* Follow the manufacturer's recommendations on the volume of product to use. If an adequate volume of an alcohol-based handrub is used, it should take 15 to 25 seconds for hands to dry.

- When washing hands with a non-antimicrobial or antimicrobial soap, wet hands first with warm water, apply three to five ml of detergent to hands and rub hands together vigorously for at least 15 seconds, covering all surfaces of the hands and fingers. Rinse hands with warm water and dry thoroughly with a disposable towel. Use towel to turn off the faucet. *(IB)*

➤ **Surgical hand antisepsis**

- Surgical hand antisepsis, using either an alcohol-based handrub or an antimicrobial soap, is recommended before donning sterile gloves when performing surgical procedures. *(IB)*
- To reduce the number of bacteria that may be released from the hands of surgical personnel while minimizing skin damage related to surgical hand antisepsis, decontaminate hands without using a brush. *(IB)*

➤ **Selection of hand hygiene agents**

- Provide personnel with efficacious hand hygiene products that have low irritancy potential, particularly when used multiple times per shift. *(IB)*
- To maximize acceptance of hand hygiene products by health personnel, solicit input from caregivers regarding the feel, fragrance, and skin tolerance of any products under consideration. Cost of hand hygiene products should not be the primary factor influencing product selection. *(IB)*
- Prior to making purchasing decisions, evaluate the dispenser systems of various product manufacturers or distributors to ensure

that dispensers function adequately and deliver an appropriate volume of product. *(II)*

- Do not add soap to a partially empty soap dispenser. This practice of "topping off" dispensers may lead to bacterial contamination of soap. *(IA)*

➤ **Skin care**

- Provide HCWs with hand lotions or creams in order to minimize the occurrence of irritant contact dermatitis associated with hand antisepsis or handwashing. *(IA)*
- Solicit information from manufacturers regarding any effects that hand lotions, creams, or alcohol-based hand antiseptics may have on the persistent effects of antimicrobial soaps being used in the institution. *(IB)*

➤ **Other Aspects of Hand Hygiene**

- Do not wear artificial fingernails or extenders when providing patient care. *(IA)*
- Keep natural nails less than 1/4 inch long. *(II)*
- Wear gloves when it can be reasonably anticipated that contact with blood or other potentially infectious materials, mucous membranes, and non-intact skin will occur. *(IC)*
- Remove gloves after caring for a patient. Do not wear the same pair of gloves for the care of more than one patient, and do not wash gloves between patients. *(IB)*
- Change gloves during patient care if moving from a contaminated body site to a clean body site. *(II)*
- No recommendation on wearing rings in healthcare settings. *(UI)*

➤ **HCW educational and motivational programs**

- As part of an overall program to improve hand hygiene practices of HCWs, educate personnel regarding the types of patient care activities that can result in hand contamination and the advantages and disadvantages of various methods used to clean their hands. *(II)*

- Monitor HCW adherence with recommended hand hygiene practices; provide personnel with information regarding their performance. *(IA)*
- Encourage patients and their families to remind HCWs to decontaminate their hands. *(II)*

➤ **Administrative measures**

- Make improved hand hygiene adherence an institutional priority and provide appropriate administrative support and financial resources. *(IB)*
- Implement a multidisciplinary program designed to improve adherence of health personnel to recommended hand hygiene practices. *(IB)*
- As part of a multidisciplinary program to improve hand hygiene adherence, provide HCWs with a readily accessible waterless antiseptic agent such as an alcohol-based handrub. *(IA)*

➤ **Outcome or process measurements**

- Develop and implement a system for measuring improvements in adherence of HCWs workers to recommended hand hygiene practices:

    Monitor and record adherence as the number of hand hygiene episodes performed by personnel/number of hand hygiene opportunities, by ward or by service; provide feedback to personnel regarding their performance.

    Monitor the volume of alcohol-based handrub (or detergent used for handwashing or hand antisepsis) used/1000 patient-days.

Monitor adherence to policies dealing with wearing of artificial nails.

When outbreaks of infection occur, assess the adequacy of HCW hand hygiene.

References/Resources

- Association for Professionals in Infection Control and Epidemiology. APIC Text of Infection Control and Epidemiology. 2000, chapter 28, 1-2.
- Association for Professionals in Infection Control and Epidemiology. APIC guideline for handwashing and hand antisepsis in healthcare settings. 1995, An J Infect Control 23:251-269.
- Centers for Disease Control and Prevention, Healthcare Infection Control Practices Advisory Committee (HICPAC). Draft Guideline for hand hygiene in healthcare settings. November 2001. Federal Register.
- Rutala, WA. Disinfection, sterilization, and antisepsis: principles and practices in healthcare facilities. Washington, DC: Association for Professionals in Infection Control and Epidemiology, Inc. 2000.

Immunizations of HCW, Children, Adult

Overview

- Immunization is the most effective means of preventing certain infectious diseases. Vaccinations against diphtheria, tetanus, pertussis, measles, mumps, rubella, varicella, poliomyelitis, Hepatitis B, *Haemophilus influenzae* type b, and pneumococcal invasive disease are routinely administered in the United States, usually in childhood.
- Individuals without a history of adequate protection against these diseases, immunizations appropriate to their age and previous immunization status should be evaluated for administration and the action taken should be documented in the medical record.
- Immunization schedules change frequently; immunization providers should obtain the most current recommendations from the appropriate agencies (e.g., ACIP and AAP—see References/ Resources).

Purpose

- Provide basic information regarding immunizations in a variety of table formats. Refer to References/Resources for details and updates.

Risk Factors

- Immunizations are not available for all infectious agents.
- Time for effective development of antibody postimmunization may be insufficient to offer protection.

- Simultaneous administration of certain vaccines may be contraindicated.
- If certain vaccines (e.g., MMR and varicella) are given with immune globulin (IG, formerly called immune serum globulin and immunoglobulin) preparations, antibody response can be diminished.
- Existing personal/health conditions may increase risk of an adverse outcome and/or prevent antibody response.

Strategies for Prevention and Control

- A complete medical history and evaluation should include:
  - Present medical therapies.
  - Drug allergies.
  - Any chronic diseases or current significant health issues (e.g., pregnancy, contraindications, immunocompromised condition).
  - Immunization history.
- Every medical encounter should be treated as an opportunity for updating immunizations.
- Public, patient, and caregiver education regarding vaccines should be provided routinely.
- As with all healthcare treatment, patients should be provided complete information about benefits and risks of immunizations; some immunizations may require informed consent (e.g., Hepatitis B vaccine in HCWs).
- Immunization/antibody response may be measured by laboratory testing, although not routinely performed in most cases.

VACCINE RECOMMENDATIONS FOR HEALTHCARE WORKERS (HCWS)

Disease:

HEPATITIS A

Vaccine Manufacturer:

Inactivated virus vaccine;
Havrix® SmithKline Beecham (800) 672 - 8900;
Vaqta®; Merck and Co. (800) 672 - 6372

Primary Dose/Booster and Route:

1 mL, IM (deltoid)/Booster: 1 mL ;
Six to 12 months after primary dose

Use in Immunocompromised Adults (IA) or Pregnancy (PR):

IA. Because hepatitis A vaccine is inactivated, no special precautions for vaccinating the immunocompromised

PR. It is not known whether hepatitis A vaccine can cause fetal harm when administered to a pregnant woman or can affect reproduction capacity. The risk associated with vaccination should be weighed against the risk for hepatitis A in women at high risk for exposure to hepatitis A.

Contraindications:

Hepatitis A vaccine should not be administered to persons with a history of hypersensitivity reactions to Alum or, in the case of Havrix, to the preservative 2 - phenoxyethanol.

Comments:

Can be given with IgG, although the ultimate antibody titer obtained is likely to be lower than when the vaccine is given alone.

Hepatitis A vaccine may be considered in food handlers who work in healthcare facilities and the staffs of neonatal intensive care units, day care centers, and institutions for developmentally disabled.

Disease:

HEPATITIS B

Vaccine Manufacturer:

Inactivated virus vaccine;
Recombivax HB®, Recombivax HB®
Merck and Co. (800) 672 - 6372

Primary Dose/Booster and Route:

1 mL, IM (deltoid)/Booster: 1 mL/
One and six months after primary dose.

Use in Immunocompromised Adults (IA) or Pregnancy (PR):

IA. For those undergoing hemodialysis and other immunosuppressed persons, higher vaccine doses/increased number of doses required (Recombivax HB 40 ug/mL).

Those with HIV infection have an impaired response to HBV vaccine. Immunogenicity of higher doses is unknown. The anti-HB surface antigen response of such persons should be tested after they are vaccinated, and those who have not responded should reinitiate the series.

PR. No contraindication.

Contraindications:

Anaphylactic reaction to common baker's yeast or vaccine components.

Comments:

Serologic testing for anti-HBsAg recommended for > 30 years, and younger adults with occupational risk of HBV infection. Duration of protection from vaccine is at least seven years among healthy adults. No current recommendations for booster. Postexposure prophylaxis for non-immune adults: series of HBV vaccine combined w/ single dose (0.06 mL/kg or 5 mL for adults) of HBIG given at a different site.

Disease:

HEPATITIS B

Vaccine Manufacturer:

Engerix-B® SmithKline Beecham (800) 366-8900

Primary Dose/Booster and Route:

1 mL, IM (deltoid)/Booster: 1 mL/
One to six months after primary dose.

Alternate: 1 mL, 1 and two months, plus additional dose at 12 months; may be used for HCWs w/ recent exposure.

Use in Immunocompromised Adults (IA) or Pregnancy (PR):

IA. See Recombivax.
PR. See Recombivax.

Contraindications:

See Recombivax

Comments:

See Recombivax

Disease:

INFLUENZA, Inactivated virus vaccine

Vaccine Manufacturer:

Connaught; (800) 822 - 2463
Lederle; (800) 533-3753
Parke-Davis; (800) 223-0432
Wyeth-Ayerst; (800) 950-5099

Primary Dose/Booster and Route:

0.5 mL, IM (deltoid), yearly
Booster: None.

Use in Immunocompromised Adults (IA) or Pregnancy (PR):

IA. Vaccination recommended.

PR. Pregnant women w/ medical conditions that increase risks of complications from influenza should be vaccinated. Administering vaccine after the first trimester is a reasonable precaution to minimize concern over the theoretical risk of teratogenicity. However, delaying vaccination of those in the first trimester of pregnancy when influenza season begins is undesirable.

Contraindications:

Persons w/ history of anaphylactic reaction after eating eggs should not be given inactivated influenza vaccine. Persons w/ acute febrile illnesses should not be vaccinated until their illness has resolved.

Comments:

HCWs w/ contact with high-risk patients and household members (including children) of high-risk persons should be vaccinated.

Amantadine hydrochloride and rimantadine can prevent influenza A (not B) or can be used to reduce symptoms if started within 72 hours of symptoms. They are not substitutes for vaccine.

Disease:

RUBELLA (GERMAN MEASLES), Live virus vaccine

Vaccine Manufacturer:

MMR II ® (measles, mumps, rubella); M-R Vax II® (measles/rubella); Meruvax® (rubella); Biavax® (mumps/rubella)
Merck (800) 672 - 6372

Primary Dose/Booster and Route:

0.5 mL, SC/Booster: 0.5 mL, SC,
No less than one month after the primary dose.

Use in Immunocompromised Adults (IA) or Pregnancy (PR):

IA. Non–HIV-infected persons: Replication of vaccine viruses can be enhanced in those w/ immune deficiency diseases and with immunosuppression, e.g., leukemia, lymphoma, generalized malignancy or therapy w/ alkylating agents, antimetabolites, radiation or large doses of steroids (excluding asymptomatic HIV-infected); these should not be given live virus vaccines. Leukemic patients who have not received chemotherapy for at least three months may receive live virus vaccines.

Asymptomatic HIV-infected persons ($CD_4 \geq 200$) in need of MMR should receive it.

Severely immunocompromised (e.g., $CD_4 < 200$ for adults) HIV-infected persons should not receive MMR or other measles-containing vaccines pending further ACIP evaluation; should receive immune globulin regardless of prior vac-cination status if exposed to measles.

PR. Contraindicated during pregnancy or for women considering becoming pregnant within the next three months after vaccination.

Contraindications:

Pregnancy (or possibility of, within three months of vaccination).

Anaphylactic reactions to egg ingestion (see Comments column) and neomycin.

Known altered immunodeficiency (hematologic and solid tumors; congenital immunodeficiency; and long-term immunosuppressive therapy) (see Use in Immunocompromised Adults column).

Avoid subsequent dose in patients with previous episode of thrombocytopenia in close temporal proximity to vaccination (i.e., within six weeks after).

MMR contains hydrolyzed gelatin as a stabilizer; persons with a history of anaphylactic reaction to gelatin or gelatin-containing products should be vaccinated with extreme caution.

Comments:

Protocols have been developed for vaccination of those with a history of anaphylactic reactions to egg ingestion; however, predictive value of such skin testing and need for special protocols when vaccinating egg-allergic persons with such vaccines is unclear at this time.

Antibody response may be blunted when administered in close proximity of immunoglobulin/blood and blood products. Postpartum vaccination of rubella-susceptible women with rubella or MMR vaccine should not be delayed because of anti-Rho(D) IG (human) or any other blood product received during the last trimester of pregnancy or delivery.

Disease:

RUBEOLA (MEASLES), Live virus vaccine

Vaccine Manufacturer:

Attenuvax®, (measles); M-R Vax II® (measles/rubella);
MMR II®* (measles/mumps/rubella)
Merck (800) 672 - 6372

Primary Dose/Booster and Route:

0.5 mL, SQ Booster: 0.5 mL, SQ

No less than one month after primary dose

Use in Immunocompromised Adults (IA) or Pregnancy (PR):

IA. See Rubella. Also, severely immunocompromised pts. and symptomatic HIV-infected pts. exposed to measles should receive IG regardless of prior vaccine status (0.5 mL/kg body weight to a maximum dose of 15 mL).

PR. Live measles vaccine, when given as a component of MR or MMR, should not be given to women known to be pregnant or who are considering becoming pregnant within the next six months. Women who are given monovalent measles vaccine should not become pregnant for at least 30 days post vaccination.

Contraindications:

See Rubella.

Comments:

Combined vaccine, MMR II, is preferred. HCWs starting job should have proof of two doses or evidence of immunity (titer). If not, vaccine should be given on employment and 2nd dose ≥ 1 mo. later. Recommend revaccination of HCWs born ≥ 1957 w/ direct patient contact and w/o titer. Vaccination may also be considered for HCWs born < 1957.

Persons who received measles vaccine of unknown type or attenuated vaccine with IG or measles IG, and those vaccinated with live virus vaccine before their first birthday should be considered unvaccinated.

Disease:

MUMPS, Live virus vaccine

Vaccine Manufacturer:

Mumpvax®, Merck (800) 672 - 6372, MMR II®, Biovax®

Primary Dose/Booster and Route:

MMR II® is preferred, 0.5 mL, SC

Booster: 0.5 mL no less than one month after the primary dose

Use in Immunocompromised Adults (IA) or Pregnancy (PR):

IA. See Measles.

PR. See Measles.

Contraindications:

See Measles.

Comments:

Most born <1957 are likely to have been infected naturally and can be considered immune even if they did not have clinically recognizable mumps disease. Persons who received killed mumps vaccine (available from 1950 to 1978) might benefit from vaccination with live mumps vaccine.

Disease:

TETANUS and DIPHTHERIA, Toxoids "For Adult Use" (Td)

Vaccine Manufacturer:

Connaught Labs, (800) 822 - 2463; Lederle Labs, (914) 732 - 5000 Massachusetts Public Health Biologic Labs, (617)-522 - 3700; Wyeth-Ayerst, (800) 321-2304

Primary Dose/Booster and Route:

0.5 mL, IM, followed by second dose four to eight weeks after first dose; third dose should be given six to 12 months after the second dose.

Booster: 0.5 mL, IM, should be given 10 years after completion of the initial series and once every 10 years thereafter.

Use in Immunocompromised Adults (IA) or Pregnancy (PR):

IA. Recommended.

PR. Although no evidence exists that tetanus and diphtheria toxoids are teratogenic, waiting until the second trimester of pregnancy to administer these vaccines is a reasonable precaution.

Contraindications:

Only contraindication is history of a neurologic or severe hypersensitivity reaction after a previous dose. Those with an Arthrus-type hypersensitivity reaction. or temp. of 103°F after a dose usually have high tetanus antitoxin levels and should not be given even emergency doses of Td more often than every 10 years, even with an unclean/major wound. If contraindication to Td exists for person w/o immunization and they have an unclean or large wound, only passive immunization should be given using tetanus immunoglobulin (TIG).

Comments:

Td is the preparation of choice for adults rather than DT because of decreased side effects.

Disease:

VARICELLA (CHICKEN-POX), Live virus vaccine

Vaccine Manufacturer:

Varivax®, Merck (800) 672 - 6372

Primary Dose/Booster and Route:

0.5 mL, SC

Booster: 0.5 mL, SC, four to eight weeks after the first dose.

Use in Immunocompromised Adults (IA) or Pregnancy (PR):

IA. Contraindicated (see section).

PR. Contraindicated. Possible effects on fetal development are unknown. However, natural varicella is known to sometimes cause fetal harm. If vaccination is given to post pubertal females, pregnancy should be avoided for one month post-vaccination. For susceptible persons with a pregnant family member, vaccination is not contraindicated. If pregnancy occurs within one month or at time of vaccination, counseling about potential effects on the fetus should be provided. Owing to lower virulence of vaccine strain compared with wild-type virus, the risk to fetus, if any, should be even lower. Generally, the decision to terminate pregnancy should not be based on vaccine administration. Contact Varivax® Pregnancy Registry (800-986-8999) if varicella virus vaccine is inadvertently administered three months before or any time during pregnancy.

Contraindications:

History of hypersensitivity to any component of vaccine including gelatin; history of anaphylactic reaction. to neomycin; blood dyscrasia, leukemia, lymphomas (any), malignant neoplasms affecting bone marrow or lymphatic system; those receiving immunosuppressive therapy or immunsuppressant doses of corticosteroids; primary or acquired immunodeficiency states, including AIDS or other clinical manifestations of infection with HIV, cellular immune deficiencies, and hypo/dysgammaglo-bulinemic states; family hx of congenital or hereditary immunodeficiency, unless immune competence of the potential vaccine recipient can be demonstrated; pregnancy; active untreated TB; any febrile respiratory illness or active febrile infection.

Comments:

Vaccination of susceptible HCWs, teachers of young children, resident/staff in institutional setting, family contacts of immunosuppressed persons, college students, inmates and staff of correctional facilities, military personnel, and susceptible international travelers is recommended. Routine postvaccination testing for immunity is not necessary for management of HCWs who may be exposed to varicella, because 99% become seropositive after the 2nd dose; however, seroconversion does not always result in full protection. Testing vaccinees for titer immediately after exposure to VZV may be considered to identify those still at risk for varicella; those with positive antibody are unlikely to develop varicella. HCWs w/o titer can be retested in five to six days; if seropositive are unlikely to develop disease. HCWs who remain seronegative may be furloughed or monitored daily to determine clinical status and furloughed at onset of varicella symptoms. It is not known whether immediate vaccination after natural exposure will prevent infection. Vaccination should be deferred at least five months after blood [except washed red blood cells (RBCs)] or plasma transfusion or administration of immune globulin or VZIG.

VZIG or other immune globulins should not be given for at least three weeks after vaccination unless the benefits of use outweighs the benefit of vaccine. Avoid use of salicylates for six weeks after vaccination (Reye's syndrome has been reported after the use of salicylates during natural varicella infection).

Note: The following applies to the chart on the facing page

This schedule indicates the recommended ages for routine administration of currently licensed childhood vaccines, as of December 1, 2001, for children through age 18 years. Any dose not given at the recommended age should be given at any subsequent visit when indicated and feasible. Indicates age groups that warrant special effort to administer those vaccines not previously given. Additional vaccines may be licensed and recommended during the year. Licensed combination vaccines may be used whenever any components of the combination are indicated and the vaccine's other components are not contraindicated. Providers should consult the manufacturers' package inserts for detailed recommendations.

1. Hepatitis B vaccine (Hep B). All infants should receive the first dose of hepatitis B vaccine soon after birth and before hospital discharge; the first dose may also be given by age 2 months if the infant's mother is HBsAg-negative. Only monovalent hepatitis B vaccine can be used for the birth dose. Monovalent or combination vaccine containing Hep B may be

continued on page 226

Recommended Childhood Immunization Schedule
United States, 2002

Range of recommended ages | Catch-up vaccinations | Preadolescent Assessment

Age → / Vaccine ↓	Birth	1 Mo.	2 Mo.	4 Mo.	6 Mo.	12 Mo.	15 Mo.	18 Mo.	24 Mo.	4-6 Yrs.	11-12 Yrs.	13-18 Yrs.
Hepatitis B	Hep B #1	(only if mother has)	Hep B #2			Hep B #3					Hep B series	
Diptheria, Tenanus Pertussis			DTP	DTP	DTP		DTP			DTP	Td	
Haemophilus Influenza type b			HiB	HiB	HiB	HiB						
Inactivated Polio			IPV	IPV		IPV				IPV		
Measles, Mumps, Rubella						MMR #1				MMR #2	MMR #2	
Varicella						Varicella				Varicella		
Pneumococcal			PCV	PCV	PCV	PCV			PCV		PPV	
Hepatitis A										Hepatitis A Series		
Influenza									Influenza (yearly)			

used to complete the series; four doses of vaccine may be administered if combination vaccine is used. The second dose should be given at least four weeks after the first dose, except for Hib-containing vaccine which cannot be administered before age 6 weeks. The third dose should be given at least 16 weeks after the first dose and at least eight weeks after the second dose. The last dose in the vaccination series (third or fourth dose) should not be administered before age 6 months. Infants born to HBsAg-positive mothers should receive hepatitis B vaccine and 0.5 mL hepatitis B immune globulin (HBIG) within 12 hours of birth at separate sites. The second dose is recommended at age 1-2 months and the vaccination series should be completed (third or fourth dose) at age 6 months. Infants born to mothers whose HBsAg status is unknown should receive the first dose of the hepatitis B vaccine series within 12 hours of birth. Maternal blood should be drawn at the time of delivery to determine the mother's HBsAg status; if the HBsAg test is positive, the infant should receive HBIG as soon as possible (no later than age 1 week). **2. Diphtheria and tetanus toxoids and acellular pertussis vaccine (DTaP).** The fourth dose of DTaP may be administered as early as age 12 months, provided 6 months have elapsed since the third dose and the child is unlikely to return at age 15-18 months. Tetanus and diphtheria toxoids (Td) is recommended at age 11-12 years if at least 5 years have elapsed since the last dose of tetanus and diphtheria toxoid-containing vaccine. Subsequent routine Td boosters are recommended every 10 years. **3. *Haemophilus influenzae* type b (Hib) conjugate vaccine.** Three Hib conjugate vaccines are licensed for infant use. If PRP-OMP (PedvaxHIB® or ComVax® [Merck]) is administered at ages 2 and 4 months, a dose at age 6 months is not required. DTaP/Hib combination products should not be used for primary immunization in infants at age 2, 4, or 6 months, but can be used as boosters following any Hib vaccine. **4. Inactivated poliovirus vaccine (IPV).** An all-IPV schedule is recommended for routine childhood poliovirus vaccination in the United States. All children should receive four doses of IPV at age 2 months, 4 months, 6-18 months, and 4-6 years. **5. Measles, mumps, and rubella vaccine (MMR).** The second dose of MMR is recommended routinely at age 4-6 years but may be administered during any visit, provided at least four weeks have elapsed since the first dose and that both doses are administered beginning at or after age 12 months. Those who have not previously received the second dose should complete the schedule by the visit at 11-12 years. **6. Varicella vaccine.** Varicella vaccine is recommended at any visit at or after age 12 months for susceptible children (i.e., those who lack a reliable history of chickenpox). Susceptible persons aged >13 years should receive two doses, given at least four weeks apart. **7. Pneumococcal vaccine.** The heptavalent **pneumococcal conjugate vaccine** (PCV) is recommended for all children aged 2 - 23 months and for certain children aged 24-59 months. **Pneumococcal polysaccharide vaccine** (PPV) is recommended in addition to PCV for certain high-risk groups. **8. Hepatitis A vaccine.** Hepatitis A vaccine is recommended for use in selected states and regions, and for certain high-risk groups; consult your local public health authority. **9. Influenza vaccine.** Influenza vaccine is recommended annually for children age >6 months with certain risk factors (including but not limited to asthma, cardiac disease, sickle cell disease, HIV, and diabetes, and can be administered to all others wishing to obtain immunity. Children aged =12 years should receive vaccine in a dosage appropriate for their age (0.25 mL if age 6-35 months or 0.5 mL if aged =3 years). Children aged =8 years who are receiving influenza vaccine for the first time should receive two doses separated by at least 4 weeks.

Vaccine Recommendations for Adults— Considerations by Risk Group

Risk Group	Vaccines Considered*	Additional Considerations
General Risk Groups		
Healthy adults		
<25 yrs old	Td, MMR, varicella†, Hep. B	
25–64 years old	Td, Rubella (women only)	
≥65 years	Td, influenza, pneumococcal	
Pregnant women	———	MMR contraindicated; test for rubella Ab and HbsAg
Immigrants and refugees	Review all immunizations	PPD
Groups by Place of Residence		
Nursing home	Td, influenza, pneumococcal	PPD
Institution mentally disabled	Hep. B; review all vaccines	Hepatitis A
Prison	Hepatitis B	PPD
Homeless	Review all vaccines	PPD

Vaccine Recommendations for Adults— Considerations by Risk Group

Risk Group	Vaccines Considered*	Additional Considerations
Groups by Lifestyle		
Homosexual/ bisexual males	Hepatitis B, Hepatitis A	
Intravenous drug users	Hepatitis B, Hepatitis A Td	
Prostitutes, those w/ multiple partners or STDs	Hepatitis B	
Groups by Occupation		
College students	MMR, hepatitis B, Td influenza, varicella†	Meningococcal vaccine**
Food handlers	Hepatitis A	
HCWs	Hepatitis B, MMR, Td, influenza, varicella†	
Day care workers	MMR, influenza, hepatitis A, varicella†	
Laboratory workers	Hep. B; review all vaccines	
Veterinarians, animal handlers, rural, and field workers	Rabies, plague, anthrax	

Vaccine Recommendations for Adults— Considerations by Risk Group

Risk Group	Vaccines Considered*	Additional Considerations
Groups by Type of Injury		
Wounds	Td	Tetanus immune globulin (if no prior tetanus vaccination series)
Animal bites	Td	Rabies vaccine, rabies immune globulin (as indicated)
Snake and spider bites	Td	Specific antivenoms
Groups by Immunocompromised Status		
HIV (asymptomatic, $CD^4 > 200/mm^3$)	Td, inactivated polio vaccine, MMR, *H.* influenzae b (Hib), Hepatitis B, pneumococcal, influenza; efficacy of measles vaccine in HIV-infected persons unknown	Oral polio vaccine and varicella vaccine are contraindicated

Vaccine Recommendations for Adults— Considerations by Risk Group

Risk Group	Vaccines Considered*	Additional Considerations
AIDS (CD^4 <200/mm^3)	Same as asymptomatic HIV group except avoid MMR or measles-containing vaccines until further recommendations by ACIP	Same as asymptomatic HIV group; + measles immunoglobulin (0.5 mL/kg, max. 15 mL) indicated within six days after measles exposure regardless of history of measles or vaccine
Splenic disorders	Hib, pneumococcal, meningococcal	
Diabetes	Pneumococcal, influenza, Td	
Renal failure/dialysis	Pneumococcal, influenza, hep. B	
Alcoholism/cirrhosis	Pneumococcal, influenza, hep. B and A (chronic liver disease)	PPD
Immunosuppressive therapy (including organ transplant)	Pneumococcal, influenza	

Vaccine Recommendations for Adults— Considerations by Risk Group

Risk Group	Vaccines Considered*	Additional Considerations
International travel	Td, MMR, polio, typhoid, varicella, influenza, hepatitis A	Yellow fever, Japanese encephalitis, hepatitis B, meningococcal, rabies as indicated.

* Consult product information regarding specific indications, contraindications, dosage, adverse effects, and route of administration.

† When considered non-immune.

** Meningococcal vaccination of college students is not routinely recommended, but may be considered as an adjunct to chemoprophylaxis during outbreaks caused by serogroups represented in the vaccine, and for students traveling to countries recognized as having high rates of meningococcal disease.

Guidelines for Spacing the Administration of Immune Globulin Preparations* and Vaccines Containing Live Measles, Mumps, or Rubella Virus

Simultaneous Administration		Nonsimultaneous Administration		
Immunobiologic Combination	Recommended Minimum Interval Between Doses	Immunobiologic Administered		Recommended Minimum Interval Between Doses
		First	Second	
Immune globulin and vaccine	Should generally not be administered simultaneously.† If simultaneous administration of MMR, MR, and monovalent measles vaccine is unavoidable, administer at different sites and revaccinate or test for seroconversion after the recommended interval.	Immune globulin	Vaccine	Dose related
		Vaccine	Immune globulin	Two weeks

* Blood products containing large amounts of immune globulin [such as serum immune globulin, specific immune globulins (e.g., TIG and HBIG), intravenous immune globulin (IGIV), whole blood, packed red cells, plasma, and platelet products].

† The duration of interference of immune globulin preparations with the immune response to the measles component of the MMR, MR, and monovalent measles vaccine is dose related.

Suggested Intervals Between Administration of Immune Globulin Preparations for Various Indications and Vaccines Containing Live Measles Virus*

Indication	Dose (including mg IgG/kg)	Months Before Measles Vaccine
Tetanus (TIG) prophylaxis	250 U (10 mg IgG/kg), IM	3
Hepatitis A (IG) prophylaxis		
Contact prophylaxis	0.02 mL/kg (3.3 mg IgG/kg), IM	3
International travel	0.06 mL/kg (10 mg IgG/kg), IM	3
Hepatitis B prophylaxis (HBIG)	0.06 mL/kg (10 mg IgG/kg), IM	3
Rabies immune globulin (HRIG)	20 IU/kg (22 mg IgG/kg), IM	4
Varicella prophylaxis (VZIG)	125 U/10 kg (20–40 mg IgG/kg), IM (maximum 625 U)	5
Measles prophylaxis (IG)		
Standard nonimmunocompromised contact	0.25 mL/kg (40 mg IgG/kg), IM	5
Immunocompromised contact	0.50 mL/kg (80 mg IgG/kg), IM	6

Suggested Intervals Between Administration of Immune Globulin Preparations for Various Indications and Vaccines Containing Live Measles Virus*

Indication	Dose (including mg IgG/kg)	Months Before Measles Vaccine
Blood Transfusion		
RBCs, washed	10 mL/kg (negligible IgG/kg), IV	0
RBCs, adenine-saline added	10 mL/kg (10 mg IgG/kg), IV	3
Packed RBCs (Hct 65%)†	10 mL/kg (60 mg IgG/kg), IV	6
Whole blood cells (Hct 35– 50%)†	10 mL/kg (80–100 mg IgG/kg), IV	6
Plasma/platelet products	10 mL/kg (160 mg IgG/kg), IV	7
Replacement therapy for immune deficiencies	300–400 mg/kg, IV,§ (as IGIV)	8
Treatment of:		
Immune thrombocytopenic purpura¶	400 mg/kg, IV (as IGIV)	8
Immune thrombocytopenic purpura¶	1,000 mg/kg, IV (as IGIV)	10
Kawasaki disease	2 g/kg, IV (as IGIV)	11

* This table is not intended for determining the correct indications and dosage for the use of immune globulin preparations. Unvaccinated persons may not be fully protected against measles during the entire suggested time interval, and additional doses of immune globulin and/or measles vaccine may be indicated after measles exposure. The concentration of measles antibody in a particular immune globulin preparation can vary by lot. The rate of antibody clearance after receipt of an immune globulin preparation also can vary. The recommended time intervals are extrapolated from an estimated half-life of 30 days for passively acquired antibody and an observed interference with the immune response to measles vaccine for five months after a dose of 80 mg IgG/kg.

† Assumes a serum IgG concentration of 16 mg/mL.

§ Measles vaccination is recommended for most HIV-infected children who do not have evidence of severe immunosuppression, but it is contraindicated for patients who have congenital disorders of the immune system.

¶ Formerly referred to as idiopathic thrombocytopenic purpura.

SPACING OF VACCINES ALREADY GIVEN												
Vaccine to be given	Measles	Mumps	Rubella	MMR	Hep. B	Hep.A	Varicella	ISG	HBIG	Tetanus	Td/Dp	Inactive flu
Measles	—	30 days	30 days	30 days	30 days	30 days	30 days	12 mos	3 mo	30 days	30 days	2 wk
Mumps	30 days	—	30 days	30 days	30 days	30 days	30 days	12 mos	3 mo	30 days	30 days	2 wk
Rubella	30 days	30 days	—	30 days	30 days	30 days	30 days	12 mos	3 mo	30 days	30 days	2 wk
MMR	30 days	30 days	30 days	—	30 days	30 days	30 days	12 mos	3 mo	30 days	30 days	2 wk
Hep. B	30 days	30 days	30 days	30 days	—	None	30 days	None	None	30 days	30 days	2 wk
Hep. A	30 days	30 days	30 days	30 days	30 days	—	30 days	30 days	30 days	None	None	2 wk
Varicella	30 days	30 days	30 days	30 days	30 days	30 days	—	30 days	30 days	None	None	2 wk
ISG	2 wk	2 wk	2 wk	2 wk	None	None	None	—	None	None	None	None
HBIG	2 wk	2 wk	2 wk	2 wk	None	None	None	None	—	None	None	None
Tetanus	30 days	30 days	30 days	30 days	None	None	None	None	None	—	—	30 days
Td/Dp	30 days	30 days	30 days	30 days	None	None	30 days	None	None	—	—	30 days
Flu	2 wk	2 wk	2 wk	2 wk	2 wk	2 wk	2 wk	2 wk	2 wk	2 wk	2 wk	—

* Consult physician to determine level of risk.

** Should not be given to pregnant adolescents or those considering pregnancy within three months of vaccinations.

*** Should not be given to pregnant adolescents or those considering pregnancy within one month of vaccination.

2/4/2002; SUMMARY OF ADOLESCENT/ADULT IMMUNIZATION RECOMMENDATIONS

AGENT: **Tetanus and Diphtheria Toxoids Combined (Td)**

Indications: All adults.

All adolescents should be assessed at 11-12 or 14-16 years of age and immunized if no dose was received during the previous five years.

Primary Schedule:

Two doses four to eight weeks apart, third dose six to 12 months after the second. No need to repeat doses if the schedule is interrupted.

Dose: 0.5 mL intramuscular (IM)

Booster: At 10 year intervals throughout life

Contraindications:

Neurologic or severe hypersensitivity reaction to prior dose.

Comments:

WOUND MANAGEMENT: Patients with three or more previous tetanus toxoid doses: (a) give Td for clean, minor wounds only if more than 10 years since last dose; (b) for other wounds, give Td if over five years since last dose. Patients with less than three or unknown number of prior tetanus toxoid doses; give Td for clean, minor wounds and Td and TIG (Tetanus Immune Globulin) for other wounds.

AGENT: **Influenza Vaccine**

Indications:

a. Adults 50 years of age and older.

b. Residents of nursing homes or other facilities for patients with chronic med. conditions.

c. Persons ≥ 6 months of age with chronic cardiovascular or pulmonary disorders, including asthma.

d. Persons ≥ 6 months of age with chronic metabolic diseases (including diabetes), renal dysfunction, hemoglobinopathies, immunosuppressive or immunodeficiency disorders.

e. Women in their second or third trimester of pregnancy during influenza season.

f. Persons 6 mo.-18 years of age receiving long-term aspirin therapy.

g. Groups, including household members and caregivers, who can infect high-risk persons.

Primary Schedule:

Dose: 0.5 mL intramuscular (IM)

Given annually each fall and winter.

Contraindications:

Anaphylactic allergy to eggs.

Acute febrile illness.

Comments:

Depending on season and destination, persons traveling to foreign countries should consider vaccination.

Any person ≥ 6 months of age who wishes to reduce the likelihood of becoming ill with influenza should be vaccinated.

Avoiding subsequent vaccination of persons known to have developed GBS within six weeks of a previous vaccination seems prudent; however, for most persons with a GBS history who are at high risk for severe complications, many experts believe the established benefits of vaccination justify yearly vaccination.

AGENT: **Pneumococcal, Polysaccharide Vaccine (PPV)**

Indications:

a. Adults ≥ 65 years of age.

b. Persons ≥ 2 years with chronic cardiovascular or pulmonary disorders including congestive heart failure, diabetes mellitus, chronic liver disease, alcoholism, CSF leaks, cardiomyopathy, COPD or emphysema.

c. Persons ≥ 2 years with splenic dysfunction or asplenia, hematologic malignancy, multiple myeloma, renal failure, organ transplantation or immunosuppressive conditions, including HIV infection.

d. Alaskan Natives and certain American Indian populations.

Primary Schedule:

One dose for most people*

Dose: 0.5 mL intramuscular (IM) or subcutaneous (SC)

* Persons vaccinated prior to age 65 should be vaccinated at age 65 if five or more years have passed since the first dose. For all persons with functional or anatomic asplenia, transplant patients, patients with chronic kidney disease, immunosuppressed or immunodeficient persons, and others at highest risk of fatal infection, a second dose should be given - at least five years after first dose.

Contraindications:

The safety of PPV during first trimester of pregnancy has not been evaluated. The manufacturer's package insert should be reviewed for additional information.

Comments:

If elective splenectomy or immunosuppressive therapy is planned, give vaccine two weeks ahead, if possible.

When indicated, vaccine should be administered to patients with unknown vaccination status. All residents of nursing homes and other long-term care facilities should have their vaccination status assessed and documented.

AGENT: **Measles and Mumps Vaccines****

Indications:

a. Adults born after 1956 without written documentation of immunization on or after the first birthday.

b. HCWs born after 1956 that are at risk of exposure to patients with measles should have documentation of two doses of vaccine on or after the first birthday or of measles seropositivity.

c. HIV-infected persons w/o severe immunosuppression.

d. Travelers to foreign countries.

e. Persons entering post-secondary educational institutions (e.g., college).

Primary Schedule:

At least one dose. (Two doses of measles-containing vaccine if in college, in healthcare profession, or traveling to a foreign country with second dose at least one month after the first).

Dose: 0.5 mL subcutaneous (SC)

Contraindications:

a. Immunosuppressive therapy or immunodeficiency including HIV-infected persons with severe immunosuppression.

b. Anaphylactic reaction to neomycin.

c. Pregnancy.

d. Immune globulin preparation or blood/ blood product received in preceding three to 11 mos.

e. Untreated, active TB.

Comments:

Women should be asked if they are pregnant before receiving vaccine, and advised to avoid pregnancy for 28 days after immunization.

AGENT: **Rubella Vaccine****

Indications:

a. Persons (especially women) without documentation of immunization on or after the first birthday or of seropositivity.

b. HCWs who are at risk of exposure to patients with rubella and who may have contact with pregnant patients should have at least one dose.

Primary Schedule:

One dose.

Dose: 0.5 mL subcutaneous (SC)

Contraindications:

Same as for measles and mumps vaccines.

Comments:

Women should be asked if they are pregnant before receiving vaccine, and advised to avoid pregnancy for 28 days after immunization.

AGENT: **Hepatitis B Vaccine**

Indications:

a. Persons with occupational risk of exposure to blood or blood-contaminated fluids.

b. Clients and staff of institutions for developmentally disabled.

c. Hemodialysis patients.

d. Recipients of clotting-factor concentrates.

e. Household contacts and sex partners of those chronically infected with HBV.

f. Family members of adoptees from countries where HBV infection is endemic, if adoptees are $HBsAg^+$.

g. Certain international travelers.

h. Injecting drug users.

i. Men who have sex with men.

j. Heterosexual men and women with multiple sex partners or recent episode of a sexually transmitted disease.

k. Inmates of long-term correctional facilities.

l. All unvaccinated adolescents.

Primary Schedule:

Three doses: second dose one to two months after the first, third dose four to six months after the first.

No need to start series over if schedule interrupted. Can start series with one manufacturer's vaccine and finish with another.

*Dose (**Adult**):* intramuscular (IM); Recombivax HB®: 10 g/1.0 mL (green cap)

Engerix-B®: 20 g/1.0mL (orange cap)

*Dose (**Adolescents 11-19 years**):* intramuscular (IM)

Recombivax HB®: 5 g/0.5 mL (yellow cap)

Engerix-B®: 10 g/0.5 mL (light blue cap)

*Two doses (**Only for Adolescents 11-15 years**):* intramuscular (IM), four to six months apart

Restricted to Recombivax HB®: 10 g/1.0 mL (green cap)

Booster: None presently recommended

Contraindications:

Anaphylactic allergy to yeast.

Comments:

a. Persons with serologic markers of prior or continuing hepatitis B virus infection do not need immunization.

b. For hemodialysis patients and other immunodeficient or immunosuppressed patients, vaccine dosage is doubled or special preparation is used.

c. *Pregnant women should be seroscreened for HBsAg and, if positive, their infants should be given postexposure prophylaxis beginning at birth.*

d. Postexposure prophylaxis: consult ACIP recommendations, or state or local immunization program.

AGENT: **Polio-virus Vaccine: IPV - Inactivated Vaccine; OPV - Oral (live) Vaccine**

Indications:

Routine vaccination of those ≥18 years of age residing in the U.S. is not necessary. Vaccination recommended for the following high-risk adults:

a. Travelers to areas or countries where poliomyelitis is epidemic or endemic.

b. Members of communities or specific population groups with disease caused by wild polioviruses.

c. Laboratory workers who handle specimens that may contain polioviruses.

d. HCWs who have close contact with patients who may be excreting wild polioviruses.

e. Unvaccinated adults whose children will be receiving OPV.

Primary Schedule:

Unimmunized adolescents/adults: IPV is recommended - two doses at four to eight week intervals, third dose six to 12 months after second (can be as soon as two months) Dose: 0.5 mL subcutaneous (SC) or intramuscular (IM).

Partially immunized adolescents/adults: Complete primary series with IPV (IPV schedule shown above). OPV is no longer recommended for use in the U.S.

Contraindications:

IPV: Anaphylactic reaction following previous dose or to streptomycin, polymyxin B, or neomycin.

Comments:

In instances of potential exposure to wild poliovirus, adults who have had a primary series of OPV or IPV may be given one more dose of IPV.

Although no adverse effects have been documented, vaccination of pregnant women should be avoided. However, if immediate protection is required, pregnant women may be given IPV in accordance with the recommended schedule for adults.

AGENT: Varicella Vaccine

Indications:

a. Persons of any age without a reliable history of varicella disease or vaccination, or who are seronegative for varicella.

b. Susceptible adolescents and adults living in households with children.

c. All susceptible HCWs.

d. Susceptible family contacts of immunocompromised persons.

e. Susceptible persons in the following groups who are at high risk for exposure:

- persons who live or work in environments in which transmission of varicella is likely (e.g., teachers of young children, day care employees, residents, and staff in institutional settings) or can occur (e.g., college students, inmates and staff of correctional institutions, military personnel).
- nonpregnant women of childbearing age
- international travelers

Primary Schedule:

For persons < 13 years of age, one dose.

For persons 13 years of age and older, two doses separated by four to eight weeks. If > eight weeks elapse following the first dose, the second dose can be administered without restarting schedule.

Contraindications:

Dose: 0.5 mL subcutaneous (SC)

a. Anaphylactic allergy to gelatin or neomycin.

b. Untreated, active TB.

c. Immunosuppressive therapy or immunodeficiency (including HIV infection).

d. Family history of congenital or hereditary immunodeficiency in first-degree relatives, unless the immune competence of the recipient has been clinically substantiated or verified by a laboratory.

e. Immune globulin preparation or blood/blood product received in preceding five mos.

f. Pregnancy.

Comments:

Women should be asked if they are pregnant before receiving vaccine and advised to avoid pregnancy for one month following each dose of vaccine.

AGENT: **Hepatitis A Vaccine**

Indications:

a. Persons traveling to or working in countries with high or intermediate endemicity of infection.

b. Men who have sex with men.

c. Injecting and non-injecting illegal drug users.

d. Persons who work w/ HAV-infected primates or with HAV in a research laboratory setting.

e. Persons w/ chronic liver disease.

f. Persons w/ clotting factor disorders.

g. Consider food handlers, where determined to be cost-effective by health authorities or employers.

Primary Schedule:

HAVRIX®: Two doses, separated by Six to 12 months.

Adults (19 years of age and older)—Dose: 1.0 mL intramuscular (IM);

Persons 2- 8 years of age—Dose: 0.5 mL (IM).

VAQTA®: *Adults (19 years of age and older):* Two doses, separated by six months. *Dose:* 1.0 mL intramuscular (IM);

Persons 2-18 years of age: Two doses, separated by six to 18 months; Dose: 0.5 mL (IM)

Contraindications:

A history of hypersensitivity to alum or the preservative 2 – phenoxyethanol.

Comments:

The safety of hepatitis A vaccine during pregnancy has not been determined, though the theoretical risk to the developing fetus is expected to be low. The risk of vaccination should be weighed against the risk of hepatitis A in women who may be at high risk of exposure to HAV.

References/Resources

- American Academy of Pediatrics Policy statement: Varicella vaccine update (RE9941), Pediatrics 2000; 105:136-141.
- American Academy of Pediatrics. In: Pickering LK, ed. 2000 Red Book: Report of the Committee on Infectious Diseases. 25th ed. 2000; AAP press, Elk Grove Village, IL.
- APIC Position Paper: Immunization. Am J Infect Control 1999; 27:52 - 3.
- Association for Professionals in Infection Control and Epidemiology. APIC Text of Infection Control and Epidemiology. 2000, chapters 31,33,35,36,37,40,49,50,79,81,82.

- Centers for Disease Control and Prevention. Control and Prevention of Meningococcal Disease and Control and Prevention of Serogroup C Meningococcal Disease: Evaluation and Management of Suspected Outbreaks. MMWR 1997; 46:RR-5.
- Ibid. HICPAC guideline for infection control in healthcare personnel. AJIC 1998; 26(3): 289–354.
- Ibid. Poliomyelitis Prevention. MMWR 2000; 49:RR-5.
- Ibid. Preventing Pneumococcal Disease Among Infants and Young Children. MMWR 2000; 49:RR-9.
- Ibid. Prevention and Control of Meningococcal Disease and Meningococcal Disease and College Students. MMWR 2000; 49:RR-7.
- Ibid. Prevention and Control of Influenza. MMWR 2000; 49:RR-3.
- Ibid. Prevention of Hepatitis A Through Active or Passive Immunization. MMWR 1999; 48:RR-12.
- Ibid. Public Health Service guidelines for immunization of healthcare workers. MMWR 1997; 46(RR-18): 23.
- Ibid. Recommendations for the Use of Lyme Disease Vaccine Recommendations of the Advisory Committee on Immunization Practices (ACIP) MMWR, 1999; 48:RR-7.
- Ibid. Human Rabies Prevention — United States, 1999. MMWR, 1999; 48: RR-1 Recommendations of the Advisory Committee on Immunization Practices (ACIP)
- Immunization Action Coalition at www.immunize.org
- National Immunization Program website www.cdc.gov/nip

Isolation and Precautions

Overview

- Isolation technique has evolved and private rooms for infected patients are used less frequently and only for patients with highly-transmissible or epidemiologically important infections or for those unable to assist with maintaining IC measures.
- Current strategies for precautions are reflected in the CDCs Hospital Infection Control Practices Advisory Committee (HICPAC) recommendations. The guideline uses a two-tiered system: Standard Precautions when caring for all patients, and Transmission-Based Precautions for interrupting at least one of the five main modes of transmission—contact, droplet, airborne, common vehicle, and vector-borne—in patients with known or suspected infections.

Purpose

- Although there are generic and specific suggestions contained within the Transmission-Based Precautions guidelines, they may not fully address the unique needs and circumstances of every healthcare setting, the individual patient, or the specific condition. The purpose of this section is to provide the ICP with References/Resources to assist in assessment and policy development.
- Modifications should be based on the principles of epidemiology and disease transmission. Other sections of this handbook should be referenced to obtain this guidance.
- Note that modifications may also be directed by federal, state, or local regulations. The ICP should include these additional regulations as appropriate in policy development.

Risk Factors

- Sources of microorganisms may be patients, personnel, or on occasion, visitors, and may include persons with acute disease, persons in the incubation period of a disease, those who are colonized by an infectious agent but have no apparent disease, or persons who are chronic carriers of an infectious agent.
- Other sources of microorganisms can be the patient's endogenous flora, which may be difficult to control, and inanimate environmental objects that have become contaminated, including equipment and medications.

Strategies for Prevention

- An effective IC program reduces the risk of infection transmission through the use of Standard Precautions and appropriate application of Transmission-Based Precautions as applicable for presumed or confirmed infectious disease or condition.
- Refer to Precautions/Protective Equipment Task Matrix (following).
- Review the HICPAC Guidelines grid for Empiric Isolation and table for Type/Duration of Precautions for more details. (Refer to References/Resources at the end of this section.) HICPAC Guidelines for Isolation Precautions in Hospital have been established to provide evidence based recommendations for isolation and barrier precautions.
  - **Category IA** *(IA)*. Strongly recommended for implementation and strongly supported by well-designed experimental, clinical, or epidemiological studies.
  - **Category IB** *(IB)*. Strongly recommended for implementation and supported by some experimental, clinical, or epidemiological studies and a strong theoretical rationale.
  - **Category IC** *(IC)*. Required by state or federal regulations, rules, or standards.

- **Category II** *(II)*. Suggested for implementation and supported by suggestive clinical or epidemiological studies or a theoretical rationale.
- **No recommendation; unresolved issue** *(UI)*. Practices for which evidence is insufficient or no consensus regarding efficacy exist.

➤ **Administrative Controls:**

- Education.
- Develop a system to ensure that hospital patients, personnel, and visitors are educated about use of precautions and their responsibilities for adherence to them. *(II)*
- Adherence to Precautions.
- Periodically evaluate adherence to precautions, and use findings to direct improvements. *(IB)*

➤ **Standard Precautions** (SP) - Use SP, or the equivalent, for the care of all patients. *(IB)*

- **Handwashing**

  Wash hands after touching blood, body fluids, secretions, excretions, and contaminated items, whether or not gloves are worn. Wash hands immediately after gloves are removed, between patient contacts, and when otherwise indicated to avoid transfer of microorganisms to other patients or environments. It may be necessary to wash hands between tasks and procedures on the same patient to prevent cross-contamination of different body sites. *(IB)*

  Use plain (non-antimicrobial) soap for routine handwashing. *(IB)*

  Use an antimicrobial agent or a waterless antiseptic agent for specific circumstances (e.g., control of outbreaks or hyperendemic infections), as defined by the infection control program. *(IB) [See Contact Precautions for additional recommendations on using antimicrobial and antiseptic agents.]*

- **Gloves**

  Wear gloves (clean, nonsterile gloves are adequate) when touching blood, body fluids, secretions, excretions, and contaminated items. Put on clean gloves just before touching mucous membranes and non-intact skin.

  Change gloves between tasks and procedures on the same patient after contact with material that may contain a high concentration of microorganisms. Remove gloves promptly after use, before touching noncontaminated items and environmental surfaces, and before going to another patient, and wash hands immediately to avoid transfer of microorganisms to other patients/environments. *(IB)*

- **Mask, Eye Protection, Face Shield**

  Wear a mask and eye protection or a face shield to protect mucous membranes of the eyes, nose, and mouth during procedures and patient care activities that are likely to generate splashes or sprays of blood, body fluids, secretions, and excretions. *(IB)*

- **Gowns**

  Wear a clean, nonsterile gown to protect skin and prevent soiling of clothing during procedures and patient care activities that are likely to generate splashes or sprays of blood, body fluids, secretions, or excretions.

  Select a gown that is appropriate for the activity and amount of fluid likely to be encountered.

Remove a soiled gown as promptly as possible, and wash hands to avoid transfer of microorganisms to other patients or environments. *(IB)*

- **Patient Care Equipment**

  Handle used patient care equipment soiled with blood, body fluids, secretions, and excretions in a manner that prevents skin and mucous membrane exposures, contamination of clothing, and transfer of microorganisms to other patients and environments.

  Ensure that reusable equipment is not used for the care of another patient until it has been cleaned and reprocessed appropriately. Ensure that single-use items are discarded properly. *(IB)*

- **Environmental Controls**

  Ensure that the hospital has adequate procedures for the routine care, cleaning, and disinfection of environmental surfaces, beds, bedrails, bedside equipment, and other frequently touched surfaces. Also ensure that these procedures are being followed. *(IB)*

- **Linen**

  Handle, transport, and process used linen soiled with blood, body fluids, secretions, and excretions in a manner that prevents skin and mucous membrane exposures, contamination of clothing, and transfer of microorganisms to other patients and environments. *(IB)*

- **Occupational Health and Bloodborne Pathogens**

  Take care to prevent injuries when using needles, scalpels, and other sharp instruments or devices; when handling sharp instruments after procedures; when cleaning used instruments; and when disposing of used needles.

Never recap or manipulate used needles or use any other technique that involves directing the point of a needle toward any part of the body; rather, use either a one-handed "scoop" technique or a mechanical device designed for holding the needle sheath.

Do not remove used needles from disposable syringes by hand, and do not bend, break, or otherwise manipulate used needles by hand.

Place used disposable syringes and needles, scalpel blades, and other sharp items in appropriate puncture-resistant containers, which should be located as close as practical to the area in which the items were used. Place reusable syringes and needles in a puncture-resistant container for transport to the reprocessing area. *(IB)*

Use mouthpieces, resuscitation bags, or other ventilation devices as an alternative to mouth-to-mouth resuscitation methods in areas where the need for resuscitation is predictable. *(IB)*

- **Patient Placement**

  Place a patient who contaminates the environment or who does not (or cannot) assist in maintaining appropriate hygiene or environmental control in a private room.

  If a private room is not available, consult with infection control professionals regarding patient placement or other alternatives. *(IB)*

➤ **Airborne Precautions (A)**

- In addition to Standard Precautions, use Airborne Precautions, or the equivalent, for patients known or suspected to be infected with microorganisms transmitted by airborne droplet nuclei (small-particle residue [5 micron or smaller in size] of evaporated droplets containing microorganisms that remain suspended in the air and that can be dispersed widely by air currents within a room or over a long distance). *(IB)*

- **Patient Placement**

  Place the patient in a private room that has: (1) monitored negative air pressure in relation to the surrounding areas, (2) six to 12 air changes/hour, and (3) appropriate discharge of air outdoors or monitored high-efficiency filtration of room air before the air is circulated to other areas in the hospital.

  Keep the room door closed and the patient in the room. When a private room is not available, place the patient in a room with a patient who has active infection with the same microorganism, unless otherwise recommended, but with no other infection.

  When a private room is not available and cohorting is not desirable, consultation with infection control professionals is advised before patient placement. *(IB)*

- **Respiratory Protection**

  Wear respiratory protection when entering the room of a patient with known or suspected infectious pulmonary tuberculosis.

  Susceptible persons should not enter the room of patients known or suspected to have measles (rubeola) or varicella (chickenpox) if other immune caregivers are available.

  If susceptible persons should enter the room of a patient known or suspected to have measles (rubeola) or varicella, they should wear respiratory protection.

  Persons immune to measles (rubeola) or varicella need not wear respiratory protection. *(IB)*

- **Patient Transport**

  Limit the movement and transport of the patient from the room to essential purposes only.

If transport or movement is necessary, minimize patient dispersal of droplet nuclei by placing a surgical mask on the patient, if possible. *(IB)*

- Additional Precautions for Preventing Transmission of Tuberculosis. (See section on Tuberculosis.)

➤ **Droplet Precautions (D)**

- In addition to Standard Precautions, use Droplet Precautions, or the equivalent, for a patient known or suspected to be infected with microorganisms transmitted by droplets (large-particle droplets [larger than 5 micron in size] that can be generated by the patient during coughing, sneezing, talking, or the performance of procedures). *(IB)*

- **Patient Placement**

  Place the patient in a private room.

  When a private room is not available, place the patient in a room with a patient(s) who has active infection with the same microorganism but with no other infection (cohorting).

  When a private room is not available and cohorting is not achievable, maintain spatial separation of at least three feet between the infected patient and other patients and visitors.

  Special air handling and ventilation are not necessary, and the door may remain open. *(IB)*

- **Masks**

  In addition to Standard Precautions, wear a mask when working within three feet of the patient. (Logistically, some hospitals may want to implement wearing a mask to enter the room.) *(IB)*.

- **Patient Transport**

  Limit the movement and transport of the patient from the room to essential purposes only.

If transport or movement is necessary, minimize patient dispersal of droplets by masking the patient, if possible. *(IB)*

➤ Contact Precautions (C)

- In addition to Standard Precautions, use Contact Precautions, or the equivalent, for specified patients known or suspected to be infected or colonized with epidemiologically important microorganisms that can be transmitted by direct contact with the patient (hand or skin-to-skin contact that occurs when performing patient care activities that require touching the patient's dry skin) or indirect contact (touching) with environmental surfaces or patient care items in the patient's environment. *(IB)*

- **Patient Placement**

  Place the patient in a private room.

  When a private room is not available, place the patient in a room with a patient(s) who has active infection with the same microorganism but with no other infection (cohorting).

  When a private room is not available and cohorting is not achievable, consider the epidemiology of the microorganism and the patient population when determining patient placement.

  Consultation with infection control professionals is advised before patient placement. *(IB)*

- **Gloves and Handwashing**

  In addition to wearing gloves as outlined under Standard Precautions, wear clean, nonsterile gloves when entering the room.

  During the course of providing care for a patient, change gloves after having contact with infective material that may contain high concentrations of microorganisms (fecal material and wound drainage).

Remove gloves before leaving the patient's environment and wash hands immediately with an antimicrobial agent or a waterless antiseptic agent.

After glove removal and handwashing, ensure that hands do not touch potentially contaminated environmental surfaces or items in the patient's room to avoid transfer of microorganisms to other patients or environments. (IB.)

- **Gowns**

  In addition to wearing gowns as outlined under Standard Precautions, wear a clean, nonsterile gown when entering the room if substantial contact with the patient, environmental surfaces, or items in the patient's room is anticipated, or if the patient is incontinent, has diarrhea, an ileostomy, a colostomy, or wound drainage not contained by a dressing.

  Remove the gown before leaving the patient's environment. After gown removal, ensure that clothing does not contact potentially contaminated environmental surfaces to avoid transfer of microorganisms to other patients or environments. *(IB)*

- **Patient Transport**

  Limit the movement and transport of the patient from the room to essential purposes only.

  If the patient is transported out of the room, ensure that precautions are maintained to minimize the risk of transmission of microorganisms to other patients and contamination of environmental surfaces or equipment. *(IB)*

- **Patient Care Equipment**

  When possible, dedicate the use of non-critical patient care equipment to a single patient (or cohort of patients infected or colonized with the pathogen requiring precautions) to avoid sharing between patients.

If use of common equipment or items is unavoidable, then adequately clean and disinfect them before use for another patient. *(IB)*

- Additional Precautions for Preventing the Spread of Vancomycin Resistance (Refer to Section 7 - Antimicrobial Utilization).

Note: This legend applies to the following charts

* Infection control professionals are encouraged to modify or adapt this table according to local conditions. To ensure that appropriate empiric precautions are always implemented, hospitals should have systems in place to evaluate patients routinely according to these criteria as part of their preadmission and admission care.

† Patients with the syndromes or conditions listed may present with atypical signs or symptoms (e.g., pertussis in neonates and adults may not have paroxysmal or severe cough). The clinician's index of suspicion should be guided by the prevalence of specific conditions in the community, as well as clinical judgment.

‡ The organisms listed under the Potential Pathogens column are not intended to represent the complete, or even most likely diagnoses, but rather possible etiologic agents that require additional precautions beyond Standard Precautions until they can be ruled out.

§ These pathogens include enterohemorrhagic *Escherichia coli* 0157:H7, *Shigella,* hepatitis A, and rotavirus.

¶ Resistant bacteria judged by the infection control program, based on current state, regional, or national recommendations, to be of special clinical or epidemiological significance.

CLINICAL SYNDROMES OR CONDITIONS WARRANTING ADDITIONAL EMPIRIC PRECAUTIONS TO PREVENT TRANSMISSION OF EPIDEMIOLOGICALLY IMPORTANT PATHOGENS PENDING CONFIRMATION OF DIAGNOSIS*

Clinical Syndrome or Condition†	Potential Pathogens‡	Empiric Precautions
Diarrhea		
Acute diarrhea with a likely infectious cause in an incontinent or diapered patient.	Enteric pathogens§	Contact
Diarrhea in an adult with a history of recent antibiotic use.	*Clostridium difficile*	Contact
Meningitis		
Rash or exanthems, generalized, etiology unknown.	*Neisseria meningitidis*	Droplet
Petechial/ecchymotic with fever.	*Neisseria meningitidis*	Droplet
Vesicular	Varicella	Airborne and contact
Maculopapular with coryza and fever.	Rubeola (measles)	Airborne
Respiratory infections		
Cough/fever/upper lobe pulmonary infiltrate in an HIV-negative patient or a patient at low risk for HIV infection	*Mycobacterium tuberculosis*	Airborne

CLINICAL SYNDROMES OR CONDITIONS WARRANTING ADDITIONAL EMPIRIC PRECAUTIONS TO PREVENT TRANSMISSION OF EPIDEMIOLOGICALLY IMPORTANT PATHOGENS PENDING CONFIRMATION OF DIAGNOSIS*

Clinical Syndrome or Condition†	Potential Pathogens‡	Empiric Precautions
Cough/fever/pulmonary infiltrate in any lung location in an HIV-infected patient or a patient at high risk for HIV infection	*Mycobacterium tuberculosis*	Airborne
Paroxysmal or severe persistent cough during periods of pertussis activity.	*Bordetella pertussis*	Droplet
Respiratory infections, particularly bronchiolitis and croup, in infants and young children.	Respiratory syncytial or parainfluenza virus	Contact
Risk of multidrug-resistant microorganisms. History of infection or colonization with multidrug-resistant organisms.¶	Resistant bacteria	Contact
Skin, wound, or urinary tract infection (UTI) in a patient with a recent hospital or nursing home stay in a facility where multidrug-resistant organisms are prevalent.	Resistant bacteria	Contact
Skin or wound infection. Abscess or draining wound that cannot be covered.	*Staphylococcus aureus*, group A streptococcus	Contact

CDC/HICPAC Recommendations Type and Duration of Precautions— Selected Infections/Conditions		
Infection/Condition	Precaution	
	Type*	Duration†
Abscess Draining, major[1] Draining, minor or limited[2]	 C S	 DI
Acquired immunodeficiency syndrome[3]	S	
Actinomycosis	S	
Adenovirus- infants and young children	D, C	DI
Amebiasis	S	
Anthrax Cutaneous Pulmonary	 S S	
Antibiotic-associated colitis (see *Clostridium difficile*)		
Arthropod-borne viral encephalitides (eastern, western, Venezuelan equine encephalomyelitis: St. Louis, California encephalitis)	S[4]	
Arthropod-borne viral fevers (dengue, yellow fever, Colorado tick fever)	S[4]	
Ascariasis	S	
Aspergillosis	S	
Babesiosis	S	
Blastomycosis, North Am.,- -cutan. or pulm.	S	
Botulism	S	
Bronchiolitis (see resp. infec. in infants and young children)		

CDC/HICPAC Recommendations Type and Duration of Precautions— Selected Infections/Conditions		
Infection/Condition	Precaution	
	Type*	Duration†
Brucellosis (undulant, Malta, Mediterranean fever)	S	
Campylobacter gastroenteritis (see gastroenteritis)		
Candidiasis, all including mucocutaneous	S	
Cat-scratch fever (benign inoculation lymphoreticulosis)	S	
Cellulitis, uncontrolled drainage	C	DI
Chancroid (soft chancre)	S	
Chickenpox (varicella; see F[5] for exposure)	A, C	F[5]
Chlamydia trachomatis Conjunctivitis Genital Respiratory	 S S S	
Cholera (see gastroenteritis)		
Closed-cavity infection Draining, limited or minor Not draining	 S S	
Clostridium *C. botulinum* *C. difficile* *C. perfringens* Food poisoning Gas gangrene	 S C S S S	 DI
Coccidioidomycosis (valley fever) Draining lesions Pneumonia	 S S	
Colorado tick fever	S	

CDC/HICPAC Recommendations Type and Duration of Precautions - Selected Infections/Conditions		
Infection/Condition	Precaution	
	Type*	Duration†
Congenital rubella	C	F[6]
Conjunctivitis Acute bacterial Chlamydia Gonococcal Acute viral (acute hemorrhagic)	 S S S C	 DI
Coxsackievirus dis. (see enteroviral infec.)		
Creutzfeldt-Jacob disease	S[7]	
Croup (see resp. infec. infants and children)		
Cryptococcosis	S	
Cryptosporidiosis (see gastroenteritis)		
Cysticercosis	S	
Cytomegalovirus infection, neonatal or immunosuppressed	S	
Decubitus ulcer, infected Major[1] Minor or limited[2]	 C S	 DI
Dengue	S[4]	
Diarrhea acute-infective etiology suspected (see gastroenteritis)		
Diphtheria Cutaneous Pharyngeal	 C D	 CN[8] CN[8]
Ebola viral hemorrhagic fever	C[9]	DI
Echinococcosis (hydatidosis)	S	
Echovirus (see enteroviral infection)		

CDC/HICPAC Recommendations Type and Duration of Precautions - Selected Infections/Conditions		
Infection/Condition	**Precaution**	
	Type*	**Duration†**
Encephalitis or encephalomyelitis (see specific etiologic agents)		
Endometritis	S	
Enterobiasis (pinworm, oxyuriasis)	S	
Enterococcus species (see multidrug-resist. organisms if epidemiologically significant or vancomycin resistant)		
Enterocolitis, *Clostridium difficile*	C	DI
Enteroviral infections Adults Infants and young children	 S C	 DI
Epiglottitis due to *H. influenzae*	D	U[24 h]
Epstein-Barr virus infection, including infectious mononucleosis	S	
Erythema infectiosum (also see parvovirus B19)	S	
Escherichia coli gastroenteritis (see gastroenteritis)		
Food poisoning Botulism Clostridium perfringens or welchii Staphylococcal	 S S S	
Furunculosis-staphylococcal Infants and young children	C	DI
Gangrene (gas gangrene)	S	

CDC/HICPAC Recommendations Type and Duration of Precautions - Selected Infections/Conditions		
Infection/Condition	**Precaution**	
	Type*	**Duration†**
Gastroenteritis		
Campylobacter species	S[10]	
Cholera	S[10]	
Clostridium difficile	C	DI
Cryptosporidium species	S[10]	
Escherichia coli		
Enterohemorrhagic 0157:H7	S[10]	
Diapered or incontinent	C	DI
Other species	S[10]	
Giardia lamblia	S[10]	
Rotavirus	S[10]	
Diapered or incontinent	C	DI
Salmonella species (including *S. typhi*)	S[10]	
Shigella species	S[10]	
Diapered or incontinent	C	DI
Vibrio parahaemolyticus	S[10]	
Viral (if not covered elsewhere)	S[10]	
Yersinia enterocolitica	S[10]	
German measles (rubella)	D	F[22]
Giardiasis (see gastroenteritis)		
Gonococcal ophthalmia neonatorum (gon. ophthalmia, acute conj.of newborn)	S	
Gonorrhea	S	
Granuloma inguinale (donovanosis, granuloma venereum)	S	
Guillian-Barré syndrome	S	
Hand, foot, and mouth disease (see enteroviral infection)		
Hantavirus pulmonary syndrome	S	
Helicobacter pylori	S	

CDC/HICPAC Recommendations Type and Duration of Precautions - Selected Infections/Conditions		
Infection/Condition	Precaution	
	Type*	Duration†
Hemorrhagic fevers (for example, Lassa and Ebola)	C[9]	DI
Hepatitis, viral Type A Diapered or incontinent patients Type B–HBsAg positive Type C and other non-A, non-B Type E	 S C S S S	 F[11]
Herpangina (see enteroviral infection)		
Herpes simplex (*Herpesvirus hominis*) Encephalitis Neonatal[12] (see F[12] for neonatal exp.) Mucocutaneous, disseminated or primary, severe Mucocutaneous, recurrent (skin, oral, genital)	 S C C S	 DI DI
Herpes zoster (varicella-zoster) Localized in immunocompromised patient or disseminated Localized in normal patient	 A, C S[13]	 D[13]
Histoplasmosis	S	
HIV infection[3]	S	
Hookworm disease (ancylostomiasis, uncinariasis)	S	
Impetigo	C	U[24 h]
Infectious mononucleosis	S	
Influenza	D[14]	DI
Kawasaki syndrome	S	

CDC/HICPAC Recommendations Type and Duration of Precautions - Selected Infections/Conditions		
Infection/Condition	**Precaution**	
	Type*	**Duration†**
Lassa fever	C[9]	DI
Legionnaires' disease	S	
Leprosy	S	
Leptospirosis	S	
Lice (pediculosis)	C	$U^{24\ h}$
Listeriosis	S	
Lyme disease	S	
Lymphocytic choriomeningitis	S	
Lymphogranuloma venereum	S	
Malaria	S[4]	
Marburg virus disease	C[9]	DI
Measles (rubeola), all presentations	A	DI
Meloidiosis, all forms	S	
Meningitis		
Aseptic (nonbacterial or viral meningitis [also see enteroviral infections])	S	
Bacterial, gram-neg. entericneonates	D	$U^{24\ h}$
Fungal	S	
Haemophilus influenzae, known or suspected	D	$U^{24\ h}$
Listeria monocytogenes	S	
Neisseria meningitidis (meningococcal) known or suspected	S	
Pneumococcal		
Tuberculosis[15]		
Other diagnosed bacterial		
Meningococcal pneumonia	D	$U^{24\ h}$

CDC/HICPAC Recommendations Type and Duration of Precautions - Selected Infections/Conditions		
Infection/Condition	Precaution	
	Type*	Duration†
Meningococcemia (mening. sepsis)	D	U[24 h]
Molluscum contagiosum	S	
Mucormycosis	S	
Multidrug-resistant org., infec. or coloniz. [16] Gastrointestinal Respiratory Pneumococcal Skin, wound or burn	 C C S C	 CN CN CN
Mumps (infectious parotitis)	D	F[17]
Mycobacteria, nontuberculosis (atypical) Pulmonary Wound	 S S	
Mycoplasma pneumonia	D	DI
Necrotizing enterocolitis	S	
Nocardiosis, draining lesions or other type	S	
Norwalk agent gastro. (see viral gastroent.)		
Orf	S	
Parainfluenza virus infection, respiratory in infants and young children	C	DI
Parvovirus B19	D	F[18]
Pediculosis (lice)	C	U[24 h]
Pertussis (whooping cough)	D	F[19]
Pinworm infection	S	
Plague -Bubonic Plague - Pneumonic	S D	
Pleurodynia (see enteroviral infection)		

CDC/HICPAC Recommendations Type and Duration of Precautions - Selected Infections/Conditions		
Infection/Condition	**Precaution**	
	Type*	**Duration†**
Pneumonia		
Adenovirus	D, C	DI
Bacterial not listed elsewhere (including gram negative bacterial)	S	
Burkholderia cepacia in cystic fibrosis	S[20]	
(CF) pts, including resp. tract coloniz.	S	
Chlamydia	S	
Fungal	S	
Haemophilus influenzae	D	U[Y]
Adults	S	
Infants and children (any age)	D	U[72 h]
Legionella		
Meningococcal	D	DI
Multidrug-resistant bacterial (see	S[21]	
multidrug-resistant organisms)	S[20]	
Mycoplasma (primary atyp. pneumonia)	S	
Pneumocystis carinii	D	U[72 h]
Pseudomonas cepacia (see *B. cepacia*)		
Staphylococcus aureus	S	
Streptococcus, group A		
Adults		
Infants and young children		
Viral pneumonia - other		
Adults		
Infants and young children (see resp. infectious disease, acute)		
Poliomyelitis	S	
Psittacosis (ornithosis)	S	
Q fever	S	
Rabies	S	
Rat-bite fever (*Streptobacillus moniliformis* dis., *Spirillum minus* dis.)	S	

CDC/HICPAC Recommendations Type and Duration of Precautions - Selected Infections/Conditions		
Infection/Condition	Precaution	
	Type*	Duration†
Relapsing fever	S	
Resistant bacterial infec. or colonization (see multidrug-resistant org.)		
Respiratory infectious disease, acute (if not covered elsewhere) Adults Infants and young children[3]	 S C	 DI
Respiratory syncytial virus infection (RSV), in infants, young children, and immunocompromised adults	C	DI
Reye syndrome	S	
Rheumatic fever	S	
Rickettsial fevers, tick-borne (Rocky Mountain spotted fever, tick-borne, typhus fever)	S	
Rickettsialpox (vesicular rickettsiosis)	S	
Ringworm (dermatophytosis, dermatomycosis, tinea)	S	
Ritter's disease (staph. scalded skin synd)	S	
Rocky Mountain spotted fever	S	
Roseola infantum (exanthem subitum)	S	
Rotavirus infection (see gastroenteritis)		
Rubella (German measles; also see congenital rubella)	D	F[22]
Salmonellosis (see gastroenteritis)		
Scabies	C	$U^{24\ h}$

CDC/HICPAC Recommendations Type and Duration of Precautions - Selected Infections/Conditions

Infection/Condition	Precaution	
	Type*	Duration†
Scalded skin syndrome, staphylococcal (Ritter's disease)	S	
Schistosomiasis (bilharziasis)	S	
Shigellosis (see gastroenteritis)		
Sporotrichosis	S	
Spirillum minus disease (rat-bite fever)	S	
Staphylococcal disease (S. aureus)		
Skin, wound or burn		
Major[1]	C	DI
Minor or limited[2]	S	
Enterocolitis	S[10]	
Multidrug-resistant (see multidrug-resistant organisms)		
Pneumonia	S	
Scalded skin syndrome	S	
Toxic shock syndrome	S	
Streptobacillus moniliformis disease (rat-bite fever)	S	
Streptococcal disease (group A strep.)		
Skin, wound or burn	C	$U^{24\,h}$
Major[1]	S	
Minor or limited[2]	S	
Endometritis (puerperal sepsis)	D	$U^{24\,h}$
Pharyngitis in infants and young children	D	$U^{24\,h}$
Pneumonia in infants and young children	D	$U^{24\,h}$
Scarlet fever in infants and young children		
Streptococcal disease (group B streptococcus), neonatal	S	

CDC/HICPAC Recommendations Type and Duration of Precautions - Selected Infections/Conditions		
Infection/Condition	**Precaution**	
	Type*	**Duration†**
Streptococcal disease (not group A or B) unless covered elsewhere Multidrug-resistant (see multidrug-resistant organisms)	S	
Strongyloidiasis	S	
Syphilis		
Skin and mucous membrane, including congenital, primary, secondary	S	
Latent (tertiary) and seropositivity without lesions	S	
Tapeworm disease		
Hymenolepis nana	S	
Taenia solium (pork)	S	
Other	S	
Tetanus	S	
Tinea (fungus infection dermatophytosis, dermatomycosis, ringworm)	S	
Toxoplasmosis	S	
Toxic shock syndrome (staphylococcal disease)	S	
Trachoma, acute	S	
Trench mouth (Vincent's angina)	S	
Trichinosis	S	
Trichomoniasis	S	
Trichuriasis (whipworm disease)	S	

CDC/HICPAC Recommendations Type and Duration of Precautions - Selected Infections/Conditions		
Infection/Condition	Precaution	
	Type*	Duration†
Tuberculosis		
Extrapulmonary, draining lesion (including scrofula)	S	
Extrapulmonary, meningitis[15]	S	
Pulmonary, confirmed or suspected, or laryngeal disease	A	F[23]
Skin-test positive with no evidence of current pulmonary disease	S	
Tularemia		
Draining lesion	S	
Pulmonary	S	
Typhoid (*Salmonella typhi*) fever (see gastroenteritis)		
Typhus, endemic and epidemic	S	
UTI (including pyelonephritis), with or without urinary catheter	S	
Varicella (chickenpox)	A, C	F[5]
Vibrio parahaemolyticus (see gastroenteritis)		
Vincent's angina (trench mouth)	S	
Viral diseases		
Respiratory (if not covered elsewhere)	S	
Adults		
Infants and young children (see respiratory infectious disease, acute)		
Whooping cough (pertussis)	D	F[19]
Wound infections		
Major[1]	C	DI
Minor or limited[2]	S	

CDC/HICPAC Recommendations Type and Duration of Precautions - Selected Infections/Conditions		
Infection/Condition	Precaution	
	Type*	Duration†
Yersinia enterocolitica gastroenteritis (see gastroenteritis)		
Zoster (varicella-zoster) Localized in immunocompromised patient, disseminated Localized in normal patient	A, C S[13]	DI[13]
Zygomycosis (phycomycosis, mucormycosis)	S	

Abbreviations:

Type of precautions:

A = airborne;

C = contact;

D = droplet;

S = standard;

when A, C, and D are specified, also use S.

† Duration of precautions: CN, until off antibiotics and culture negative; DH, duration of hospitalization; DI, duration of illness (with wound lesions, DI means until they stop draining); U, until time specified in hours after initiation of effective therapy; F, see footnote number.

1 No dressing or dressing does not contain drainage adequately.

2 Dressing covers and contains drainage adequately.

3 Also see syndromes or conditions listed on pp.142–144.

4 Install screens in windows and doors in endemic areas.

5 Maintain precautions until all lesions are crusted. The average incubation period for varicella is 10–16 days, with a range of

10–21 days. After exposure, use varicella-zoster immune globulin (VZIG) when appropriate, and discharge susceptible patients if possible. Place exposed susceptible patients on Airborne Precautions beginning 10 days after exposure and continuing until 21 days after last exposure (up to 28 days if VZIG has been given). Susceptible persons should not enter the room of patients on precautions if other immune caregivers are available.

6 Place infant on precautions during any admission until one year of age, unless nasopharyngeal and urine cultures are negative for virus after age three months.

7 Additional special precautions are necessary for handling and decontamination of blood, body fluids and tissues, and contaminated items from patients with confirmed or suspected disease. See latest College of American Pathologists (Northfield, Ill.) guidelines or other References/Resources.

8 Until two cultures taken at least 24 hours apart are negative.

9 Call state health department and CDC for specific advice about management of a suspected case. During the 1995 Ebola outbreak in Zaire, interim recommendations were published (see article for reference). Pending a comprehensive review of the epidemiologic data from the outbreak and evaluation of the interim recommendations, the 1988 guidelines for management of patients with suspected viral hemorrhagic infections (see article for reference) will be reviewed and updated if indicated.

10 Use Contact Precautions in infants and children <6 years of age for duration of illness.

11 Maintain precautions in infants and children <3 years of age for duration of hospitalization; in children 3–14 years of age, until two weeks after onset of symptoms; and in others until one week after onset of symptoms.

12 For infants delivered vaginally or by C-section and if mother has active infection and membranes have been ruptured for more than 4–6 hours.

13 Persons susceptible to varicella are also at risk for developing varicella when exposed to patients with herpes zoster lesions; therefore, susceptible people should not enter the room if other immune caregivers are available.

14 *The Guideline for prevention of nosocomial pneumonia* (see article for References/Resources) recommends surveillance, vaccination, antiviral agents, and use of private rooms with negative air pressure as much as feasible for patients for whom influenza is suspected or diagnosed. Many hospitals encounter logistical difficulties and physical plant limitations when admitting multiple patients with suspected influenza during community outbreaks. If sufficient private rooms are unavailable, consider cohorting patients, or at the very least, avoid room sharing with high-risk patients. See Guideline for prevention of nosocomial pneumonia (see article for References/Resources) for additional prevention and control strategies.

15 Patient should be examined for evidence of current (active) pulmonary tuberculosis. If evidence exists, additional precautions are necessary (see section on Tuberculosis).

16 Resistant bacteria judged by the infection control program, based on current state, regional, or national recommendations, to be of special clinical and epidemiologic significance.

17 For nine days after onset of swelling.

18 Maintain precautions for duration of hospitalization when chronic disease occurs in an immunodeficient patient. For patients with transient aplastic crisis or redcell crisis, maintain precautions for seven days.

19 Maintain precautions until five days after patient is placed on effective therapy.

20 Avoid cohorting or placement in the same room with a CF patient who is infected or colonized with B. cepacia. Persons with CF who visit or provide care and are not infected or colonized with B. cepacia may elect to wear a mask when within three feet of a colonized or infected patient.

21 Avoid placement in the same room with an immunocompromised patient.

22 Until seven days after onset of rash.

23 Discontinue precautions only when TB patient is on effective therapy, is improving clinically, and has three consecutive negative sputum smears collected on different days, or TB is ruled out. Also see section on Tuberculosis.

References/Resources

- Association for Professionals in Infection Control and Epidemiology. APIC Text of Infection Control and Epidemiology. 2000, chapter 29 1-12.
- Centers for Disease Control and Prevention, Public Health Service, U.S. Department of Health and Human Services, Guideline for isolation precautions in hospitals. 1996, Am J Infect Control 24:24-52.

PRECAUTIONS/PROTECTIVE EQUIPMENT TASK MATRIX

✔ Use routinely ✘ Follow isolation/precautions
C If contamination with blood/OPIM occurs or is likely
SS If splashing/spraying with blood/OPIM occurs or is likely
FP Facial Protection LC Lab coat/cover gown
H Heavy-duty utility gloves preferred
HW Handwashing GL Gloves
MR Mask or Respirator
FRG Fluid Resistant Gown

Task	Example	HW	GL	MR	FP	LC	FRG
Transporting patient	Pushing wheelchair/ stretcher	✔		If pt. is in airborne isolation, have pt. wear a mask			
Entering non-isolation room	Delivering food tray	C					
	Giving pt. education, taking history, registering pt., getting signature	C		H			
Entering airborne isolation room	Delivering food tray	✔	✘	✘	SS	✘	
	Giving pt. education, taking history, registering pt., getting signature	✔	✘	✘	SS	✘	
Pt. exam, **no** contact with blood/OPIM	Taking vital signs, adjusting IV fluid rate	✔	✘	✘	SS	✘	

PRECAUTIONS/PROTECTIVE EQUIPMENT TASK MATRIX

✔ Use routinely ✘ Follow isolation/precautions
C If contamination with blood/OPIM occurs or is likely
SS If splashing/spraying with blood/OPIM occurs or is likely
FP Facial Protection LC Lab coat/cover gown
H Heavy-duty utility gloves preferred
HW Handwashing GL Gloves
MR Mask or Respirator
FRG Fluid Resistant Gown

Task	Example	HW	GL	MR	FP	LC	FRG
Exam and contact with blood/OPIM or mucous membranes, nonintact skin	Performing wound/ostomy care, catheter care, feeding tube change, mouth care, suturing	✔	✔	✔	✔	✔	SS
Noninvasive radiology or cardiology procedures	Performing EKG, EEG, EMG, external ultrasound, placing electrodes, chest X-rays	✔	✘/C	✘		✘	SS
Performing radiology or cardiology invasive procedures	Placing internal ultrasound or endoscopic probe, performing barium enemas	✔	✔	✘	SS	✘	SS

PRECAUTIONS/PROTECTIVE EQUIPMENT TASK MATRIX

✔ Use routinely ✘ Follow isolation/precautions
C If contamination with blood/OPIM occurs or is likely
SS If splashing/spraying with blood/OPIM occurs or is likely
FP Facial Protection LC Lab coat/cover gown
H Heavy-duty utility gloves preferred
HW Handwashing GL Gloves
MR Mask or Respirator
FRG Fluid Resistant Gown

Task	Example	HW	GL	MR	FP	LC	FRG
Performing vascular access	Drawing venous blood, finger sticks	✔	✔	✘	SS	✔	SS
	Manipulating and inserting IVs	✔	✔	✘	SS	✔	SS
	Drawing arterial blood, transfusing blood	✔	✔	✘	SS	✔	SS
	Inserting central venous or arterial lines	✔	✔ Sterile	✔ Surgical mask	SS	✔ Sterile	SS Sterile
Administering medication	Administering eye, ear, nose, mouth drops/ tablets, nebulization	✔	✘	✘	SS	✘	SS
	Performing IM subcutaneous injections	✔	✘/C	✘	SS	✘	SS
	Placing rectal suppositories, enemas	✔	✔	✘/C	SS	✘/C	SS

PRECAUTIONS/PROTECTIVE EQUIPMENT TASK MATRIX

✔ Use routinely   ✘ Follow isolation/precautions   H Heavy-duty utility gloves preferred
C If contamination with blood/OPIM occurs or is likely   HW Handwashing   GL Gloves
SS If splashing/spraying with blood/OPIM occurs or is likely   MR Mask or Respirator
FP Facial Protection   LC Lab coat/cover gown   FRG Fluid Resistant Gown

Task	Example	HW	GL	MR	FP	LC	FRG
Performing respiratory care	Performing intubation or extubation	✔	✔	✘/SS	SS	✘/SS	SS
	Performing CPR	✔	✔	✘/SS	SS	✘/SS	SS
	Suctions, placing, and caring for trach	✔	✔	✘/SS	SS	✘/SS	SS
Performing operative procedures	Intraoperative procedures	✔	✔ Sterile	✔	SS	✔ Sterile	SS Sterile
Performing bedside invasive procedures	Performing cardiac cath, bone marrow biopsy, joint taps, endoscopy, lumbar puncture	✔	✔ Sterile	✘	SS	✔ Sterile	SS Sterile
Handling specimens	Agitation, vortexing, pipetting	✔	✔	✘	SS	✔	SS

PRECAUTIONS/PROTECTIVE EQUIPMENT TASK MATRIX

✔ Use routinely ✘ Follow isolation/precautions
C If contamination with blood/OPIM occurs or is likely
SS If splashing/spraying with blood/OPIM occurs or is likely
FP Facial Protection LC Lab coat/cover gown
H Heavy-duty utility gloves preferred
HW Handwashing GL Gloves
MR Mask or Respirator
FRG Fluid Resistant Gown

Task	Example	HW	GL	MR	FP	LC	FRG
Obtaining specimens	Swabbing wounds, aspiration	✔	✔	✘/C	SS	✘/SS	SS
	Swabbing throats, collecting urine, stool	✔	✘/C	✘	SS	✘/C	SS
Transporting specimens	Touching primary collection container	✔	✔				
	Touching secondary collection container	✔					
Handling waste or contaminated equipment	Handling soiled linen at point of generation	✔	✔/H	✘		✘/C	
	Placing sharps into sharps containers	✔					
	Cleaning contaminated equipment	✔/H	✔/H	✘	✔	✔	SS
	Cleaning blood/ body fluid spills	✔	✔/H	✘	✔	✔	SS

Laundry Handling

Overview

- Although soiled linen may harbor large numbers of pathogenic organisms, the risk of actual disease transmission is negligible. Rather than rigid rules and recommendations, common-sense hygienic practices for handling, processing, and storage of linen are recommended to reduce the risk of cross-infection. Many healthcare facilities utilize offsite contract services to process linen. Regardless of the use of in-house or offsite contract services, appropriate procedures are required to minimize potential nosocomial and occupational risks associated with soiled linen handling.

Purpose

- Development of Infection Control policies for laundry handling will protect healthcare workers from exposure to potentially infectious materials during collection, handling, and sorting of soiled linens.

Risk Factors

- The risk of actual disease transmission by linen is negligible. However, theoretically agitation of soiled linen could result in airborne contamination.

Strategies for Prevention and Control

- Use of personal protective equipment, handwashing, containment of linen, hazard communication, and ergonomics will decrease potential disease transmission and worker injury.

- Laundry handling practices that minimize agitation to prevent microbial aerosolization. Bagging soiled linen at the location of use, separation, and appropriate transport and storage of clean linen will create minimal risks to patients.
- Handwashing facilities should be readily available and utilized by workers handling linen.
- Personal Protective Equipment such as gloves should be worn if laundry is soiled with blood or body fluids. Laundry personnel sorting linen should always wear gloves and other appropriate Personal Protective Equipment.
- Soiled linen should be handled as little as possible with minimum agitation and be placed in bags at the point of generation.
- Soiled linen should not be sorted or rinsed in patient care areas.
- Linens should be placed in bags that prevent leakage, and bags should be closed securely to prevent opening during transport.
- Loose soiled pieces of laundry should not be tossed into laundry chutes.
- Double bagging of linen is not necessary unless the primary bag leaks.
- Foreign materials (e.g., needles) should not be placed in soiled linen. Removal of solid objects (e.g., feces) or use of protective disposable pads will reduce risks of contamination.
- Clean and soiled linen should be transported in separate, covered containers.
- Clean linen should be handled with clean hands away from clothing or surfaces to avoid contamination.
- Clean linen should be stored in protected areas until distributed for patient use.

- Clean and soiled processing areas should be physically separated and/or have negative air pressure in the soiled linen area relative to clean.
- Wash water temperatures of 160°F (71°C) or lower temperatures of 71°-77°F (22° - 50°C) (with carefully controlled laundry chemicals such as bleach) are effective in sanitizing linens.
- Healthcare workers should be trained in the collection, transport, sorting, and washing of soiled linen.

References/Resources

- Centers for Disease Control and Prevention, Healthcare Infection Control Practices Advisory Committee (HICPAC). Draft Guideline for Environmental Infection Control in Healthcare Facilities, 2001. 2001, Federal Register.
- McDonald LL., Linen Services. APIC Text of Infection Control and Epidemiology. 2000: 75; 1-4.
- "Laundry," Issues in Healthcare Settings, www.cdc.gov/ncidod/hip/Sterile/laundry.htm

Reuse and Reprocessing of SUDs

Overview

- The U.S. Food and Drug Administration (FDA) released its final guidance on August 14, 2000 pertaining to the practice of reusing medical devices that are intended to be used only once. The goal of the new Single Use Devices (SUDs) reuse policy is to protect the public health by assuring that the practice of reprocessing and reusing SUDs is based on good science, while ensuring that the regulatory requirements are equitable to all parties. Under the final guidance, hospitals that reprocess SUDs may be subject to the requirements of the Food, Drug, and Cosmetic Act, including premarket notification and approval; registration and listing; submission of adverse events reports under the Medical Device Reporting (MDR) regulation; good manufacturing practice under the Quality System regulation; device labeling; device tracking; and corrections, removals, and recalls.

Purpose

- Provide the ICP with basic understanding of SUDs by offering definitions and direction to establish policies/procedures for addressing the use of SUDs in the healthcare setting in order to reduce infection and safety risks.

Definitions

- **Class I Medical Device:** A medical device for which general controls provide reasonable assurance of the safety and effectiveness of the device. If there is insufficient evidence to reasonably ensure safety and effectiveness, the device is not life-supporting or life-sustaining, its use is not substantially important in preventing impairment of human health, and/or its use "does not present a potential unreasonable risk of illness or injury."

- **Class II Medical Device:** A medical device for which general controls alone do not provide reasonable assurance of device safety and effectiveness but for which there is sufficient information to establish special controls (e.g., performance standards, guidelines, patient registries, postmarket surveillance) to provide that assurance.
- **Class III Medical Device:** A medical device for which neither general controls nor special controls provide reasonable assurance of device safety and effectiveness and the device is life-supporting, life-sustaining, or its use "is of substantial importance in preventing impairment of human health" or "presents a potential risk of illness or injury."
- **Opened-but-unused Device:** A device whose sterility is compromised before being introduced onto the sterile field and which is not contaminated with blood and/or other potentially infectious materials (OPIM) external to the sterile field.
- **Reprocessing:** Includes all operations to render a contaminated reusable or single-use device patient ready. Single-use devices to be reprocessed may be either used or unused. The steps may include cleaning, functional testing, repackaging, relabeling, disinfection, or sterilization.
- **Resterilization:** The application of a process intended to remove or destroy all viable forms of microbial life, including bacterial spores. Because sterility is not an absolute, the accepted sterility assurance level (SAL) is usually defined as 10^{-6}.
- **Reuse:** The repeated or multiple uses of any medical device whether marketed as reusable or single use. Repeated/multiple use may be on the same patient or on different patients with applicable reprocessing of the device (cleaning, disinfection, or sterilization) between uses.

- **Single-use device (SUD):** A single-use device, also referred to as a disposable device, is intended to be used on one patient during a single procedure. It is not intended to be reprocessed (cleaned, disinfected, or sterilized) and used on another patient. The labeling may or may not identify the device as single use or disposable and does not include instructions for reprocessing. SUDs examples include surgical saw blades, surgical drills, laparoscopy scissors, orthodontic (metal) braces, electrophysiology catheters, electro-surgical electrodes and pencils, respiratory therapy and anesthesia breathing circuits, endotracheal tubes, balloon angioplasty (PTCA) catheters, and biopsy forceps.
- **Third-party Reprocessor:** A business establishment, separate from the user facility and the device manufacturer, one of whose primary businesses is to reprocess single-use/disposable medical devices.

Risk Factors

- Reprocessing of medical devices labeled for single use has grown steadily in recent years, as has the complexity of devices being reprocessed.
- This trend has intensified concern about patient safety, informed consent, the ethics of this practice, and the equitable regulation of the original manufacturer and reprocessors.
- Evidence suggests that some SUDs can be safely reprocessed if appropriate cleaning, testing, and sterilization procedures are carefully followed.
- SUDs reprocessing is not invariably safe, and relatively little is known/reported about the practice of reprocessing SUDs in healthcare institutions or by third party reprocessors.
- Because the demonstrated health risks from SUDs reprocessing are small, the new FDA guidance may have only a limited impact on public health.

Strategies for Prevention and Control

- Policies/procedures related to SUDs should be developed.
- A multidisciplinary team, including personnel from the OR, reprocessing, purchasing, IC, risk management, legal affairs, and others as appropriate for the facility should be assembled to review policies/procedures.
- Published documents, regulations, and guidelines should be readily available for reference.
- Manufacturer literature for item(s) being considered for reprocessing should be obtained.
- A cost-benefit analysis for reprocessing each SUD item under consideration should be completed.
- Reprocessing protocol specific to each device should be developed including, but not limited to:
  - Number of times the item can be reprocessed,
  - Tracking and record keeping methods,
  - Patient consent form (if recommended by facility legal counsel),
  - Appropriate patient charge when the reprocessed SUD item is used, and
  - Criteria for evaluating/testing SUD item post-reprocessing (e.g., color, shape, size, motion, flexibility, tensile strength).
- Quality assessment indicators to evaluate patient outcome should be defined and monitored.
- A recall process should be developed.
- Training and competency programs should be developed and implemented prior to initiation of reprocessing.

References/Resources

- Association for Professionals in Infection Control and Epidemiology. APIC Text of Infection Control and Epidemiology. 2000, chapter 55 pp.1-6, 58 pp.1-7.
- FDA Reuse Homepage at: www.fda.gov/cdrh/reuse/index.shtml
- Ulatowski TA, Reuse of single-use devices in Rutala, WA. Disinfection, sterilization, and antisepsis: principles and practices in healthcare facilities. 2001, Washington, DC: Association for Professionals in Infection Control and Epidemiology, Inc., 16-27.
- U.S. Department of Health and Human Services, Food and Drug Administration, Center for Devices and Radiological Health. Labeling reusable medical devices for reprocessing in healthcare facilities: FDA reviewer guidance. Rockville, MD: FDA, Center for Devices and Radiological Health, Office of Device Evaluation, March 1995.
- U.S. Department of Health and Human Services, Food and Drug Administration, Center for Devices and Radiological Health, Division of Enforcement III, Office of Compliance. Guidance for Industry and for FDA Staff, Enforcement Priorities for Single-Use Devices Reprocessed by Third Parties and Hospitals. August 14, 2000, Washington, DC: U.S. Government Printing Office.
- U.S. Department of Health and Human Services, Food and Drug Administration, Center for Devices and Radiological Health, Guidance for Hemodialyzer Reuse Labeling, October 6, 1995, available at http://www.fda.gov/cdrh/ode/dilreuse.pdf

- U.S. Department of Health and Human Services, Food and Drug Administration, Center for Devices and Radiological Health, User Facility Reporting Bulletin, A quarterly bulletin to assist hospitals, nursing homes, and other device user facilities. Summer 2000, Issue No. 31.
- United States General Accounting Office, Single-use medical devices, little available evidence of harm from reuse, but oversight warranted. Medical Device Reprocessing GAO Report to Congressional Requesters June 2000, GAO/HEHS-00-123.

Scrubs and Surgical Apparel

Overview

- Clothing, known as surgical scrub suits or scrubs, consists of a wide variety of apparel. Because this type of attire commonly replaces the more traditional uniform, its original function as an ensemble worn by surgical personnel no longer prevails. Scrubs and related apparel are used for many applications in healthcare inside and outside of the operating room.

Purpose

- Although the use of scrubs and apparel has not been scientifically associated with infection transmission, certain guidelines are recommended regarding the use of these garments in the healthcare setting.

Definitions

- **Cover gown** – a garment (laboratory coat or jacket) worn over scrubs to prevent their contamination.
- **PPE** – personal protective equipment worn to protect from exposure to hazardous agents, e.g., bloodborne pathogens; per the OSHA Bloodborne Pathogen Standard, the "employer provide, at no cost to the employee, appropriate personal protective equipment" and "that the type and characteristics will depend upon the task and degree of exposure anticipated."
- **Scrubs** – a set of clothing that began in the operating room setting around 1900; modern scrubs include apparel in a wide selection of sizes, colors, and prints with relative ease of laundering and

maintenance; Scrubs are less expensive than conventional healthcare uniforms.

- **Uniform** – defined by Webster as the official or distinctive clothes or outfit worn by members of a particular group when on duty.

Risk Factors

- Concerns for airborne contamination from scrubs and surgical apparel contributing to risk of surgical site infection were the rationale for establishing guidelines.
- Studies demonstrated a reduction in dissemination of skin squames/airborne bacteria arising from perineum, thighs, and feet was achieved by wearing specially designed trouser-like clothing.
- AORN suggests that scrubs in the operating room "promote high-level cleanliness and hygiene within the practice setting."
- There is no scientific evidence that the use of scrubs or related apparel (e.g., cover gowns) contributes to either the cause or the prevention of infections associated with healthcare facilities.
- A detailed study reported no significant difference in the infection rate between the use versus non-use of cover gowns in a neonatal intensive-care unit.
- There is no scientific evidence to suggest that home laundering versus institutional laundering poses any increased risk of infection transmission.
- There are no scientific data supporting or regulations requiring healthcare employers to provide scrubs for personnel for infection prevention reasons.
- There are no reports that scrub apparel worn home has been responsible for the transmission of infections of any kind.

Strategies for Prevention and Control

- To reduce risk of exposure to bloodborne pathogens per OSHA, "scrubs are usually worn in a manner similar to street clothing, and normally should be covered by appropriate gowns, aprons, or laboratory coats when splashes to skin or clothing are anticipated."
- Traditional scrubs are generally not made of a barrier-type, liquid-resistant material; they may not provide adequate protection if used as PPE.
- Apparel selection should include consideration for the "type and characteristics" commensurate with "the task and degree of exposure anticipated" to protect the wearer, including quality of the material and design.
- Policies/procedures should include information per OSHA related to pull-over scrubs (as opposed to scrubs with snap closures); if scrubs become minimally contaminated, the employee should be trained to remove the pull-over scrub in such a way as to avoid contact with the outer surface, e.g., rolling up the garment as it is pulled toward the head for removal; if the amount of blood exposure is such that the blood penetrates the scrub and contaminates the inner surface; it may be prudent to train employees to cut such a contaminated scrub to aid removal and prevent exposure to the face.
- OSHA holds employers responsible for laundering any clothing, including scrubs, worn by healthcare workers that become contaminated with blood or other potentially infectious body fluids, regardless of who owns the scrubs.
- AORN's current position states that the use of cover gowns "depends on the culture of each perioperative setting, the perioperative manager's assessment of priorities, and state regulatory laws".

- The varied application of scrubs and related apparel in healthcare settings raises issues and challenges best resolved by a multidisciplinary healthcare group with representatives from administration, nursing, medicine, materials management, human resources, infection control, and other affected departments.

References/Resources

- Association for Professionals in Infection Control and Epidemiology. APIC Text of Infection Control and Epidemiology. 2000, chapter 53 pp.1-11, 75 pp.1-4.
- Association of Operating Room Nurses. Recommended practices for surgical attire: standards and recommended practices. Denver: AORN; 1995. p. 141-142.
- Association of Operating Room Nurses. www.aorn.org
- Belkin NL. APIC State-of-the-art report: Use of scrubs and related apparel in healthcare facilities. Am J Infect Control 1997; 25:401-404.
- Centers for Disease Control and Prevention, Healthcare Infection Control Practices Advisory Committee (HICPAC). Draft guideline for environmental infection control in healthcare facilities, 2001. 2001, Federal Register
- Department of Labor and Department of Health and Human Services (US), Occupational Safety and Health Administration. OSHA Instruction CPL 2 - 2.69. Enforcement procedures for the occupational exposure to bloodborne pathogens. November 27, 2001
- Department of Labor and Department of Health and Human Services (US), Occupational Safety and Health Administration.
- 29 CFR Part 1910.1030, Occupational Exposure to Bloodborne Pathogens; Needlesticks and Other Sharps Injuries; Final Rule, Federal Register/Vol.66, No. 12/January 18, 2001.

- Pelke S, Ching D, Easa D, Melish ME. Gowning does not affect colonization or infection rates in a neonatal intensive care unit. Arch Pediatr Adolesc Med 1994; 148:1016-20
- Webster's New World Dictionary. 3rd Ed. New York: Simon and Schuster; 1990. p. 64.

Service and Companion Animal Considerations

Overview

- The presence of service and companion animals in healthcare settings is increasing as animal therapy and visitation have been found to improve patients' psychosocial well-being. Service animals are trained to perform tasks for the benefit of a person with a disability, assisting many persons to achieve greater functional independence.
- Although all types of animals may potentially carry zoonotic pathogens transmissible to humans or pose safety concerns, ensuring that animals are healthy, clean, vaccinated, and well trained can minimize risks.

Purpose

- Development of Infection Control policies will guide procedures to reduce infection and safety risks posed by service and companion animals in healthcare settings.

Risk Factors

- Bites and Scratches
- Ectoparasites and Endoparasites
- Allergens and odors
- Elimination exposures
- Immunocompromised patients
- Offending cultural/religious beliefs

References/Resources

- Centers for Disease Control and Prevention. HICPAC Guideline (Draft) for Environmental Infection Control in Healthcare Facilities, 2001, 92 - 95.
- Duncan, S., APIC State of the Art Report: the implications of service animals in healthcare settings. Am J Infect Control 2000, 28: 170-80.
- www.deltasociety.org

Section III

HEALTHCARE ASSOCIATED INFECTIONS

Pressure Ulcers

Overview

- Development of a pressure ulcer is a concern in the care of patients in healthcare facilities as well as home care.
- Prevalence of pressure ulcers increases in the elderly, quadriplegic, critical care, and orthopedic patients. Prevention of pressure ulcers can be accomplished by continuous assessment of risk factors and tissue management.
- Once a pressure ulcer has developed, the rate of bacterial colonization of the wound is high, increasing the risk for infection. Complications of infected ulcers can include: bacteremia, sepsis, advancing cellulitis, and osteomyelitis.
- Education and quality improvement are integral to an effective pressure ulcer treatment program for healing and prevention of infection.

Purpose

- Prevention of pressure ulcer development will reduce associated infections and complications.

Definition

- Pressure Ulcer: Any lesion caused by unrelieved pressure resulting in damage of underlying tissue usually over bony prominences which are graded by stages to classify tissue damage.

Strategies for Prevention and Control

- Animal assessments should be performed and include: current immunization record, name of veterinarian, date of most recent visit, evidence of ectoparasites treatment (e.g., fleas, ticks), and absence of dermatalogic lesions.
- An evaluation of patients/staff should be performed to identify cultural considerations and allergies.
- Policies should be developed to restrict animals from food preparation areas, operation rooms, laundries, clean storage areas, medication preparation areas, isolation and protective environments, and patient eating areas.
- Pet sleeping and eating areas should be designated.
- Visiting animals should be supervised (e.g., contained with leash/cages) at all times.
- ICPs should develop policies for:
  - Handwashing/hand hygiene after contact with pets, pet food, or pet waste.
  - Supervision protocol assigning responsibility for feeding, walking, and cleaning.
  - Protocol for clean-up and disposal of pet waste.
  - Procedure for exposure management.
- Case-by-case consideration should be given to pet visitation with immunocompromised adults and children.
- Turtles, rodents, ferrets, skunks, and raccoons are not good candidates for pet therapy due to a high likelihood of colonization with enteric pathogens (e.g., turtles), rabies (e.g., skunks and raccoons) and/or behavioral issues (e.g., biting).
- Staff training should include education of the role of Service animals and the "Americans with Disabilities Act" of 1990.

Risk Factors

- Extrinsic:
  - Pressure
  - Poor nutrition
  - Wetness/dampness
  - Improper positioning
  - Poor hygiene
  - Improper lifting techniques
  - Shearing/ friction
  - Medications (psychotropic drugs anticoagulants, sedatives)
  - Use of restraints
  - Casts/braces
- Intrinsic:
  - Incontinence
  - Decreased mobility
  - Impaired circulation
  - Postcerebrovascular accident status
  - Diabetes
  - Abnormal body weight
  - Depression or confusion
  - Advanced age
  - Use of steroids
  - Infection at other body sites

Strategies for Prevention and Control

- The goal of tissue management should always be prevention of pressure ulcer formation. Accomplishment of this begins with thorough and accurate skin assessment and identification of risk factors.
- Management of tissue loads (i.e., pressure, friction, and shearing) is vital components of prevention. Patients who present with or develop pressure ulcers should have treatment plans that promote healing, prevent infection, and control colonization of the wound.
- Identification of infected ulcers includes the presence of serosanguinous drainage, inflammation, purulence, pain, induration, or erythema in the surrounding tissue. A positive tissue culture that lacks these signs and symptoms may indicate colonization of the pressure ulcer. Staging (I, II, III, or IV) of the ulcers will assist with treatment options.
- Initial and ongoing skin assessment and pressure relief should be performed.
- Clean gloves must be used for each patient and should be changed between clean and dirty procedures for the same patient; hands should be washed hands after removing gloves.
- When treating multiple ulcers on the same patient, treat the most contaminated ulcer last.
- Wounds should be cleansed with normal saline.
- Debridement should be performed when indicated using a sterile sharp, mechanical, or enzymatic means.
- Cultures should not be routinely performed. If culture is indicated, swabs should not be used (due to potential colonization and possible trauma to wound). Needle aspiration or biopsy should be done if a culture is clinically indicated.

- If pressure ulcers are not healing or continues to produce exudates after two to four weeks of meticulous care, a two week trial of topical antibiotics may be indicated. Antibiotics should be broad spectrum (effective against gram negative, gram positive, and anaerobic bacteria). Topical antibiotics will have no effect on deep wound or systemic infections.
- If patient has signs of bacteremia, sepsis, advancing cellulitis, or osteomyelitis, systemic intravenous antibiotics may be needed. Blood cultures may be indicated.
- Ulcers should be protected from exogenous sources of contamination (e.g., feces) and trauma.
- Clean dressings should be used (sterile dressings are rarely indicated). Dressings should be kept in original packaging in clean, dry place; discard if wet or dirty.
- Pressure ulcer education programs should include principles of cleansing and infection control.
- Continuous quality improvement program should include patients, families, and caregivers.

References/Resources

- Association for Professionals in Infection Control and Epidemiology. APIC Text of Infection Control and Epidemiology. 2000, chapters 35,37,46.
- U.S. Department of Health and Human Services. Clinical Practice Guidelines, Treatment of pressure ulcers, Dec. 1994.

Respiratory Tract Infections

Overview

- Respiratory infections may occur in the healthcare setting. Nosocomial pneumonia is the second most frequent infection and has the greatest mortality. Recognition of populations most at risk and preventative measures are key to decreasing the risk of infection.

Purpose

- Evidence-based guidelines should be followed to reduce the significant morbidity and mortality associated with lower respiratory tract infections, particularly pneumonia.

Risk Factors

- Risk for nosocomial pneumonia can be easily divided by type of patient.
- The most important risk factor for nosocomial pneumonia is mechanical or tracheal incubation, which gives a threefold to 21-fold increased risk compared to the unventilated patient.
  - Patients Without Mechanical Ventilation

    Chronic lung disease

    Severity of illness/trauma

    Upper abdominal or thoracic surgery

    Duration of surgery

    Age

    Poor nutritional state or hypoalbuminemia

    Immunosuppressive therapy

Depressed level of consciousness

Impaired airway reflexes or difficulty handling secretions

Duration of hospitalization

Large volume aspiration

Nasoenteric tube

Neuromuscular disease

Male gender

- Mechanically ventilated patients

    Duration of mechanical ventilation

    Chronic lung disease

    Severity of lung disease

    Age

    Severe head trauma or intracranial pressure monitor

    Barbiturate therapy after head trauma

    Gross aspiration of gastric contents

    Reintubation or self-extubation

    Upper abdominal or thoracic surgery

    Ventilator circuit changes at intervals of < 48 hour

    Supine head position

    Fall–winter season

    Prior antibiotic therapy

    Nasoenteric tube

    Bronchoscopy

    Shock

    Blunt trauma

    Stress ulcer with macroscopic bleeding

- Common etiologic agents
  - *Pseudomonas* species
  - *Enterobacter* species
  - *Staphylococcus* aureus
  - *Klebsiella* species
  - *Acinetobacter* species

Strategies for Prevention and Control

- Hands should be washed after removing gloves and between patients.
- Aseptic technique should be used for respiratory tract manipulation.
- Proper disinfection and maintenance of respiratory equipment should be performed (Refer to Section 2 - Disinfection and Sterilization).
- Supine head positions should be avoided. The head of bed should be elevated (30–45°) for patients whenever possible.
- Drainage of ventilator tubing condensate should maintain flow away from the patient.
- Ventilator circuit should be changed at intervals ≥ 48 hours
- Gastric acidity should be maintained by using nonalkalinizing gastric cytoprotective agent in patients at risk of stress bleeding.
- Antibiotic use should be limited to clinical necessity.
- Nutritional status of severely ill patients should be assessed and optimized.
- The duration of immunosuppression (e.g., use of granulocyte colony-stimulating factor) should be limited to as short as clinically possible.

- Nasogastric tubes should be removed as soon clinically possible.
- Surveillance for pneumonia should be performed and feedback provided to personnel.
- Specific measures – Legionnaires' disease
  - Hyperchlorinate or superheat hospital water system or use.
  - Routinely clean water supply system.
  - Consider use of sterile water by immunosuppressed patients.
  - Properly design, place, and maintain cooling towers.
  - Do not routinely culture for *Legionella* spp.
- Specific measures – Aspergillosis
  - Remove granulocytopenic patients from vicinity of construction (refer to Section 2 – Construction and Renovation).
  - Place severely granulocytopenic patients in a protected environment (PE) with HEPA filtered air under positive pressure.
  - Have granulocytopenic patients wear a clean mask when leaving a protected environment.
  - Routinely maintain hospital air-handling systems and rooms of immunosuppressed patients.
- Specific measures - Respiratory syncytial virus infection (RSV)
  - Consider routine pre-admission screening of high-risk patients (e.g., < 2 years of age, congenital pulmonary/cardiac disease, immunosuppression).
  - Use private rooms, cohorting of patients and nursing personnel during hospital outbreaks of RSV infection.
  - Wash hands and wear gloves and a gown when caring for infected patients.

- Specific measures – Influenza
  - Vaccinate high-risk patients and their care providers before influenza season.
  - Use amantadine/rimantadine for chemoprophylaxis and treatment of patients and personnel during influenza A outbreaks.

References/Resources

- Association for Professionals in Infection Control and Epidemiology. APIC Text of Infection Control and Epidemiology. 2000, chapters 35, 88, 98, 100, 105, 111, 116.
- Centers for Disease Control and Prevention. Guidelines for prevention of nosocomial pneumonia. MMWR 1997; 46 (RR-1):1–79.
- Centers for Disease Control and Prevention, Healthcare Infection Control Practices Advisory Committee (HICPAC). Draft guideline for environmental infection control in healthcare facilities, 2001. 2001, Federal Register.
- George DL. Nosocomial pneumonia. In: Mayhall CG, editor. Hospital epidemiology and infection control. Baltimore: Williams and Wilkins; 1996. p 175–192.

Surgical Site Infections

Overview

- Approximately 27 million surgical procedures are performed annually in the U.S.; about 25% of these occur in the inpatient or hospital setting. Surgical site infections (SSIs), the third most common healthcare associated infection, have associated morbidity and mortality leading to increased LOS and related resource expenditures. Nearly 2/3 of SSIs are confined to the incision site and 1/3 involves organs or spaces accessed during the operation.
- The risk for SSI is influenced by characteristics of the patient, operation, personnel, and healthcare environment. Advances in infection control practices including improved OR ventilation, sterilization methods, barriers, surgical technique, and availability of antimicrobial prophylaxis have decreased SSIs.
- Despite these efforts, continued occurrences may be related to increased numbers of surgical patients who are elderly and/or have chronic, debilitating or immunocompromising diseases, an increase in prosthetic implants, and organ transplants.

Purpose

- Evidence-based guidelines should be used to help key parties establish a systematic and practical approach to reduce rates of SSIs in the patient populations served. The team to develop specific preventative actions and evaluation techniques should include surgeons, perioperative nurses, ICPs, anesthesiologists and CRNAs, healthcare epidemiologists, and others involved in the care of surgical patients and related support activities.

Risk Factors

- Patient factors include:
  - Age
  - Nutritional status
  - Diabetes
  - Smoking
  - Obesity
  - Coexistent infections at a remote body site
  - Colonization with microorganisms
  - Altered immune response
  - Length of preoperative stay
- Operative related factors consist of:
  - Duration of surgical scrub
  - Skin antisepsis
  - Preoperative shaving
  - Preoperative skin prep
  - Duration of operation
  - Antimicrobial prophylaxis
  - Operating room ventilation
  - Inadequate sterilization of instruments
  - Foreign material in the surgical site
  - Surgical drains
  - Surgical technique

    Poor hemostasis

    Failure to obliterate dead space

    Tissue trauma

- Pathogens implicated in SSIs depend upon site of procedure; the most common include*:
  - *Staphylococcus aureus*
  - Coagulase-negative staphylococci
  - *Enterococcus* spp.
  - *Escherichia coli*
  - *Pseudomonas aeruginosa*
  - *Enterobacter* spp.
  - *Proteus mirabilis*
  - *Klebsiella pneumoniae*
  - Other *Streptococcus* spp.
  - *Candida albicans*
  - Group D streptococci (non-enterococci)
  - Other gram-positive aerobes
  - *Bacteroides fragilis*

* Pathogens representing < 2% are excluded

Strategies for Prevention and Control

- Recommended practices are from the Centers for Disease Control and Prevention (CDC)/Healthcare Infection Control Practices Advisory Committee (HICPAC) *Guideline for Prevention of SSI* 1999. Each recommendation is categorized on the basis of existing scientific data, theoretical rationale, applicability, and economic impact. The system for categorizing recommendations is as follows:
  - **Category IA** *(IA)*. Strongly recommended for implementation and strongly supported by well-designed experimental, clinical, or epidemiological studies.

- **Category IB** *(IB)*. Strongly recommended for implementation and supported by some experimental, clinical, or epidemiological studies and a strong theoretical rationale.
- **Category IC** *(IC)*. Required by state or federal regulations, rules, or standards.
- **Category II** *(II)*. Suggested for implementation and supported by suggestive clinical or epidemiological studies or a theoretical rationale.
- **No recommendation;** unresolved issue *(UI)*. Practices for which evidence is insufficient or no consensus regarding efficacy exist.

➤ **Preoperative preparation of the patient**

- Whenever possible, identify and treat all infections remote to the surgical site before elective operation, and postpone elective operations on patients with remote site infections until the infection has resolved. *(IA)*
- Do not remove hair preoperatively unless the hair at or around the incision site will interfere with the operation. *(IA)*
- If hair is removed, remove immediately before the operation, preferably with electric clippers. *(IA)*
- Adequately control serum blood glucose levels in all diabetic patients and particularly avoid hyperglycemia perioperatively. *(IB)*
- Encourage tobacco cessation. At minimum, instruct patients to abstain for at least 30 days before elective operation from smoking cigarettes, cigars, pipes, or any other form of tobacco consumption. *(IB)*
- Do not withhold necessary blood products from surgical patients as a means to prevent SSI. *(IB)*
- Require patients to shower or bathe with an antiseptic agent on at least the night before the operative day. *(IB)*

- Thoroughly wash and clean at and around the incision site to remove gross contamination before performing antiseptic skin preparation. *(IB)*
- Use an appropriate antiseptic agent for skin preparation. *(IB)*
- Apply preoperative antiseptic skin preparation in concentric circles moving toward the periphery. The prepared area should be large enough to extend the incision or create new incisions or drain sites, if necessary. *(II)*
- Keep preoperative hospital stay as short as possible while allowing for adequate preoperative preparation of the patient. *(II)*
- No recommendation to taper or discontinue systemic steroid use (when medically permissible) before elective operation. *(UI)*
- No recommendation to enhance nutritional support for surgical patients solely as a means to prevent SSI. *(UI)*
- No recommendation to preoperatively apply mupirocin to nares to prevent SSI. *(UI)*
- No recommendation to provide measures that enhance wound space oxygenation to prevent SSI. *(UI)*

➤ **Hand/forearm antisepsis for surgical team members**

- Keep nails short and do not wear artificial nails. *(IB)*
- Perform a preoperative surgical scrub for at least two to five minutes using an appropriate antiseptic. Scrub the hands and forearms up to the elbows. *(IB)*
- After performing the surgical scrub, keep hands up and away from the body (elbows in flexed position) so that water runs from the tips of the fingers toward the elbows. Dry hands with a sterile towel and don a sterile gown and gloves. *(IB)*
- Clean underneath each fingernail prior to performing the first surgical scrub of the day. *(II)*

- Do not wear hand or arm jewelry. *(II)*
- No recommendation on wearing nail polish. *(UI)*

➤ **Management of infected or colonized surgical personnel**

- Educate and encourage surgical personnel who have signs and symptoms of a transmissible infectious illness to report conditions promptly to their supervisory and occupational health service personnel. *(IB)*
- Develop well-defined policies concerning patient care responsibilities when personnel have potentially transmissible infectious conditions. These policies should govern (a) personnel responsibility in using the health service and reporting illness, (b) work restrictions, and (c) clearance to resume work after an illness that required work restriction. The policies also should identify persons who have the authority to remove personnel from duty. *(IB)*
- Obtain appropriate cultures from, and exclude from duty, surgical personnel who have draining skin lesions until infection has been ruled out or personnel have received adequate therapy and infection has resolved. *(IB)*
- Do not routinely exclude surgical personnel who are colonized with organisms such as *S. aureus* (nose, hands, or other body site) or group A *Streptococcus*, unless such personnel have been linked epidemiologically to dissemination of the organism in the healthcare setting. *(IB)*

➤ **Antimicrobial prophylaxis**

- Administer a prophylactic antimicrobial agent only when indicated, and select it based on its efficacy against the most common pathogens causing SSI for a specific operation and published recommendations. *(IA)*
- Administer by the intravenous route the initial dose of prophylactic antimicrobial agent, timed such that a bactericidal

concentration of the drug is established in serum and tissues when the incision is made. Maintain therapeutic levels of the agent in serum and tissues throughout the operation and until, at most, a few hours after the incision is closed in the operating room. *(IA)*

- Before elective colorectal operations [in addition to above], mechanically prepare the colon by use of enemas and cathartic agents. Administer non-absorbable oral antimicrobial agents in divided doses on the day before the operation. *(IA)*
- For high-risk cesarean section, administer the prophylactic antimicrobial agent immediately after the umbilical cord is clamped.*(IA)*
- Do not routinely use vancomycin for antimicrobial prophylaxis. *(IB)*

➤ **Intraoperative ventilation**

- Maintain positive-pressure ventilation in the operating room with respect to the corridors and adjacent areas. *(IB)*
- Maintain a minimum of 15 air changes per hour, of which at least three should be fresh air. *(IB)*
- Filter all air, recirculated and fresh, through the appropriate filters per the American Institute of Architects' recommendations. *(IB)*
- Introduce all air at the ceiling, and exhaust near the floor. *(IB)*
- Do not use UV radiation in the operating room to prevent SSI. *(IB)*
- Keep operating room doors closed except as needed for passage of equipment, personnel, and the patient. *(IB)*
- Consider performing orthopedic implant operations in operating rooms supplied with ultraclean air. *(II)*
- Limit the number of personnel entering the operating room to necessary personnel. *(II)*

➤ **Intraoperative cleaning and disinfection of environmental surfaces**

- When visible soiling or contamination with blood or other body fluids of surfaces or equipment occurs during an operation, use an EPA-approved hospital disinfectant to clean the affected areas before the next operation. *(IB)*
- Do not perform special cleaning or closing of operating rooms after contaminated or dirty operations. *(IB)*
- Do not use tacky mats at the entrance to the operating room suite or individual operating rooms for infection control. *(IB)*
- Wet vacuum the operating room floor after the last operation of the day or night with an EPA-approved hospital disinfectant. *(II)*
- No recommendation on disinfecting environmental surfaces or equipment used in operating rooms between operations in the absence of visible soiling. *(UI)*

➤ **Intraoperative microbiologic sampling**

- Do not perform routine environmental sampling of the operating room. Perform microbiologic sampling of operating room environmental surfaces or air only as part of an epidemiologic investigation. *(IB)*

➤ **Intraoperative sterilization of surgical instruments**

- Sterilize all surgical instruments according to published guidelines. *(IB)*
- Perform flash sterilization only for patient care items that will be used immediately (e.g., to reprocess an inadvertently dropped instrument). Do not use flash sterilization for reasons of convenience, as an alternative to purchasing additional instrument sets, or to save time. *(IB)*

- **Intraoperative Surgical attire and drapes**
  - Wear a surgical mask that fully covers the mouth and nose when entering the operating room if an operation is about to begin, is already under way, or if sterile instruments are exposed. Wear the mask throughout the operation. *(IB)*
  - Wear a cap or hood to fully cover hair on the head and face when entering the operating room. *(IB)*
  - Do not wear shoe covers for the prevention of SSI. *(IB)*
  - Scrubbed surgical team member should wear sterile gloves. Put on gloves after donning a sterile gown. *(IB)*
  - Use surgical gowns and drapes that are effective barriers when wet (i.e., materials that resist liquid penetration). *(IB)*
  - Change scrub suits that are visibly soiled, contaminated, and/or penetrated by blood or other potentially infectious materials. *(IB)*
  - No recommendations on how or where to launder scrub suits, on restricting use of scrub suits to the operating suite, or for covering scrub suits when out of the operating suite. *(UI)*
- **Intraoperative asepsis and surgical technique**
  - Adhere to principles of asepsis when placing intravascular devices (e.g., central venous catheters), spinal, or epidural anesthesia catheters or when dispensing and administering intravenous drugs. *(IA)*
  - Assemble sterile equipment and solutions immediately prior to use. *(II)*
  - Handle tissue gently, maintain effective hemostasis, minimize devitalized tissue and foreign bodies (i.e., sutures, charred tissues, necrotic debris), and eradicate dead space at the surgical site. *(IB)*
  - Use delayed primary skin closure or leave an incision open to heal by second intention if the surgeon considers the surgical site to be heavily contaminated (e.g., Class III and Class IV). *(IB)*

- If drainage is necessary, use a closed suction drain. Place a drain through a separate incision distant from the operative incision. Remove the drain as soon as possible. *(IB)*

➤ **Postoperative incision care**

- Protect with a sterile dressing for 24 to 48 hours postoperatively an incision that has been closed primarily. *(IB)*
- Wash hands before and after dressing changes and any contact with the surgical site. *(IB)*
- When an incision dressing should be changed, use sterile technique. *(II)*
- Educate the patient and family regarding proper incision care, symptoms of SSI, and the need to report such symptoms. *(II)*
- No recommendation to cover an incision closed primarily beyond 48 hours nor on the appropriate time to shower or bathe with an uncovered incision. *(UI)*

➤ **Surveillance**

- Use CDC definitions of SSI without modification for identifying SSI among surgical inpatients and outpatients. *(IB)* (Refer to Section 1 - Acute Care Nosocomial Surveillance.)
- For inpatient case finding (including read-missions), use direct prospective observation, indirect prospective detection, or a combination of both direct and indirect methods for the duration of the patient's hospitalization. *(IB)*
- When post-discharge surveillance is performed for detecting SSI following certain operations (e.g., coronary artery bypass graft), use a method that accommodates available resources and data needs. *(II)*
- For outpatient case-finding, use a method that accommodates available resources and data needs. *(IB)*

- Assign the surgical wound classification upon completion of an operation. A surgical team member should make the assignment. *(II)*
- For each patient undergoing an operation chosen for surveillance, record those variables shown to be associated with increased SSI risk (e.g., surgical wound class, ASA class, and duration of operation). *(IB)*
- Periodically calculate operation-specific SSI rates stratified by variables shown to be associated with increased SSI risk (e.g., NNIS risk index). *(IB)*
- Report appropriately stratified, operation-specific SSI rates to surgical team members. The optimum frequency and format for such rate computations will be determined by stratified case-load sizes (denominators) and the objectives of local, continuous quality improvement initiatives. *(IB)*
- No recommendation to make available to the infection control committee coded surgeon-specific data. *(UI)*

References/Resources:

- American Association for the Advancement of Medical Instrumentation Sterilization in Healthcare Facilities (STBK8-1-293). Arlington, VA: AAMI; 1998.
- Association for Professionals in Infection Control and Epidemiology. APIC Text of Infection Control and Epidemiology. 2000, chapter 53 pp.1-11.
- Association of Operating Room Nurses. Standards, Recommended Practices, and Guidelines. Denver: AORN; 2000.

- Centers for Disease Control and Prevention, Healthcare Infection Control Practices Advisory Committee (HICPAC). Guideline for the Prevention of Surgical Site Infections, 1999, Am J Infect Control 1999; 27:97-119.
- Herwaldt LA, et al. Infection control guidelines for the operating suite. In: Abrutyn E, Goldman D, Scheckler W, Eds. Saunders Infection Control Reference Service. Philadelphia: WB Saunders; 1998:555–573.
- Patchen Dellinger E, Ehrenkranz NG. Surgical infections. In: Bennett J, Brachman PS, Eds. Hospital Infections. 4th ed. Philadelphia: Lippencott-Raven; 1998; 571–586.

Urinary Tract Infections

Overview

- The urinary tract is the most common site of healthcare acquired infections. The risk of urinary tract infection (UTI) increases significantly with instrumentation of the urinary tract i.e., catheterization. Complications of UTIs include bacteremia, septic shock, and death especially in the elderly. Treatment of UTIs increases costs due to; prolonged hospital stays, use of antimicrobials, diagnostic tests, and procedures. Common etiologic agents of UTIs include: *E. coli, Klebsiella, Enterobacter, Proteus,* as well as gram positive bacteria: *Staphylococcus aureus* and Enterococci.

Purpose

- Prevention of UTIs should involve education of healthcare personnel and caregivers on identification of symptomatic and asymptomatic bacteriuria.

Risk Factors

- Indwelling urinary catheters
- Urologic instrumentation
- Advanced age
- Female gender
- Severe underlying illness

Strategies for Prevention

- The primary prevention strategy for UTIs is to avoid indwelling catheterization whenever possible.
- Intermittent catheterization should be used whenever possible.
- Condom catheter use should be considered for cooperative male patients.
- If indwelling catheterization should be used, the duration of catheterization should be assessed and minimized as practical.
- Antibiotic use in asymptomatic patients should be considered carefully due to increasing emergence of multi-drug resistant organisms; this practice has not been shown to be effective in decreasing morbidity associated with UTIs.
- Utilization of indwelling catheters should be assessed daily and be monitored for proper aseptic insertion and prompt removal.
- Catheters should be inserted using clean aseptic technique.
- Indwelling catheters should be secured after insertion to avoid urethral traction.
- Closed sterile drainage systems should be used.
- The collection bag should be placed in order to maintain gravity drainage.
- Urine specimens should be obtained from catheter or collection port, not drainage bag.
- Catheters should not be changed at arbitrary fixed intervals; the bag and catheter should only be changed if there is poor urine flow, leaks in the system, or the there is the presence odor or obstruction.
- Caregivers should perform handwashing before and after inserting or handling catheters and bags.

References/Resources

- Kunin C. Urinary Tract Infection, APIC Text of Infection Control and Epidemiology, 2000, 92:1-5
- Wong, E. in Consultation with Hooton, T. Guidelines for Prevention of Catheter Associated Urinary Tract Infections, 1991.

Vascular Device Related Infections

Overview

- Intravascular catheters are indispensable in modern-day medical practice and they provide necessary vascular access. However, their use puts patients at risk for local and systemic infectious complications, including local site infection, bloodstream infection (BSI), septic thrombophlebitis, endocarditis, and other metastatic infections (e.g., lung abscess, brain abscess, osteomyelitis, endophthalmitis).
- To decrease patient morbidity/mortality and associated resources, efforts should be multidisciplinary, involving healthcare professionals who insert and maintain intravascular catheters, healthcare managers who allocate resources, and patients who are capable of assisting in the care of their catheters.

Purpose

- This section provides principles, practices, and control methods to reduce infection and associated safety risks in healthcare settings (hospital, outpatient, home) related to vascular devices. Implementation of specific strategies to reduce the incidence of these infections will help to improve patient outcome and reduce healthcare costs.

Definitions

- **Administration sets** - Include the area from the spike of tubing entering the fluid container to the hub of the vascular access device. However, a short extension tube may be connected to the catheter and may be considered a portion of the catheter to facilitate aseptic technique when changing administration sets.

- **Catheter-Related Bloodstream Infection** (CR-BSI) – Bacteremia/fungemia in a patient with an intra-vascular catheter with at least one positive blood culture and with clinical manifestations of infections (i.e., fever, chills, and/or hypotension) and no apparent source for the bloodstream infection except the catheter or any of the following:
  - A positive, semiquantitative (>15 CFU/catheter segment),or quantitative (>10^3 CFU/catheter segment catheter) culture whereby the same organism (species and antibiogram) is isolated from the catheter segment and peripheral blood;
  - Simultaneous quantitative blood cultures with a >5:1 ratio (central venous catheter (CVC) vs. peripheral);
  - Differential time period of CVC culture vs. peripheral blood culture positivity of > two hours.
- **Clinical exit site infection or tunnel infection** -Tenderness, erythema, or site induration >2 cm from the catheter site along the subcutaneous tract of a tunneled (e.g., Hickman or Broviac) catheter, in the absence of concomitant bloodstream infection.
- **Exit Site Infection** - Erythema or induration within 2 cm of the catheter exit site, in the absence of bloodstream infection, and w/o concomitant purulence
- **Infusate-Related Bloodstream Infection** - Concordant growth of the same organism from the infusate and blood cultures (preferably percutaneously drawn) with no other source of infection.
- **Localized Catheter Colonization** - Significant growth of a microorganism (>15 CFU) from the catheter tip, subcutaneous segment of the catheter, or catheter hub.

- **Pocket Infection** - Purulent fluid in the subcutaneous pocket of a totally implanted intravascular catheter that may or may not be associated with spontaneous rupture and drainage or necrosis of the overlaying skin, in the absence of concomitant bloodstream infection.

Risk Factors

- Patient related
  - Extremes of age
  - Granulocytopenia
  - Immunosuppressive chemotherapy
  - Loss of skin integrity (e.g., burns, psoriasis)
  - Severity of underlying illness
  - Presence of distant infection
  - Catheter composition (plastic > steel)
  - Size of catheter
  - Number of catheter lumens
  - Location of catheter (central > peripheral; femoral > jugular/subclavian)
  - Type of placement (cutdown > percutaneous; emergency > elective)
  - Duration of placement
  - Alteration in patient's cutaneous microflora
- Suboptimal handwashing practices of hospital personnel.
- Common etiologic agents
  - *S. epidermidis, S. aureus, Klebsiella* sp., *Serratia marcescens, Candida* sp., *Pseudomonas* sp., *Corynebacteria, Enterobacter* sp., *and Acinetobacter* sp.

- Signs of local inflammation present in only about 50% of the cases; semiquantitative culturing of the catheter tip most widely used for diagnosis (positive: ≥15 colonies on agar plate; 76–96% specificity, and 16–31% positive predictive value for catheter-associated sepsis).

Strategies for Prevention

- Recommended practices are from the Centers for Disease Control and Prevention (CDC)/Healthcare Infection Control Practices Advisory Committee (HICPAC) [**draft**] guideline. Each recommendation is categorized on the basis of existing scientific data, theoretical rationale, applicability, and economic impact. The CDC/HICPAC system for categorizing recommendations is as follows:
  - **Category IA** *(IA)*. Strongly recommended for implementation and strongly supported by well-designed experimental, clinical, or epidemiological studies.
  - **Category IB** *(IB)*. Strongly recommended for implementation and supported by some experimental, clinical, or epidemiological studies and a strong theoretical rationale.
  - **Category IC** *(IC)*. Required by state or federal regulations, rules, or standards.
  - **Category II** *(II)*. Suggested for implementation and supported by suggestive clinical or epidemiological studies or a theoretical rationale.
  - **No recommendation; unresolved issue** *(UI)*. Practices for which evidence is insufficient or no consensus regarding efficacy exist.

- General recommendations for all intravascular catheters in adult and pediatric patients.
  - **Handwashing**

    Observe proper hand hygiene either by washing hands with conventional antiseptic-containing soap and water or with waterless alcohol-based gels or foams.

    Observe hand hygiene before and after palpating catheter insertion sites, as well as before and after inserting, replacing, or dressing an intravascular catheter. *(IA)*

    Use of gloves does not obviate the need for hand hygiene. *(IA)*
  - Minimize manipulation of the system (entry into the system for blood drawing, medication administration, etc.)
  - Ensure appropriate aseptic techniques for catheter insertion, maintenance, and removal as outlined below.
- **Healthcare worker education and training**
  - Educate healthcare workers regarding indications for intravascular catheter use, proper procedures for the insertion and maintenance of intravascular catheters, and appropriate infection control measures to prevent intravascular catheter related infections. *(IA)*
  - Assess competence and compliance with guidelines periodically for all individuals who insert and manage intravascular catheters. *(IA)*
  - Ensure appropriate nursing staff-to-patient ratios in ICUs. *(IB)*
- **Catheter insertion**
  - Maintain aseptic technique for the insertion and care of intravascular catheters. *(IA)*
  - Wear clean or sterile gloves when inserting an intravascular catheter as required by the OSHA Bloodborne Pathogens Standard. *(IC)*
  - Wearing clean gloves is acceptable for the insertion of peripheral intravascular catheters if aseptic technique can be maintained.

Sterile gloves should be worn for the insertion of arterial and central catheters. *(IA)*

- Wear clean or sterile gloves when changing the dressing on intravascular catheters. *(IC)*
- Do not routinely use cutdown procedures as a method to insert catheters. *(IA)*
- Disinfect clean skin with an appropriate antiseptic before catheter insertion and at the time of dressing changes. A 2% chlorhexidine-based preparation is preferred. Alternatively, tincture of iodine, an iodophor, or 70% alcohol could be used. *(IA)* No recommendation for the use of chlorhexidine in infants less than 2 months of age. *(UI)*
- Allow the antiseptic to remain on the insertion site and to dry before inserting the catheter. Allow povidone iodine to remain on the skin for at least two minutes, or longer if it is not yet dry before inserting the catheter. *(IB)*
- Do not apply organic solvents (e.g., acetone or ether) to the skin before insertion of catheters or during dressing changes. *(IB)*

➤ **Catheter site maintenance**

- Use either a sterile gauze or sterile transparent semi-permeable dressing to cover the catheter site. *(IA)*
- Well-healed tunneled CVC sites may not require dressings. *(II)*
- If the patient is diaphoretic, or if the site is bleeding or oozing, a gauze dressing is preferred. *(II)*
- Replace catheter site dressing if the dressing becomes damp, loosened, or visibly soiled. *(IB)*
- Change dressings regularly for adult and adolescent patients; the frequency of such changes should be determined individually depending on the circumstances of the patient, but should be done at least weekly. *(II)*

- Do not use topical antibiotic ointment or creams on insertion sites because of their potential to promote fungal infections and antimicrobial resistance. *(IA)*
- Do not submerge the catheter under water. Showering may be permitted if precautions can be taken to reduce the likelihood of introducing organisms into the catheter, e.g., use an impermeable covering for the catheter and connecting device during the shower. *(II)*

➤ **Selection and replacement of intravascular catheters**

- Select the catheter, the insertion technique, and the insertion site with the lowest risk of complications (infectious and noninfectious) for the anticipated type and duration of intravenous [IV] therapy. *(IA)*
- Remove any intravascular catheter that is no longer essential. *(IA)*
- Do not routinely replace central venous or arterial catheters solely for the purposes of reducing the incidence of infection. *(IB)*
- Replace peripheral venous catheters every 96 hours in adults to prevent phlebitis. *(IB)*
- In pediatric patients, leave peripheral venous catheters in place until IV therapy is completed, unless a complication occurs. *(IB)*
- Replace all catheters inserted under emergency conditions within 48 hours when adherence to aseptic technique cannot be ensured. *(II)*
- Use clinical judgment to determine when to replace a catheter that could be a source of infection. For example, do not routinely replace catheters in patients whose only indication of infection is fever. Venous catheters do not necessarily need to be replaced routinely in patients who are bacteremic or fungemic if the source of infection is unlikely to be the catheter. *(II)*
- Replace all CVCs if the patient is hemodynamically unstable and CR-BSI is suspected. *(II)*

- Do not use guidewire techniques to replace catheters for which there is a clinical suspicion for CR-BSI. *(IB)*

➤ **Replacement of administration sets, needleless systems, and parenteral fluids**

- Replace administration sets, including secondary sets and add-on devices, no more frequently than at 96-hour intervals, unless CR-BSI is suspected or documented. *(IA)*
- Replace tubing used to administer blood, blood products, or lipid emulsions within 24 hours of initiating the infusion. *(II)*
- Needleless intravascular devices

  Change the needleless components at least as often as administration set. *(II)*

  Change caps no more frequently than every 96 hours or according to manufacturers' recommendations. *(II)*

  Minimize leaks and breaks in the system by making sure that all components of the system are compatible. *(II)*

  Minimize contamination risk by using aseptic technique when accessing needleless systems. *(IB)*

- Parenteral fluids

  Complete the infusion of lipid emulsions within 24 hours of hanging the emulsion. *(IB)*

  Complete infusions of blood within four hours of hanging the blood. *(IC)*

  No recommendation for the hang time of other parenteral fluids. *(UI)*

➤ **Intravenous injection ports**

- Clean injection ports with 70% alcohol or an iodophor before accessing the system. *(II)*
- Cap all stopcocks when not in use. *(IB)*

➤ **Preparation and quality control of intravenous admixtures**

- Admix all routine parenteral fluids in the pharmacy in a laminar-flow hood using aseptic technique. *(IB)*
- Do not use any container of parenteral fluid with visible turbidity, leaks, cracks, particulate matter, or if the manufacturer's expiration date has passed. *(IB)*

  Use single-dose vials for parenteral additives or medications whenever possible. *(II)*

- If multidose vials are used:

  Refrigerate multidose vials after they are opened, if recommended by the manufacturer. *(II)*

  Cleanse the access diaphragm of multi-dose vials with 70% alcohol before inserting a device into the vial. *(II)*

  Use a sterile device to access a multi-dose vial and avoid touch contamination of the device before penetrating the access diaphragm. *(IA)*

  Discard multidose vial if sterility is compromised. *(IA)*

- Inline filters - Do not use filters routinely for infection control purposes. *(IA)*
- Intravenous therapy personnel - Designate trained personnel for the insertion and maintenance of intravascular catheters. *(IB)*
- Prophylactic antimicrobials - Do not administer intranasal or systemic antimicrobial prophylaxis routinely before insertion or during use of an intravascular catheter as a method to prevent catheter colonization or BSI. *(IA)*

➤ **Peripheral venous catheters, including midline catheters, in adult and pediatric patients**

- Select catheters based on the intended purpose and duration of use, known complications (e.g., phlebitis and infiltration), and experience at the institution. *(IB)*

- Avoid the use of steel needles for the administration of fluids and medication that may cause tissue necrosis if extravasation occurs. *(IA)*
- Use a midline catheter or PICC when the duration of IV therapy is expected to exceed six days. *(IB)*
- In adults, use an upper extremity site in preference to one on a lower extremity for catheter insertion. Replace a catheter inserted in a lower extremity site to an upper extremity site as soon as it is feasible. *(IB)*
- In pediatric patients, the hand, the dorsum of the foot, or the scalp may be used as the catheter insertion site. *(II)*
- Inspect catheter insertion site daily. *(II)*
- Remove peripheral venous catheters if the patient develops signs of phlebitis (i.e., warmth, tenderness, erythema, palpable venous cord), infection, or a malfunctioning catheter. *(IB)*
- In adults, replace short, peripheral venous catheters every 96 hours to reduce the risk of phlebitis. *(IA)*
- Do not routinely replace midline catheters as a means to reduce the risk for infection. *(IB)*
- In pediatric patients, peripheral venous catheters may be left in place until intravenous therapy is completed, unless a complication occurs. *(IB)*
- Do not routinely apply prophylactic topical antimicrobial or antiseptic ointment or cream to the insertion site of peripheral venous catheters. *(IA)*

➤ **Central venous catheters, including PICC, hemodialysis, and pulmonary artery catheters, in adult and pediatric patients**

- Use a CVC with the minimum number of ports or lumens essential for the management of the patient. *(IB)*

- Use an antimicrobial or antiseptic-impregnated CVC in adults if despite full adherence to maximal barrier precautions, there is still a high rate of CR-BSI (e.g., more than 3.3/1000 catheter days). *(IB)*
- Patients are expected to be at high risk for CR-BSI e.g., patients are receiving total parental nutrition (TPN), are neutropenic, or are in an ICU and the catheter is expected to remain in place more than four days. *(II)*
- No recommendation in other patients whose catheter is expected to stay in place more than four days. *(UI)*
- No recommendation for the use of impregnated catheters in children. *(UI)*
- Designate trained personnel with documented competence and provide adequate supervision for trainees who perform catheter insertion. *(IA)*
- Use totally implantable access devices for patients who require long-term, intermittent vascular access. For patients requiring frequent or continuous access, a PICC or tunneled central venous catheter is preferable. *(II)*
- Use a cuffed central venous catheter for dialysis if the period of temporary access is anticipated to be prolonged (e.g., more than two weeks). *(IB)*
- Use a fistula or graft instead of a central venous catheter for permanent access for dialysis. *(IB)*
- Do not use hemodialysis catheters for blood drawing or applications other than hemodialysis except during dialysis or under emergency circumstances. *(II)*
- Weigh the risk and benefits of placing a device at a recommended site to reduce infectious complications against the risk of mechanical complications (e.g., pneumothorax, subclavian artery

puncture, subclavian vein laceration, subclavian vein stenosis, hemothorax, thrombosis, air embolism, catheter misplacement). *(IA)*

- To minimize infection risk, use a subclavian site for non-tunneled CVC placement rather than a jugular or a femoral site. *(IB)*
- Place catheters used for hemodialysis and pheresis in a jugular or femoral vein rather than a subclavian vein to avoid venous stenosis if catheter access is needed. *(IA)*
- Use sterile technique including the use of a cap, mask, sterile gown, sterile gloves, and a large sterile sheet for the insertion of CV catheters or guidewire exchange. *(IA)*
- Use a sterile sleeve to protect pulmonary artery catheters during insertion. *(IB)*
- Do not routinely replace central venous catheters or PICCs as a method to prevent catheter-related infections. *(IB)*
- Do not routinely replace hemodialysis catheters as a method to prevent catheter related infection. *(IB)*
- Do not routinely replace pulmonary artery catheters more frequently than seven days as a method to prevent catheter-related infections. *(IB)*
- Do not remove central venous catheter or PICCs solely because of fever. Use clinical judgment regarding the appropriateness of removing the catheter if there is evidence of infection elsewhere. *(II)*
- Guidewire exchange

  Do not use guidewire exchanges routinely for non-tunneled catheters. *(IB)*

  Use a guidewire exchange to replace a malfunctioning non-tunneled catheter if there is no evidence of infection and the risk of inserting a catheter into a new site is unacceptably high (e.g., due to obesity, coagulopathy). *(IB)*

Use a new set of sterile gloves prior to handling the new catheter when guide-wire exchanges are performed. *(II)*

- Designate one port exclusively for hyperalimentation if a multi-lumen catheter is used to administer parenteral nutrition. *(II)*
- Do not routinely use antibiotic lock solutions as a means of preventing CR-BSI. Use prophylactic antibiotic lock solution only in special circumstances (e.g., in treating a patient with a long-term catheter or port who has a history of multiple CR-BSIs despite optimal aseptic technique). *(II)*
- Replace catheter site dressing when the dressing becomes damp, loosened, or soiled, or when inspection of the site is necessary. *(IA)*
- Replace dressings used on short-term central catheter sites every two days for gauze dressings and every seven days for transparent dressings, except in pediatric patients because in these patients the risk of dislodging the catheter outweighs the benefit of changing the dressing. *(IB)*
- Replace dressings used on tunneled or implanted central catheter sites no more than once per week, until the insertion site has healed. *(IB)* The frequency of catheter dressing changes over well-healed catheter exit sites is an unresolved issue.
- No recommendation for the use of chlorhexidine sponge dressings to reduce the incidence of infection. *(UI)*; do not use chlorhexidine sponge dressings in neonates less than 7 days old or of gestational age less than 26 weeks. *(II)*
- Ensure that catheter site care is compatible with the catheter material. *(IB)*
- Use a sterile sleeve for all pulmonary artery catheters. *(IB)*
- Additional recommendations for peripheral arterial catheters and pressure monitoring devices for adult and pediatric patients

  Selection of pressure monitoring system - use disposable rather than reusable transducer assemblies when possible. *(IB)*

Replacement of catheter and pressure monitoring system

Replace peripheral arterial catheters and relocate catheter insertion sites no more frequently than every five days for infection control purposes. *(IB)*

Replace disposable or reusable transducers at 96-hour intervals. Replace other components of the system, including the tubing, continuous-flush device, and flush solution, at the time the transducer is replaced. *(IB)*

Keep all components of the pressure monitoring system (including calibration devices and flush solution) sterile. (IA)

Minimize the number of manipulations of and entries into the pressure monitoring system. Use a closed-flush system (i.e., continuous flush), rather than an open system (i.e., one that requires a syringe and stopcock), to maintain the patency of the pressure monitoring catheters. *(II)*

When the pressure monitoring system is accessed through a diaphragm rather than a stopcock, wipe the diaphragm with an appropriate antiseptic before accessing the system. *(IA)*

Do not administer dextrose-containing solutions or parenteral nutrition fluids through the pressure monitoring circuit. *(IA)*

Use disposable transducers. *(IB)*

Sterilize reusable transducers according to the manufacturers' instructions if the use of disposable transducers is not feasible. *(IA)*

➤ **Umbilical catheters**

- Umbilical artery catheters should be removed and not replaced if any signs of CR-BSI, vascular insufficiency, or thrombosis occur. *(II)*
- Umbilical venous catheters should be removed and not replaced if any signs of CR-BSI or thrombosis occur. *(II)*

- No recommendation for treating through an umbilical venous catheter suspected of being infected. *(UI)*
- Umbilical venous catheters should be replaced only if mechanical malfunction of the catheter occurs. *(II)*
- Cleanse the umbilical insertion site with an appropriate antiseptic before catheter insertion. Avoid iodine-containing agents because of the potential effect on the neonatal thyroid. *(IB)*
- Do not use topical antibiotic ointment or creams on umbilical catheter insertion sites because of the potential to promote fungal infections and antimicrobial resistance. *(IA)*
- Add low doses of heparin (0.5–1.0 u/ml TPN, 5000 u q 6 hr or 12 hr) to the fluid infused through umbilical arterial catheters. *(IB)*
- Remove umbilical catheters as soon as possible when not needed or when there is any sign of vascular insufficiency to the lower extremities. Optimally, umbilical artery catheters should not be left in place over five days. *(II)*
- Umbilical venous catheters should be removed as soon as possible when not needed but can be used up to 14 days if managed aseptically. *(II)*

➤ **Surveillance for catheter-related infections**

- Monitor the catheter sites visually or by palpation through the intact dressing on a regular basis. The frequency of examination will depend on the clinical situation for the individual patient. If the patient has tenderness at the insertion site, fever without obvious source, or other manifestations suggesting local or bloodstream infection, the dressing should be removed to allow thorough examination of the site. *(IB)*
- Conduct surveillance for CR-BSI in ICUs and other patient populations suspected of having a high rate of CR-BSI to determine catheter-specific bloodstream infection rates, to monitor

trends in those rates, and to assist in identifying lapses in infection control practices. *(IA)*

- Express ICU data as the number of catheter-associated BSIs per 1000 catheter days to facilitate comparisons with national data in comparable patient populations and healthcare settings. *(IB)*
- Investigate events leading to serious, unexpected, life-threatening, or fatal outcomes. This includes any process variation for which a recurrence would carry a significant chance of a serious adverse outcome. *(IC)*
- Encourage patients to report any changes in their catheter site or any new discomfort to their healthcare provider. *(II)*
- Record the operator, date and time of catheter insertion and removal, and dressing changes in a standardized location. *(II)*
- Do not routinely culture catheter tips. *(IA)*

References/Resources

- Association for Professionals in Infection Control and Epidemiology. APIC Text of Infection Control and Epidemiology. 2000, chapter 30 pp.1-8.
- Centers for Disease Control and Prevention, Healthcare Infection Control Practices Advisory Committee (HICPAC). Draft Guideline for the Prevention of Intravascular Catheter-Related Infections, August 2001. Federal Register.
- Henderson DK. Bacteremia due to percutaneous intravascular devices. In: Mandell GL, Bennett JE, Dolin R, Eds. Principles and practice of infectious diseases. New York: Churchill Livingstone; 1995. p 2587–2599.
- Maki DG, Mermel LA. Infections due to infusion therapy. In: Bennett J, Brachman P, Eds. Hospital Infections.4th ed. Philadelphia, PA: Lippincott-Raven; 1998:689–724.

- Pearson ML, the Hospital Infection Control Practices Advisory Committee. Guidelines for prevention of intravascular device-related infections. Infect Control Hosp Epidemiol 1996; 17:438–473.
- Wilson J. Infection control in clinical practice. London: Bailliere Tindall; 1995. p 202–214.

Section IV

SPECIALIZED POPULATIONS AND SETTINGS

Adult Intensive Care Units

Overview

- It is estimated that only 5–10% of all hospital beds are in Intensive Care Units (ICUs), however infections in this population account for over 20% of all healthcare associated infections. Additionally, stable patients with long-term needs for demanding care are being treated in subacute or intermediate care facilities. Infections may increase a patient's length of stay, cause additional morbidity/mortality, and consume resources.

Purpose

- Numerous factors contribute to increased risk of infection in the ICU setting. Understanding these factors and basic preventative strategies will assist ICPs in reducing their impact, thus minimizing their effect.

Risk Factors

- Impaired host defenses – age extremes, nutritional status, genetic/acquired altered immune response.
- Severity of illness - underlying diseases including diabetes, cancer, renal failure, neutropenia, liver failure/cirrhosis, altered consciousness, devitalized tissue.
- Length of stay in ICU exceeding 48 hours.
- Therapeutic interventions - bypass natural defenses of skin/mucus membranes.
- Vascular devices: hemodialysis, Swan-Ganz, single or multi-lumen central venous, peripheral "IV," arterial lines, "permanent" access.

- All-purpose multi-lumen central venous catheters pose greater risk of infection than short-term peripheral devices.
- Long-term or permanent-access devices (e.g., Hickman, Broviac, Infusaport) are associated with lesser risk.
- Epidural catheters – longer duration increases risk of infection/abscess.

➤ Urinary catheters - indwelling catheters provide channel for organisms to access bladder; duration increases risk of infection.

➤ Surgical drains - retrograde migration of skin flora or infusion with extrinsic pathogens can result in deep/organ space infection.

➤ Oral/nasal endotracheal tube - organisms readily bypass normal clearance mechanisms; bacterial adherence and changes in oropharyngeal flora may be exacerbated by artificial airway.

➤ Gastric tubes - nasogastric tubes contribute to sinusitis; gastrostomy tubes can become colonized with organisms (e.g., MRSA) and enhance likelihood of soft tissue infection.

➤ Ventriculostomy and intracranial pressure monitoring devices.

➤ Injured tissue, perfusion deficits, and infection cause fever and tachycardia through mechanisms mediated by hormones, cytokines, and bacterial products such as endotoxins.

➤ Colonization with microorganisms.

➤ Factors listed above predispose ICU patients to colonization with "hospital organisms."

- Endogenous flora are rapidly altered in patients treated in ICU settings.
- Organisms adhere to epithelial/mucosal cells and/or invasive devices proliferate and persist at the site of attachment; biofilm/slime formation may contribute to persistence.

- Colonization is often a prerequisite for most nosocomial infections (exceptions might include infusion with contaminated blood, medication, or intravenous fluids).
- Patients highly colonized with hospital organisms become *the* major reservoir of pathogens, thereby increasing the risk of transmission to others.

➤ Medications

- Use of multiple antibiotics.
- Use of stomach acid reducing agents (e.g., H2 blockers, antacids).
- Steroids/immunosuppressants.

➤ Other factors

- Poor handwashing compliance and inconsistent use of PPE (i.e., Standard Precautions).
- Lack of aseptic technique.
- Improperly cleaned, disinfected. or sterilized medical equipment including fiberoptic bronchoscopes and endoscopes, transducers for hemodynamic monitoring, urine collection system, devices to measure urine pH, dialysis machines, respiratory spirometry devices, and suction containers.
- Intrinsically or extrinsically contaminated blood, intravenous fluids, medications, and flush solutions.
- Contaminated environmental surfaces.
- Features of the room/unit that enhance potential for contamination: splash from sink onto items, poor storage design for supplies, lack of work surfaces, mixing soiled and clean items, work flow, location of handwashing stations, renovation, or construction activities.
- Staffing patterns and skills.

Strategies for Prevention and Control

- Patient Assessment
  - Scoring models to predict mortality, severity of illness, and risks of various outcomes may be useful in identifying patients at high risk of infections thus providing guidance for implementation of preventative strategies.
  - Scoring models may be useful for risk stratification and comparison of like populations.
  - Several scoring models are:

    Acute Physiology and Chronic Health Evaluation (APACHE II) - physiologic score with predictive value for mortality.

    Simplified Acute Physiology Score II - score based on the number of acute organ system failures.

    Injury Severity Score (ISS) - major anatomic scoring system for trauma patients; useful in trauma research and patient comparisons in trauma systems.

    Therapeutic Intervention Scoring System - useful as predictor for nosocomial infection when the length of stay is more than seven days.
- Refer to Sections 2 and 3 for General Prevention and Control Measures (e.g., handwashing and hand hygiene, Standard Precautions, aseptic technique, care of invasive devices, optimal cleaning, disinfection, and sterilization).
- Refer to Section 5 for Employee Health considerations.
- Refer to Section 2 - Environmental Maintenance and Construction/Renovation.
- Setting Specific Practices
  - Appropriate levels of skilled nursing personnel can affect patient outcomes; in general, the higher the RN skills mix, the lower the incidence of adverse occurrences.

- The addition of a medical intensivist in an ICU has been shown to improve clinical and educational outcomes, which may include reducing nosocomial infections.
- ICU length of stay should be kept as short as possible; length of stay is a strong predictor of ICU-related infections.
- Up-to-date, uncomplicated clinical practice guidelines/pathways, supported by evidence-based recommendations, should be used to help prevent/reduce infections and other outcomes.
- Nutritional status of ICU patients should be optimized to increase physical strength and immune defenses and to enhance recovery. Under-nutrition is associated with respiratory muscle weakness and may contribute to ventilatory dependency.
- Adopt use of improved technology/devices to reduce trauma.
- Less invasive techniques such as noninvasive ventilatory support have potential to reduce infection risks.
- Minimally invasive surgical techniques, diagnostic imaging, and interventional techniques utilizing radiographic support can diagnose/treat conditions without creating large portals of entry.
- Endotracheal tubes that allow suctioning of subglottic secretions may reduce risk of ventilator-associated pneumonia.
- Antiseptic- or antibiotic-coated invasive devices (e.g., vascular access devices and indwelling urinary catheters) may reduce infection.

➤ IC Program

- A successful infection control program requires interdisciplinary involvement including ICP, nursing, physicians, respiratory care, pharmacy, and other support functions.
- The ICP, in collaboration with ICU staff, should develop setting specific polices and procedures and a system for monitoring compliance with policies and procedures.

- Surveillance

  Concurrent surveillance plays an important role in identifying clusters and trends to help prevent outbreaks; program should use standard definitions and device days (Refer to Section 1).

  Device related infection surveillance is of particular importance in ICU settings.

- Education

  Caregivers should be provided age/condition specific education regarding infection risks and strategies to reduce risks and prevent infection.

  Caregivers should be able to demonstrate understanding and skills.

References/Resources

- Association for Professionals in Infection Control and Epidemiology. APIC Text of Infection Control and Epidemiology. 2000, chapter 45 pp.1-6.
- Atkinson S, Sieffert E, Bihari D, et al. A prospective, randomized, double blind, controlled clinical trial of enteral immunonutrition in the critically ill. Crit Care Med 1998; 26:1164-72.
- Beale RJ, Bryg DF, Bihari DJ, et al. Immunonutrition in the critically ill: A systematic review of clinical outcome. *Crit Care Med* 1999; 27:2799-2805.
- Blegan MA, Good CJ, Reed L. Nurse staffing and patient outcomes. *Nurs Res* 1998; 47:43–50.
- Carlson RW, Weiland DE, Srivathsan K. Does a full time 24-hour intensivist improve care and efficiency? *Crit Care Clin* 1996; 12:525–551.

- Fridkin SK, Welbel SF, Weinstein RA. Nosocomial infections. Infect Dis Clin North Am. 1997; 2:479–496.
- Gadek JE, Demichele SJ, Karlstad MD, et al. Effect of enteral feeding with eicosapentaenooic acid, gamma-linolenic acid, and antioxidants in patients with acute respiratory distress syndrome. Crit Care Med 1999; 27-1409-20.
- Galban C, Montejo JC, Mesejo A, et al. An immune-enhancing enteral diet reduces mortality rate and episodes of bacteremia in septic intensive care unit patients. Crit Care Med 2000; 28-643-48.
- Gaynes RP. Surveillance of nosocomial infections: A fundamental ingredient for quality. Infect Control Hosp Epidemiol 1997; 18:475–478
- Gerou E, Stephan F, and Novara A, et al. Risk factors and outcome of nosocomial infections: results of a matched case-control study of ICU patients. Am J Respir Crit Care Med 1998; 157:1151–1158
- Heyland DK, Cook DJ, Guyatt GH. Does the formulation of enteral feeding products influence infectious morbidity and mortality rates in the critically ill patient? A critical review of the evidence. Crit Care Med 1994; 22:1192 - 1202.
- Heys SD, Walker LG, Smith I, et al. Enteral nutritional supplementation with key nutrients in patients with critical illness and cancer. Ann Surg 1999; 229:467-77.
- Hurr H, Hawley HB, Czachor JS, et al. APACHE II and ISS scores as predictors of nosocomial infections in trauma patients. Am J Infect Control 1999; 27:79–83
- Iskibaski N, Plank LD, Kinya S, et al. Optimal protein requirements during the first 2 weeks after the onset of critical illness. Crit Care Med 1998; 26:1529–1535

- Kollef MH. The prevention of ventilator-associated pneumonia. NEngl J Med 1999; 340:627–633
- Shojania KG, Duncan BW, McDonald KM, et al., Eds. Making Healthcare safer: a critical analysis of patient safety practices. AHRQ Publication No. 01-E058, Rockville, MD: Agency for Healthcare Research and Quality. July 2001.

Ambulatory Care Settings

Overview

- An ambulatory care practice setting may be defined as one that provides direct health or wellness care services to patients or clients who do not remain overnight. Many patients who were once treated only in inpatient hospital settings are now treated in ambulatory care settings. The term ambulatory care may be misleading by suggesting that patients are non-acute, primarily well patients. In reality, ambulatory care settings serve a wide range of patients and provide all types of services including invasive and advanced technological procedures.
- Examples of settings include medical offices and clinics, family practice and primary care clinics, specialty clinics, mental health clinics, dental offices, emergency medical services, emergent and urgent care centers, ambulatory surgery centers, correctional facility clinics, diagnostic treatment centers, student health clinics, Indian health clinics and military clinics.
- The basic principles of communicable disease transmission and prevention are the same in ambulatory care settings as in traditional hospital settings. Prevention strategies vary somewhat based upon the patient population served and the specific setting. However, strategies may differ in ambulatory care settings, and further research should concentrate in efficacy and efficiency of recommendations in alternate settings.
- Commonly there is not a person dedicated to infection control in ambulatory settings. It is suggested that each site appoint and Infection Control Liaison (ICL) to act as the infection control advocate for the site.

Purpose

- Many of the elements are required by regulatory or accrediting bodies and/or are considered best practice by experts in Infection Control. They are based on a thorough review of current literature and community, regulatory, and accreditation standards. However, since research efforts have focused primarily on acute care facilities, most of the References/Resources and guidelines cited have been written from this perspective and may be adapted for the ambulatory setting.

Risk Factors

- Patients of higher acuity are being treated in ambulatory care settings due to a shift in care delivery from acute inpatient settings to alternative settings including ambulatory care.
- Invasive procedures and advanced technologies are being used with increasing frequency in ambulatory care settings.
- Mobility of potentially communicable patients throughout the setting.
- Waiting rooms.

Strategies for Prevention

- Patient assessment and triage
  - In all ambulatory care settings, patients are often clustered in common waiting areas. The range of potentially transmissible infections depends on the population served (the case mix) and the type of services offered. Patients may be at increased risk for droplet-borne or airborne diseases in these settings. Patients may also transmit undiagnosed diseases when first presenting to ambulatory care settings. Transmission is enhanced by close quarters in waiting areas and may be enhanced by communal toys

and movement of patients between waiting areas, exam rooms, and diagnostic areas.

- Patients should be assessed as soon as possible at each visit for signs and symptoms of potentially communicable illnesses including productive cough, diarrhea, undiagnosed rash, bleeding, or wound or eye drainage.

  Patients with these conditions should be placed in a separate exam room as soon as possible.

  Patients with coughs or respiratory symptoms should be provided with tissues and/or surgical masks and instructed to cover coughs and sneezes with a tissue, proper disposal of tissues, and handwashing. Symptom-based evaluation can allow appropriate triage and application of precautions prior to full diagnostic work-up.

  Patients with known disease or a high index of suspicion for tuberculosis (TB), chickenpox, measles, mumps, rubella, or bacterial meningitis should wear a surgical mask and be placed in a separate room with the door closed and an appropriate sign to inform staff of necessary precautions.

  In the case of suspected TB, it may be prudent to allow the room to ventilate for some time before using again. Ideally, a room with negative pressure and dedicated ventilation to outdoors or a high efficiency particulate air filtration (HEPA) unit should be used. Check with local health department for recommendations and requirements.

- Patients should be assessed for sensitivities to latex, antiseptic agents such as iodine, antibiotics, and other medications.

➤ Refer to Sections 2 and 3 for General Prevention and Control Measures (e.g., handwashing and hand hygiene, Standard Precautions, aseptic technique, care of invasive devices, optimal cleaning, disinfection, and sterilization).

- Refer to Section 5 for Employee Health considerations.
- Refer to Section 2 - Environmental Maintenance and Construction/Renovation.
- Setting specific considerations
  - Cleaning, disinfection, and sterilization practices in ambulatory care settings.

    The basic principles of cleaning, disinfection, and sterilization are the same in ambulatory care as in all other delivery settings. (Refer to Section 2 - Disinfection and Sterilization)

    Endoscopic procedures are frequently performed in ambulatory care settings and have been associated with clusters and outbreaks in ambulatory settings. (Refer to Section 2 - Disinfection and Sterilization)

    Special ambulatory care settings including dental clinics, rehabilitation centers, and dialysis centers have specific cleaning and reprocessing challenges.

    In ambulatory care settings, staff often have not received adequate training to perform appropriate reprocessing processes. A competency assessment and training procedure should be developed and implemented for personnel responsible for reprocessing.

    Consideration may be given to replacing reusable items with disposable when possible or outsourcing reprocessing.
  - Environment of Care

    A facility assessment should be performed to identify adequate workflow space, traffic flow, ventilation, temperature, and humidity for reprocessing activities, and the availability of protective equipment (i.e., latex and non-latex gloves, masks, gowns, etc.) When there are not adequate facilities for reprocessing on site, consideration should be given to the use of disposables and outsourcing to a facility having appropriate resources.

A policy outlining environment of care standards and the responsibilities of housekeeping/maintenance personnel and clinic staff should be established. There should be a designated point person or building manager assigned to oversee the environment of care.

All horizontal surfaces in clinics (including exam tables and counters) should be cleaned with an infection control approved hospital grade cleaner/disinfectant between patients. An acceptable alternative is to use disposable paper covering for each patient. Surfaces must be cleaned and disinfected when the paper covering is torn, wet, or visibly altered.

The organization should implement an integrated pest management plan (IPM) aligned with local, state, and federal requirements. The plan should address prevention and control factors for insects and vermin. This is frequently a contracted service and oversight may be a collaborative effort between the ICP/ICL and building manager.

Housekeeping and maintenance may be contracted services in ambulatory care settings. The contracts between the vendor and the facility should outline the infection control responsibilities of the vendor and clearly identify employer responsibility for employee health requirements and mandatory training requirements.

- Dietary Services

  Dietary services policies should include policies and procedures for kitchen sanitation, food handling and storage, microwave/toaster cleaning, and vending machine sanitation and maintenance.

  There should be a setting-specific procedure and assignment to monitor temperatures and clean refrigerators.

Dietary services are frequently contracted services in ambulatory care settings. The contracts between the vendor and the facility should outline the infection control responsibilities of the vendor and clearly identify employer responsibility for employee health requirements and mandatory training requirements.

- Laundry Services

  Laundry services are often minimal in ambulatory care settings. Often disposable exam gowns and table covers are used. Otherwise, policies and procedures addressing the handling, processing and storage of clean and dirty linen should be established. (Refer to Section 2 - Laundry Handling)

  Clean and dirty linen should always be stored separately to avoid recontamination of clean linen.

- Pharmacy Services

  Medications used externally or internally must be stored separately in designated and labeled areas.

  Multidose vials should be labeled.

  Aseptic technique should be used when withdrawing solution from the vial.

  Multidose vials should be discarded when empty, when suspected or known contamination has occurred, or when the manufacturer's expiration date has been reached. Refer to manufacturer's guidelines for each product.

  If sample medications are provided to patients, a tracking log should be implemented in the event a recall is required.

  Medication Refrigerators

    There should be a setting-specific procedure and assignment to monitor temperatures and clean refrigerators and freezers. In areas where refrigerators/freezers are not used on a daily basis, there should be a method to ensure temperature stability. This may include sophisticated methods such as audible alarms or a simple method such as placing a penny on top of a frozen cup of water. If the penny sinks, there has been a failure in temperature maintenance.

Refrigerated storage should be dedicated based on type of item to be stored (e.g. separate medications, food, clinical specimens).

Some items such as Varicella vaccines may require freezer storage and necessitate the purchase of additional equipment in the ambulatory care setting.

Manufacturer labels should be reviewed for storage requirements for all medications.

- Pathology Services

  Pathology services may be a combination of contracted and onsite specimen collection and testing.

  Laboratory tests performed outside of an accredited laboratory must be in compliance with the Clinical Laboratory Improvement Amendments of 1988 (CLIA '88) as well as any local or state requirements.

  Specimen collection (e.g., venipuncture, urine, and swab specimens) and transport must be in compliance with OSHA Bloodborne Pathogens Final Rule and applicable state regulations.

  Specimen refrigerators must be labeled with the Biohazard Symbol as required by OSHA.

  Only specimens may be stored in these refrigerators.

  There should be a setting-specific procedure and assignment to monitor temperatures and clean refrigerators on a routine basis.

➤ IC Program

- Many other functions interface with infection control issues in the ambulatory care setting. Examples of functions include but are not limited to quality improvement, customer satisfaction, safety, risk management, and staff development.

- Often the ICP/ICL may be assigned more than one of these functions. It is beneficial to establish an ongoing communication link and collaboration between these areas and others in order to maximize resources and impact change more effectively and efficiently.
- The ICP/ICL should actively participate in patient/family and caregiver education. Individual instruction, pamphlets, videotapes, leaflets, newsletter, bulletin boards, and Web sites may be used to instruct patients/families and caregivers on such topics as handwashing, immunizations, reporting communicable illnesses, disposal of sharps used in the home, food safety, signs and symptoms of infection, and disease specific information.

➤ Education

- Patients and caregivers should be provided with written and verbal instructions that outline general infection control and hygiene principles and specific precautions to take while performing dressing change, intravenous (IV) therapy, or other treatments in the home.
- Such instructions should include:

  The most common ways organisms can be spread (e.g., contact with body fluids, open skin contact touching contaminated objects, use of needles and other sharps, sneezing, and coughing).

References/Resources

➤ Committee on Infectious Diseases and Committee on Practice and Ambulatory Medicine. Infection Control in Physicians' Offices (RE9962). American Academy of Pediatrics-Pediatrics 105(6): 1361-1369, 2000.

- Craven PC: Spread of infection in the infectious diseases office, Infect Dis Clin Pract 3(1): 67-69, and 1994.
- Drummond DC, Skidmore AG: Sterilization and disinfection in the physician's office, Can Med Assoc J 145(8): 937-942, 1991.
- Goodman RA, Solomon SL: Transmission of infectious diseases in outpatient healthcare settings, JAMA 265(18): 2377-2380, 1991.
- Haim L, Booth JH, and Greaney K: Recommendations for optimizing an infection control practitioner's effectiveness in an ambulatory care setting, JHQ 16(2): 31-34, 1994.
- Herwaldt LA et al. Infection control in the outpatient setting. Infection Control and Hospital Epidemiology, 1998, 19(1): 41-74.
- Hurst J, Nickel K, and Hilborne LH: Are physicians' office laboratory results of comparable quality to those produced in other laboratory settings? JAMA, 279:468-71, 1998.
- Hurt N: The role of the infection control nurse in quality management in the ambulatory care setting, JHQ 15(3): 43-44, 1993.
- Ilott S: Infection control in general practice, Nurs Standard 5(6): 25-28, 1990.
- Joint Commission on Accreditation of Healthcare Organizations: Accreditation manual for ambulatory healthcare, (1).Standards, Oakbrook Terrace, Ill, current edition.
- Joint Commission on Accreditation of Healthcare Organizations: Accreditation Manual for Ambulatory Healthcare, volume 2. Scoring guidelines, Oakbrook Terrace, Ill, current edition.
- Kaczmarek RG, Moore RM, and McCrohan J et al: Multi-state investigation of the actual disinfection/sterilization of endoscopes in healthcare facilities, Am J Med 92:257-260, 1992.
- Lee TB: Surveillance in acute care and non-acute care settings: Current issues and concepts. Am J Infection Control, 1997, 25:121-124.

- Manian F, Meyer L: Comprehensive surveillance of surgical wound infections in outpatient and inpatient surgery, Infect Control Hosp Epidemiol 11(10): 515-520, 1990.
- Manian FA and Meyer L. Adjunctive use of monthly physicians questionnaires for surveillance of surgical site infections after hospital discharge and in ambulatory surgical patients: report of a seven year experience. Am J Infect Control, 1997, 25: 390-394.
- Manian FA, Meyer L: Comparison of patient telephone survey with traditional surveillance and monthly physician questionnaires in monitoring surgical wound infections, Infect Control Hosp Epidemiol 14(4): 216-218, 1993.
- Nafziger DA et al. Infection Control in Ambulatory Care in: Infectious Disease Clinics of North America, Rutala and Weber, ed. 1997, 279-297.
- Rice R, Jorden JU: Implementing an infection control program for the community-based healthcare facility, JONA 22(5): 18-21, 1992.
- Rogers WO, Waites KB and Friedberg RC: Microbiology testing and the pediatrician's office. Pediatr Infect Dis, 16:339-45, 1997.
- Stone R: The employee-safety and infection-control manual: guidelines for the ambulatory healthcare center, Nurse Practitioner 16(4): 58-63, 1991.
- Zalabak WD Jr: Developing a formal policy for the management of blood and body fluids in an outpatient setting, College Rev 7(1): 51-58, 1990.
- Zoutman D, Pearce P, and McKenzie M et al: Surgical wound infections occurring in day surgery patients, Am J Infect Control 1990 18(4): 277-282,1990.

Behavioral Health Settings

Overview

- Behavioral health (BH) treatment may be offered in outpatient, inpatient, or residential care facilities (e.g., group homes). Invasive procedures are rare in BH unless the client is being treated concomitantly for acute or chronic physiological conditions. Risk for infection is primarily related to behavioral factors.

Purpose

- Provide principles, practices, and control methods to reduce infection and related safety risks in the behavioral health setting.

Risk Factors

- Pathophysiology of mental illness may affect dependability of client as reliable historian.
- Behavior may create infection risks or harm to self or others.
  - Risk for spitting at or biting others.
  - Encopresis – unintentional defecation.
  - Enuresis – unintentional urination.
  - Pica – ingestion of non-food substances.
- During therapy course, clients may be sexually active while still infectious; treatment may be incomplete or an STD is unsuspected.
- Inadequate hygiene, nutrition, hydration, and medications may increase risk of infection.
- Mental illness and/or effects of psychotropic drugs or chemical dependency may mask disease thus delay diagnosis and treatment.

- Delivery of care is very different than acute care facilities
  - The patient/client is usually responsible for his/her own personal care.
  - Client activities may include laundry and food preparation.
  - Clients participate and interact with each other.
  - Care delivery may take place across outpatient, inpatient, and residential settings.
- Frequently physical facility design does not meet the same standards (e.g., air handling, traffic control, etc.) as acute care facilities.

Strategies for Prevention

- Patient/client assessment and triage is critical in the behavioral health setting.
- Patients should be evaluated for signs and symptoms of communicable conditions (e.g., rash, diarrhea, eye drainage, productive cough).
  - Provide box of tissues and waste bag.
  - Instruct to cover coughs and sneezes.
  - Clients with signs/symptoms should undergo treatment (e.g., ectoparasites – scabies or lice, diarrhea – bacterial, viral, parasitic, or Conjunctivitis- bacterial or viral).
  - For known disease or a high index of suspicion of chicken pox, measles, mumps, rubella, or tuberculosis (TB).
  - Consider therapy delay until the condition is treated or resolved.
  - Obtain medical clearance post-treatment.
- Refer to Sections 2 and 3 for General Prevention and Control Measures (e.g., handwashing and hand hygiene, Standard Precautions, aseptic technique, care of invasive devices, optimal cleaning, disinfection, and sterilization).

- Refer to Section 5 for Employee Health considerations.
- Refer to Section 2 - Environmental Maintenance and Construction/Renovation.
- Setting Specific Measures
  - Mental/physical impairments may require additional precautions including behavior modification techniques, close observation, etc.
  - Patients/clients with a known or suspected communicable diseases should be moved to a safe holding area and appropriate precautions taken (e.g., mask patient) until they can be transferred to a facility that is able to accommodate special needs such as negative pressure rooms.
- IC Program Aspects in BH
  - Federal, state, local regulations and accreditation agencies govern BH facilities.
  - Program administration and the ICP

    Interdisciplinary involvement in the IC program including nursing, physicians, therapists, and other support personnel.

    The ICP should have a working knowledge of epidemiology, microbiology, infection transmission, and patient care practices.

    Knowledge and experience in education and problem solving are desired.

    The services offered by the facility, duration of stay, and intensity of staff-client contact influence IC program design and implementation.
  - Surveillance

    Short-term admission and outpatient care may make infection diagnosis and infection rates impractical to calculate.

    Conversely, admissions of several weeks or more facilitate infection diagnosis and IC interventions; focus surveillance on incidence, prevalence, and trends.

Communicable disease reporting is an important aspect of behavioral health IC programs.

Nosocomial infections may be identified as they relate to care delivery or as they relate to patient behavior, e.g., a milieu infection is one that occurs in client populations after admission as a result of patient behavior.

Infections should be analyzed as rates versus raw numbers. Numerators represent the number of infections in a specific category and denominators represent days or persons at risk for developing the infection in each category.

Surveillance should be accompanied by analysis to identify improvement opportunities; action plans to address these opportunities, and evaluation of improvement efforts.

- Education
  - Caregivers should be provided age/condition specific education regarding infection risks and strategies to reduce risks and prevent infection.
  - Caregivers should be able to demonstrate understanding and skills.

References/Resources

- Association for Professionals in Infection Control and Epidemiology. APIC Text of Infection Control and Epidemiology. 2000, chapter 47, 1 - 10.
- Centers for Disease Control and Prevention, Healthcare Infection Control Practices Advisory Committee (HICPAC). Draft Guideline for Environmental Infection Control in Healthcare Facilities, 2001. 2001, Federal.

Correctional Settings

Overview

- The correctional setting is composed of a wide range of penal institutions: jails, state and federal prisons, and juvenile detention centers. Prison healthcare provides a window of opportunity for inmates to receive medical care and risk reduction information that they might not otherwise be able to obtain.
- Effective interventions help cultivate close collaboration between community health agencies and correctional healthcare services. These activities include: discharge planning with linkage to community agencies for follow up, educational programs, policy and procedure development, surveillance and screening activities, and assistance with prophylaxis, treatment, and outbreaks of communicable disease.

Purpose

- Provide principles, practices, and control methods to reduce infection and related safety risks in this unique and varied healthcare setting with the goal of promoting wellness and positive health behaviors.

Risk Factors

- In these settings, the IC program should address crowded institutions, high-risk populations, frequent inmate movement, and an environment that is primarily correctional, not medical, in intent.
- Demographics may be disproportionately poor, male, uneducated, medically underserved, and largely from minority groups.

Furthermore, over 1/3 of all inmates report some physical or mental disability.

- There is an increased prevalence of high-risk related and sex-related behaviors in this population, including needle sharing for drug injection and history of multiple sexual partners, may place inmates at a high risk for HIV and hepatitis B, C, and D.

Strategies for Prevention

- Inmate assessment
  - Visual inspection of hair and skin - scabies, pediculosis, rashes, and skin lesions.
  - STD screen - include clinical and laboratory examination for syphilis, gonorrhea, chlamydia, other inflammatory/ulcerative disease, and a Papanicolaou test for women.
  - TB - include Mantoux PPD skin test and symptoms check; chest radiograph for those who are skin test positive or symptomatic.
  - Determination of presence of risk factors for HIV infection: substance abuse, injection behaviors including tattooing and drug administration, and multiple sexual partners.
  - Dental screening - visual inspection of the oral cavity, teeth, and gums, noting the presence of any gross abnormalities or oral lesions; many infections and communicable diseases have oral manifestations, including candidiasis, syphilis chancre, Kaposi's sarcoma, herpes, and gonococcal pharyngitis.
- Refer to Sections 2 and 3 for General Prevention and Control Measures (e.g., handwashing and hand hygiene, Standard Precautions, aseptic technique, care of invasive devices, optimal cleaning, disinfection, and sterilization).
- Refer to Section 5 for Employee Health considerations.

- ➤ Refer to Section 2 - Environmental Maintenance and Construction/Renovation.
- ➤ Setting specific measures
  - Bloodborne Pathogens/Standard Precautions (SP) - the medical and non-medical staff should be well educated in SP; it should be practiced by all, including inmates assigned to handle contaminated laundry and those assigned housekeeping duties in medical areas who may have exposure to blood and OPIM. Ensure that appropriate PPE is immediately available for use where it may be needed.

    Hepatitis B vaccine should be offered to all medical and non-medical staff who are at risk of occupational exposure, including inmate workers.

    CDC recommends pre-exposure vaccination for inmates in long-term correctional facilities; NCCHC recommends a hepatitis B vaccination program for all inmates.

    Postexposure protocols for significant exposure to blood/body fluid in compliance with local and state laws regarding the testing of source blood and patient confidentiality; should address potential exposure to hepatitis B and C as well as HIV; it may require modification for inmate-inmate, staff-inmate, or staff-staff exposures.

    Safe handling and disposal of sharp instruments should consider security concerns and current regulations/guidelines.

    HIV counseling and testing services to provide early identification, treatment for HIV infection and appropriate education; HIV testing should be in compliance with state and local laws and with the informed consent, protection of confidentiality, notification process for partners, and disclosure protocol.

Integration of HIV-infected inmates, if their physical condition permits, into the general population generally provides them with equal access to all programs available to non-infected inmates; the NCCHC opposes segregated housing for asymptomatic HIV-positive inmates.

Medical conditions related to HIV infection (e.g., dementia, weakness, and chronic diarrhea) may require special housing considerations as recommended by the medical staff.

Harm reduction - although prisons have zero tolerance for sex and drugs, high-risk behaviors may occur; NCCHC supports a public health perspective by proposing a statement on HIV by making "available to inmates whatever appropriate protective devices can reduce the risk of contagion."

- Tuberculosis (TB)

  Policy/procedures should be developed including a TB Exposure Control Plan and Respirator Protection Program per regulations (OSHA) and guidelines (CDC and NIOSH).

  Those infected with HIV and TB have a 30- to 40-fold increased risk of progression from infection to disease, therefore, TB may be of concern, dependent upon demographics and location of the correctional facility.

  Screening - CDC has published guidelines for TB screening; although CDC has recommended mandatory testing program in correctional settings, recent court decisions have been split regarding inmates' refusing to be tested voluntarily or religious grounds.

  Surveillance for TB should be established, as applicable (e.g., statistics infection rate in new admits, skin test conversion rates of inmates and staff, active TB disease).

Symptomatic individuals should be tested for confirmation of disease; appropriate airborne isolation and respirators should be provided.

Chemoprophylaxis or preventive therapy is recommended for those identified with TB infection and for anergic, HIV-infected individuals who have other risk factors for TB; directly observed therapy (DOT) is preferred method of administration.

Chemotherapy for inmates with active TB disease chemotherapy should be DOT; adherence to recommendations for four-drug therapy will help prevent drug-resistant strains; follow recommendations for related testing, e.g., liver function.

Contact investigation should be performed for staff and inmates who had unprotected exposure to a person with active TB for testing/evaluation.

Inmates and medical/non-medical staff should receive accurate information on transmission, TB infection vs. disease, and symptoms of disease that is appropriate in content to each group.

There should be active collaboration with public health agencies for all aspects of the TB control program including discharged inmates with infection or disease requiring follow-up post release.

- Sexually transmitted diseases (STDs)

  Previous studies of incarcerated populations have reported high rates of STDs.

  Based upon setting, protocol to screen new admissions for STDs should be established.

  STD screen should include syphilis, gonorrhea, and chlamydia, a Papanicolaou test for women, and screening for any additional diseases to which the specific population is known to be at high risk.

Rapid screening and treatment protocols have been developed and can be effectively implemented in some correctional facilities.

STD infection in the presence of concurrent HIV may have altered manifestations and treatment requirements.

Appropriate education should be provided to inmates (e.g., safe sex practices and reproductive health).

- Vaccine preventable diseases

  Recommendations for the routine immunization of healthy and immunocompromised adults by the Advisory Committee on Immunization Practices (ACIP) should be followed.

  Influenza vaccine should be offered annually to high-risk inmates, staff, and other inmates.

  Pneumococcal vaccine should be given once to those for whom it is medically indicated; due to varied antibody response to pneumococcal disease and other vaccine preventable infections in those with symptomatic HIV infection, immunizations should be offered to HIV-infected inmates early in the course of their disease.

  Inmates may not have received the recommended childhood immunizations; outbreaks of vaccine preventable diseases may occur in this setting.

    Each correctional system should develop policies and procedures for mumps, rubella, measles, and varicella for medical/non-medical staff and for inmates.

    In the event of an exposure to or outbreak of measles, rubella, or mumps, the responsible local or state health department may place quarantine on the facility.

- Enteric diseases

  Infections of the gastrointestinal (GI) tract can occur; foodborne illness outbreaks and opportunistic infections in relation to HIV infection have been reported in correctional settings.

  Inmates with a diarrhea-associated illness may require additional precautions if unable or unwilling to maintain good hygiene; provide a single room with dedicated handwashing and toilet facilities.

  Contaminated laundry should be handled using Standard Precautions, regardless of suspected presence of any infection.

  Foodborne illness outbreaks

    A foodborne outbreak is usually recognized by the abrupt occurrence of illness associated with nausea, vomiting, and/or diarrhea in a group within a short time after eating.

    Prompt evaluation of stool and suspected foods is essential.

    Local or state health departments should be notified of the outbreak; they can provide guidance or personnel, or both to assist in an investigation.

    Appropriate food preparation and sanitation practices are necessary for prevention of foodborne illness.

    Correctional institutions may have different protocols for inmate food-handler clearance; refer to local/state regulations.

    Infection with a bloodborne pathogen or TB infection is not a reason to exclude an inmate from kitchen work.

    Inmate food-handlers should receive education on basic food sanitation and safety.

    Food handling practices including sanitation and storage should be followed (refer to 3.5) to prevent of foodborne illness.

- Ectoparasite control

  Inmates should be screened at admission for the presence of scabies and pediculosis.

  Newly admitted, infested inmates should be kept separate until 24 hours after appropriate treatment.

  If a single case is identified in a housing area, health staff should offer to screen roommates.

  If more cases are identified, all roommates should be screened for infestation.

  In a widespread outbreak, treatment of all roommates may be considered; screening of exposed staff should be provided.

  In an outbreak situation, the ICP should attempt to identify and eliminate the source and determine the pathways of transmission.

- Fungal infections

  Fungal infections (e.g., body and feet) can be a pervasive in the correctional setting.

  A fungicidal agent should routinely be used to clean shower stalls, bathroom floors, gymnasium floors, and benches.

  Shower slippers should be available to inmates.

  If prison farm workers are affected, the farm animals should be examined and treated; farmers suggest that keeping farm fences freshly painted can help prevent reinfection of the animals.

- Meningitis

  Fear and panic can occur amongst inmates and personnel in the event of a single meningitis case.

  Neisseria meningitidis, the causative organism of meningococcal meningitis, may have a healthy carrier prevalence of 25% in these populations.

If a case of meningococcal meningitis is diagnosed in the correctional setting, close contacts of the patient should be identified and observed for early signs of illness.

Chemoprophylaxis should be offered to socially intimate contacts only, such as sexual contacts or those with whom eating utensils or cigarettes are shared.

- Emerging infections - With an increase in international travel and drug trafficking, inmates may have acquired infections that are endemic in their countries of origin or travel.
- Special women's health issues

Studies have found incarcerated women to be at high risk for physical and sexual abuse, to have high rates of STD and HIV infection (outcomes of high-risk sexual behaviors), and to have a high rate of drug use.

Crisis intervention and counseling should be available for women currently or recently in an abusive relationship in order to break the cycle of abuse—drug use—high-risk sex work.

Prenatal services and parenting classes should be provided as applicable; the substance-abusing pregnant women who were fearful of punitive measures may have avoided prenatal care before incarceration.

Because of the high prevalence of risk factors associated with hepatitis B infection in this population, prenatal screening of all pregnant women for hepatitis B surface antigen should be conducted for the prevention of perinatal transmission.

If nurseries are onsite, services should be compliant with local, state, and federal regulations.

Because women in prison are subject to the same or worse overcrowded conditions as men, often have higher rates of HIV infection, and may be pregnant, communicable disease control in the female institution is more complex.

Before disease control measures are instituted, it may be necessary to verify the pregnancy status of the inmate; pregnancy test performed on the day of incarceration may not reflect an inmate's current status.

- Laundry

  Because of the likelihood of undetected infection and disease in the correctional setting, it is recommended that all laundry be handled with Standard Precautions regardless of suspected presence of any particular infection (Refer to Section 2 - Laundry Handling).

  Have a protocol for defining and handling known contaminated laundry if Standard Precautions are not used.

  Laundry bags should be clearly designated as contaminated with appropriate labels or color-coded red.

  Laundry workers should not be permitted to eat, drink, or smoke in workplace.

- Release planning should include:

  This should be initiated at the time of admission in anticipation of sudden release from facility.

  All inmates should be given information on local departments of health if any of the screening test results are positive and if further evaluation or treatment is not performed or completed while incarcerated.

  The inmate receiving treatment for an infectious disease should be given information on clinics that will be able to continue medical care after discharge.

  It is preferred that the inmate receive a specific follow-up appointment with appropriate community agencies for continued care after discharge.

Departments of health should be informed about inmates who are being discharged with communicable disease.

If it is known that an inmate who is ready for discharge is homeless, appropriate housing should be identified, if possible.

- IC Program Aspects in Correctional Settings
  - There should be a designated responsible person for infection control in large institution or system and minimally a part-time resource with infection control knowledge (e.g., medical or nursing director) in smaller facilities.
  - Written policies/procedures for screening, surveillance, and control of infectious/communicable diseases in inmates and staff; include preventive and control measures specific to the disease and appropriate treatment of the identified cases.
  - Environmental control policies/procedures for maintenance of a clean, safe, and healthy environment in compliance with state and local regulations including: medical and non-medical waste disposal, water supply, sewerage, ventilation, pest control, food handling and preparation, and laundry and housekeeping practices.
  - Written policies/procedures for compliance with regulations (e.g., OSHA) and consideration of guidelines (e.g., CDC) should be established and updated as appropriate.
  - A multidisciplinary ICC chaired by the responsible ICP should meets regularly to evaluate the policies/procedures of the IC program, evaluate surveillance outcomes and make recommendations for improvement, and address outbreaks or other urgent IC related situations.
  - Active interaction and communication with local or state departments of public health and other agencies and hospitals that may have responsibility or oversight of the correctional healthcare is recommended.

- Accreditation by the National Commission on Correctional Healthcare (NCCHC), the only national accreditation program designed specifically for correctional healthcare services, may be considered.
- Surveillance

  Communicable disease reporting is an important aspect of correctional setting IC programs.

  Nosocomial infections may be identified as they relate to care delivery or as they relate to patient behavior, e.g., a milieu infection is one that occurs in client populations after admission as a result of patient behavior.

  Infections should be analyzed as rates versus raw numbers. Numerators represent the number of infections in a specific category and denominators represent days or persons at risk for developing the infection in each category.

  Surveillance should be accompanied by analysis to identify improvement opportunities; action plans to address these opportunities, and evaluation of improvement efforts.

  Environmental surveillance

    NCCHC has set standards for environmental surveillance in the correctional setting.

    It is important for the ICP to be involved in this process, either directly with correctional staff, or by sharing surveillance reports; infection control inspections of the health-service areas should be conducted at regular intervals with prepared checklists.

    Areas to be surveyed include general housekeeping practices, proper medical supply storage, cleaning, disinfection and sterilization practices, availability of soap and paper towels for handwashing, dental clinics and instrument sterilization procedures, other operatory settings and related instrument sterilization procedures, appropriate handling and disposal of infectious waste, compliance with work practice controls (e.g., Standard Precautions), and all medical housing areas.

IC inspections in nonmedical areas may include housing areas, kitchen, other food production activities, housekeeping, laundry, beauty/barber shop, gymnasium, swimming pool, and emergency equipment.

➤ Education

- Instruction/education on hygiene should be provided to inmates and personnel.
- Handwashing is an important means of preventing the spread of infection; medical and non-medical staff and inmate workers should understand the importance of frequent and thorough handwashing and the importance of keeping their hands away from their face and mucous membranes while they are working.
- Ongoing educational programs about relevant communicable diseases should be provided for inmates and non-medical and medical staff that are appropriate to each audience: Topics should include basics of personal hygiene practices, principles of disease transmission, and harm reduction.
- Educational programs regarding infection control work practices for specific groups of workers, inmate or civilian, should be provided for: laundry, housekeeping, food services, and other areas as appropriate.
- HIV prevention education programs in correctional institutions should provide explicit information on risk reduction behaviors including needle hygiene and safer sex activities; program should be culturally and linguistically appropriate.

References/Resources

- American Public Health Association www.apha.org
- American Correctional Health Association www.corrections.com/achsa
- Association for Professionals in Infection Control and Epidemiology. APIC Text of Infection Control and Epidemiology. 2000, chapter 41, 1-9.
- Centers for Disease Control and Prevention. Assessment of sexually transmitted diseases services in city and county jails—United States, 1997. MMWR 1998; 47:429–431
- Centers for Disease Control and Prevention. Prevention and control of tuberculosis in correctional facilities: recommendations of the advisory council for the elimination of tuberculosis. MMWR 1996; 45:1–27.
- Centers for Disease Control and Prevention. Syphilis screening among women arrestees at the Cook County Jail—Chicago, 1996. MMWR 1998; 47:432–433
- Institute for Criminal Justice Healthcare Corrections Connection, Online Healthcare Network www.corrections.com/healthnet
- National Commission on Correctional Healthcare www.corrections.com/ncchc
- National Juvenile Detention Association www.corrections.com/njda/index.html
- Skolnick AA. Look behind bars for key to control of STDs. JAMA 1998;279:97–98
- Skolnick AA. Correctional and community healthcare collaborations. JAMA 1998; 279:98–99
- Steenland K, Levine AJ, Sieber K, Schulte P, Aziz D. Incidence of tuberculosis infection among New York State prison employees. Am J Pub Health 1997; 87:2012–2017.

Day Care Settings, Adult and Child

Overview

- The past several decades have seen increasing numbers of children attending childcare facilities outside of their home.
- Adult day care for the elderly, functionally disabled, and cognitively impaired has also become a necessity for caregivers.
- Day care settings can be in homes or centers caring for several children or adults.
- Infections acquired in day care settings may spread to staff, family members, and the community. Loss of work time for caregivers can have economic impact if lost time occurs due to illness of the child or adult. Children may transmit childhood illness such as chicken pox, conjunctivitis, Fifth disease, infectious diarrhea, impetigo, strep throat, or rubella. The adult participant is at increased risk for resistant strains of organisms due to history of illness. The adult also has a potential for life threatening complications when exposed to illnesses such as pneumonia, influenza, or urinary tract infections.

Purpose

- State and Federal regulations should be followed in addition to recommendations set forth by the CDC, American Public Health Association, and the Academy for Pediatrics.
- Infection Control policies/procedures, education, and monitoring should be established by each individual setting based on regulations and recommendations to reduce the risks of infection transmission.

Risk Factors

- Current health and immune status of participant and caregiver
  - Status of immunizations
  - Immature or compromised immune systems due to age, chronic illness, or lack of prior encounters with increased numbers of microorganisms
  - Incubating or acute illness
- Hygienic practices
  - Lack of handwashing by caregivers
  - Poor hygienic practices of participants (poor handwashing, "mouthing" objects) increasing risk of transmission of enteric pathogens
- Educational Level of Caregivers
  - Increased use of volunteers, students, trainees with lack of training
  - Untrained caregivers increase may lack understanding of principles and policies
- Environmental Considerations
  - Shared equipment, walkers, furniture, playpens, highchairs
  - Diapering areas, toileting facilities
- Food Preparation
  - Foodborne disease can be transmitted by improperly stored or processed food, improper sanitation, or poor hygiene habits of food preparers
  - Common eating utensils or drinking cups not properly handled or sanitized
  - Sanitation

    Sink or hand sanitizer availability

    Diapering area location

Disposal of soiled diapers/ adult briefs

Air exchange and ventilation systems

- Sharing Personal Items
  - Sharing of toys, puzzles, combs, sleeping mats, occupational therapy devices can result in transmission of microorganisms
  - Coats, sweaters, and hats stored where contact may occur can result in transmission of pediculosis or lice
- Pools and water play
  - Wading pools can become contaminated and are not intended for public use
  - Water tables used in childcare centers may become contaminated by hands

Strategies for Prevention and Control

- Assessment
  - Participants as well as caregivers should have health screenings prior to participation/employment.
  - Assessment should include immunization status of participants and caregivers. Persons not up-to-date on recommended immunization status should be referred to their physician or health department.
- Refer to Sections 3 and 4 for General Prevention and Control Measures (e.g., handwashing and hand hygiene, Standard Precautions, aseptic technique, care of invasive devices, optimal cleaning, disinfection, and sterilization).
- Refer to Sections 2 and 3 for General Prevention and Control Measures (e.g., handwashing and hand hygiene, Standard Precautions, aseptic technique, care of invasive devices, optimal cleaning, disinfection, and sterilization).
- Refer to Section 5 for Employee Health considerations.

- Refer to Section 2 - Environmental Maintenance and Construction/Renovation.
- Setting specific measures
  - Policies for participant and caregivers medical evaluation and follow up for post infectious illness should be established.
  - Policies for providing care to sick participants should be established including criteria for exclusion for communicable illnesses.
  - Hygienic practices

    Handwashing should be practiced by caregivers and participants following toileting/diapering and before food handling/preparation.

    There should be an adequate numbers of sinks at accommodating heights of children and wheelchairs.

    Soap, instant hand sanitizers, disposable tissue, and paper towels should be readily available for use by participants and caregivers.
  - Environmental considerations

    Daily routine cleaning procedures for:

    > Toys, blankets, occupational therapy manipulatives, and other shared equipment such as walkers, parallel bars, highchairs, playpens, cribs, and eating surfaces should be washable and cleaned according to an established schedule or when visibly soiled.
    >
    > Bathrooms, diapering areas, potty chairs, and commodes should be cleaned routinely and when there is visible soiling or contamination.

    Procedures for cleaning up blood and body fluid spills should be established and followed.

Disinfectants should be non-toxic and stored in areas inaccessible to participants.

Areas for diapering or toileting should be physically separated from food preparation areas.

Soiled diapers/briefs should be disposed of in covered containers and that are emptied/cleaned at least daily or when full.

- Adequate ventilation and air exchange systems can decrease odors and potential airborne illness.
- Food preparation:

Sinks and towels should be physically separated from diaper changing facilities.

Hands should be washed before food preparation, serving, and feeding.

Clean vinyl gloves should be worn when handling ready to eat and unwrapped food.

Food/formula/breast milk brought in from home should be labeled with participant name and date and appropriately stored.

Unused food/formula/breast milk should be disposed of within 24 hours.

Foods should be prepared, stored, and handled appropriately. (Refer to Section 2 - Food Handling)

Untrained persons should not prepare food.

- Sharing personal items

Each participant should have a separate area for storing personal belongings.

Separate sleeping mats, cribs, or cots should be provided and distanced by at least 18 inches.

Coats, sweaters, and hats should be stored and separated by at least 12 inches.

- Pools or water play

  Use sprinklers for water play.

  If pools are used, contact local health department for guidelines.

➤ IC Program

- Appropriate infection control resources should be available for reference.
- Surveillance

  Participants and staff should be evaluated for signs and symptoms of infections and findings documented.

  Communicable disease reporting should be performed according to local and state regulations.

➤ Educational of caregivers

- Caregivers should be provided age/condition specific education regarding infection risks and strategies to reduce risks and prevent infection.
- Caregivers should be able to demonstrate understanding and skills.
- Staff, students, volunteers, and family members who provide care should be oriented to the centers infection control policies and procedures.
- Standard Precautions should be taught to caregivers.

References/Resources

- American Academy of Pediatrics. Health appraisal guidelines for day camps and resident camps. (RE9843) Pediatrics 2000, 105(3): 643-44.
- Association for Professionals in Infection Control and Epidemiology. APIC Text of Infection Control and Epidemiology. 2000, chapter 40, 1-14.
- Department of Health and Human Services, US Public Health Service and the Centers for Disease Control and Prevention. The ABC's the safe and healthy childcare: a handbook of childcare providers. 1996.
- McFarland L, Kelso KY. Childcare. In: Olmsted RN, editor. APIC infection control and applied epidemiology: principles and practice. St. Louis, MO: Mosby; 1996. p 86-1–86-21.
- The National Adult Day Care Services Association, Guidelines for Infection Control in Adult Day Centers, 2001.
- The National Adult Day Services Association: http://www.ncoa.org/nadsa
- Yahamuchi T. Guidelines for attendees and personnel. In: Donowitz LG, editor. Infection control in the childcare center and preschool. Baltimore: Williams and Wilkins; 1991. P 19–26.

Dentistry

Overview

- Dental healthcare personnel (DHCP) are exposed to a wide variety of potentially infectious microorganisms. Reservoirs include blood, saliva, and respiratory secretions from patients and contaminated environmental surfaces and equipment. Transmission can occur through percutaneous inoculation, mucous membrane exposure including aerosol inhalation, and/or non-intact skin exposure. Confirmed transmission of HIV and HBV has been documented in dental settings.

Purpose

- Dental care provides unique exposure risks to communicable diseases that can be minimized by following recommended principles, practices, and control methods to reduce infection and safety risks in the dental and oral surgery setting.

Risk Factors

- Patient assessment and triage
  - Communicable illness

    Skin rash, open skin lesions, uncontained bleeding, productive cough, eye drainage, diarrhea

    Suspected/confirmed chickenpox, measles, mumps, rubella, TB, scabies, lice
  - Allergies

    Latex, iodine, medication
  - Mental/physical/social

Risk of spitting/biting

Understanding and ability to cooperate, e.g., pediatric, mental impairment, Alzheimer's disease

Poor oral hygiene

Language barrier

Cultural beliefs

- Medical condition

  Mitral valve prolapse

  Implant

  Stroke – risk of aspiration or choking

  Seizure disorder

  Chronic illness, medication and/or treatment that compromises immunity

➤ Procedures and techniques

- Asepsis
- Patient positioning
- Barrier use

➤ Equipment, supplies, environment

- Reusable vs. disposable
- Cleaning, disinfection, sterilization
- Unique items

  Handpieces and prophylaxis angles

  Water lines

  Suction canisters

  Dental lab items and supplies

    Impressions and wax bites

  - Rag wheels
  - Acrylic splints
- Medications
- Lasers and X-rays
- Design and storage
- Waste and sharps
- Release of item to patient (e.g., tooth)

Strategies for Prevention

➤ Patient assessment and chart documentation should be obtained for:

- Allergies (e.g., latex, iodine, and medications).
  - Substitutions should be available.
- Behavioral or medical considerations (such as biting, spitting, seizures, etc.).
  - Assistance should be obtained before beginning procedures on these patients.
- Cultural or language considerations.
  - Interpreters or family/friends can provide assistance if needed.
  - Pictures can be used to convey information.
  - Language specific materials should be available.
- Mitral valve prolapse/implant.
  - Administration of antimicrobial prophylaxis per American Heart Association and American Dental Association.

➤ Refer to Sections 3 and 4 for General Prevention and Control Measures (e.g., handwashing and hand hygiene, Standard Precautions, aseptic technique, care of invasive devices, optimal cleaning, disinfection, and sterilization).

- Refer to Sections 2 and 3 for General Prevention and Control Measures (e.g., handwashing and hand hygiene, Standard Precautions, aseptic technique, care of invasive devices, optimal cleaning, disinfection, and sterilization).
- Refer to Section 5 for Employee Health considerations.
- Refer to Section 2 - Environmental Maintenance and Construction/Renovation.
- Setting Specific Measures
  - Standard Precautions including handwashing and PPE use should be observed. (Refer to Section 2)
  - Isolation Procedures should be observed if appropriate. (Refer to Section 2 - Isolation and Precautions)
  - Procedures and techniques

    Clean and sterile aseptic techniques should be used. (Refer to Section 2 - Asepsis)

    Patients should be positioned to minimize splashing.

    Appropriate barrier techniques and equipment should be used to minimize splashing.

    Dams should be used to minimize splashing.

    PPE and splash shields should be used.

    Covers for surfaces – light handles, X-ray unit heads, knobs, switches should be used and changed between patients.

    High-velocity air evacuation should be used.
  - Sharps safety

    If needles should be recapped, devices or one-hand scoop techniques should be used.

    Sharps should be counted.

    Sharps should be disposed of in designated puncture-proof NIOSH approved containers.

- Equipment and supplies

  Informed decisions regarding reusable or disposable equipment should be made. (Refer to Section 2)

  Informed decisions regarding high-level disinfection vs. sterilization should be made (Refer to Section 2) based upon intended use.

  After each patient use, handpieces should be flushed for > 30 seconds to remove patient material from turbine and air/water lines.

  Sterilization between patients is recommended for all high-speed dental handpieces, low-speed components used intraorally, and reusable prophylaxis angles.

  Internal surfaces or high-speed handpieces, low-speed handpiece components, and prophylaxis angles may become contaminated with patient material during use.

  Manufacturer's directions should be followed for disassembly, cleaning, sterilization, and lubrication of handpieces.

  Disinfection by wiping or soaking in liquid chemical germicides is not an acceptable method for reprocessing.

  At the start of the day, handpieces should be removed and the water lines run for several minutes to reduce microbial accumulation in the lines.

  Anti-retraction valves (one-way flow check valves) should be installed to prevent fluid aspiration back into the handpiece and water lines and to reduce the risk of transfer of potentially infectious material.

  Routine maintenance of anti-retraction valves is critical; contact manufacturer of dental unit for recommendations.

  Tubing for handpieces and air/water syringes should be straight, not kinked or coiled, and not used in enclosed retraction devices. Fabric-covered tubing should not be used because it cannot be effectively cleaned.

Only sterile water/saline should be used as a coolant/irrigant when surgical procedures involve bone cutting.

Ultrasonic scaler tips and component parts and air/water syringe tips should be cleaned and sterilized between each patient use.

Handles or dental unit attachments, saliva ejectors, high-speed air evacuators, and air–water syringes should be covered with impervious barriers, changed after use, and wiped with intermediate-level disinfectant.

Proper maintenance of suction canisters, tubing, and connector/flow control assemblies is important to avoid them becoming reservoirs for microorganisms.

Disposable suction tips, tubing, and canister should be used whenever feasible.

Suction tubing from the canister to the patient should be changed between patients.

Suction canisters should be changed/emptied when 3/4 full or weekly, whichever comes first.

Disposable suction canisters may be treated with a solidifying agent before disposal into regular waste stream.

Suction canisters may be emptied into a flushing hopper provided the person performing this activity is wearing PPE.

Reusable suction canisters should be disinfected with an appropriate disinfectant (e.g., dilute bleach solution) after emptying and before reuse.

- Dental Labs

A receiving area should be designated and kept separate from the production area of the lab.

Impression cases should be disinfected as they are received, before storage, or before being returned to the patient. Containers should be sterilized or disinfected after each use.

Work surfaces and equipment should be kept free from debris and disinfected at least daily.

Instruments, attachments, and materials used with prostheses/appliances should be maintained separately from those that have already been inserted into the mouth.

Ragwheels should be washed and sterilized after each case. Brushes and other equipment should be cleaned and disinfected at least daily.

A small amount of pumice should be dispensed in small disposable containers for individual use on each case; any excess should be discarded.

A liquid disinfectant (1:20 bleach solution made fresh daily or stabilized bleach solution) may serve as a mixing medium for pumice. Adding three parts green soap will keep the pumice suspended.

Alginate impressions and wax bites should be placed into a sealable plastic bag for transport to the dental lab.

Impressions/bites should be rinsed under running tap water prior to complete immersion in an iodophor solution (refer to manufacturer's instructions for concentration) for at least ten (10) minutes. A sealable bag (e.g., Ziplock®) may be used as the immersion container.

Impressions/bites should be rinsed thoroughly with tap water after disinfection to prevent damage to the stone model. Discard used iodophor solution and soaking bag.

Splints should be completely immersed in iodophor disinfectant solution (refer to manufacturer's directions for concentration) for at least 10 minutes.

Splints should be rinsed thoroughly with tap water after disinfection. Used iodophor solution and soaking bag should be discarded after use.

Splints should be placed into a small amount of diluted mouthwash (e.g., Cepacol®) prior to delivery to the patient.

- Medications

  Patient specific unit doses are preferred.

  Proper storage and handling of multidose medications.

- Lasers and X-rays

  Appropriate PPE (e.g., wavelength specific goggles, lead apron) should be used.

  Regulatory compliance applicable to laser/X-rays should be followed.

- Release of items such as teeth/impressions to patients

  Documentation should be maintained with a signed affidavit for release.

  Teeth should be soaked in detergent and water before removing adherent patient blood/OPIM by scrubbing with a brush.

  Teeth should be disinfected in a liquid chemical germicide suitable for clinical specimen fixation, such as fresh solution of sodium hypochlorite diluted 1:10 with water, for a minimum of 20 minutes.

➤ IC Program Aspects in Dentistry

- There should be a designated resource person in dental settings who have knowledge of infection control principles and practices.
- Appropriate infection control resources should be available for reference.

- Identification of infection control resources/liaisons with local hospitals and health departments is recommended.
- Surveillance

  Active surveillance programs are usually not implemented in dental setting. However, there should be close attention to potential clusters and outbreaks that can be identified during patient assessment and follow-up appointments/calls.

➤ Education

- Caregivers should be provided age/condition specific education regarding infection risks and strategies to reduce risks and prevent infection.
- Caregivers should be able to demonstrate understanding and skills.

References/Resources

➤ Association for Professionals in Infection Control and Epidemiology. APIC Text of Infection Control and Epidemiology. 2000, chapter 42, 1 - 18.

➤ Centers for Disease Control and Prevention. Recommended Infection Control Practices for Dentistry. 1993, MMWR. 42 (RR-8): 1-10.

➤ Centers for Disease Control and Prevention, Healthcare Infection Control Practices Advisory Committee (HICPAC). Draft Guideline for Environmental Infection Control in Healthcare Facilities, 2001. 2001, Federal Register

➤ American Dental Association www.ada.org

➤ Organization for Safety and Asepsis Procedures www.osap.org

Diagnostic Services

Overview

- Diagnostic imaging services uses radioactive substances or high-frequency sound waves to visualize internal body areas for diagnostic and/or therapeutic purposes. This consultative/treatment specialty includes three major areas:
  - Diagnostic imaging by means of external radiation,
  - Nuclear medicine using radioactive materials placed into blood/body organs, and
  - Therapeutic/interventional procedures that may include invasive, percutaneous imaging guidance.
- Common examples of procedures by imaging services
  - Computed topography (CT)
  - Fluoroscopy (e.g., barium enema, cryptogram, intravenous pellagra)
  - Diagnostic radiography (e.g., chest radiography, mammography)
  - Magnetic resonance imaging (MRI)
  - Nuclear medicine (e.g., Reno gram, bone scan, gallium scan, or white blood cell scan)
  - Ultrasound (e.g., transvaginal, vascular, abdominal)
  - Interventional/invasive (e.g., angiographies, percutaneous drainage of abscess, gastrostomy tube placement, placement of peripherally inserted central catheters, and needle biopsy)

Purpose

- The ICP should have a basic understanding of the scope of diagnostic services and interventional strategies to reduce infectious outcomes associated with diagnostic services.

Risk Factors

- Radiographic procedures without vascular or percutaneous access pose a nominal risk of infection transmission (e.g., X-ray, routine barium fluoroscopy, mammography, zoography, and CT or MRI without IV contrast)
- Airborne diseases (e.g., TB and varicella)
- Bloodborne pathogens during invasive procedures
- Procedure-related transmission of microorganisms to HCW and/or between patients (e.g., monographic probes, inadvertent injection of radioactive isotope–labeled blood products with reuse of a syringe, meningitis after xylography)

Strategies for Prevention and Control

- Patient Assessment
  - Patients should be evaluated for signs/symptoms of airborne communicable diseases prior to scheduling patient appointment for diagnostic services.
- Refer to Sections 3 and 4 for General Prevention and Control Measures (e.g., handwashing and hand hygiene, Standard Precautions, aseptic technique, care of invasive devices, optimal cleaning, disinfection, and sterilization).
- Refer to Sections 2 and 3 for General Prevention and Control Measures (e.g., handwashing and hand hygiene, Standard Precautions, aseptic technique, care of invasive devices, optimal cleaning, disinfection, and sterilization).

- Refer to Section 5 for Employee Health considerations.
- Refer to Section 2 - Environmental Maintenance and Construction/Renovation.
- Setting Specific Measures
  - If a patient with an airborne communicable disease is transported to the diagnostic testing area, appropriate precautions should be followed such as masking the patient during transport.
  - Technicians should follow transmission-based precautions for patients with suspected or known airborne communicable diseases. (Refer to Section 2)
  - The use of antimicrobial prophylaxis to prevent infectious complications related to invasive procedures should be evaluated on an individual patient basis.

References/Resources

- American College of Radiology www.acr.org
- American Society for Therapeutic Radiology and Oncology www.astro.org/home.html
- Association for Professionals in Infection Control and Epidemiology. APIC Text of Infection Control and Epidemiology. 2000, chapters 62, 66.
- Centers for Disease Control and Prevention, Healthcare Infection Control Practices Advisory Committee (HICPAC). Draft guideline for the prevention of intravascular catheter-related infections, August 2001. Federal Register
- Centers for Disease Control and Prevention, Healthcare Infection Control Practices Advisory Committee (HICPAC). Draft guideline for environmental infection control in healthcare facilities, 2001. March 6, 2001, Federal Register

- Ehrlich RA, McCloskey ED, Daly JO. Patient Care in Radiography. 5th ed. St. Louis: Mosby; 1998
- Green KA, Shouldachi B, Schoer K, et al. Gadolinium-based MR contrast media: potential for growth of microbial contaminants when single vials are used for multiple patients. AJR Am J Roentgenol 1995;165:669-71.
- Society of Cardiovascular and Interventional Radiology www.scvir.org
- Society of Nuclear Medicine www.snm.org
- Society of Radiologists in Ultrasound www.sru.org
- Torres LS. Basic Medical Techniques and Patient Care in Imaging Technology. 5th ed. Philadelphia: JB Lippincott; 1997
- Trerotola SO, Kuhn-Fulton J, Johnson MS, et al. Tunneled infusion catheters: increased incidence of symptomatic venous thrombosis after subclavian versus internal jugular venous access. Radiology 2000; 217:89-93.

Dialysis

Overview

- Dialysis simulates normal kidney function by removing metabolic waste products, toxins, and fluid to maintain water and electrolyte balance.
- Acute dialysis treatment may be utilized for organ failure, treatment of septic shock, fluid overload, or overdose of a toxic substance.
- Chronic dialysis is applicable for end stage renal disease (ESRD) or renal transplant failure.
- Chronic dialysis is usually performed in the ambulatory setting or in the home.
- Treatment modalities include hemodialysis (HD) and peritoneal dialysis (PD).
  - Both treatments have three components: access to bloodstream, a semi-permeable membrane, and dialysate fluid.
  - In HD, the artificial kidney is the dialyzer or semi-permeable membrane.
  - In PD, the patient's peritoneal membrane is the dialyzer.
  - A balanced electrolyte solution (dialysate) is exposed to one side of a membrane and blood flow to the other side.
- The HD system consists of a water supply, a system for mixing purified water and concentrated dialysis fluid, and a machine to pump the fluid through the dialyzer.
  - HD patients have temporary or permanent access.
  - Temporary vascular access: a dual lumen catheter in large vein such as the subclavian, jugular, or femoral and ending in the superior vena cava.

- Permanent access: native arteriovenous fistula (surgical revision joining artery and vein) or arteriovenous graft (synthetic material, such as Gortex® or Teflon®, connects artery and vein).
- Patients with PD modality may use Continuous Ambulatory Peritoneal Dialysis (CAPD) with gravity exchange and/or an automated cycler machine during nighttime hours with the last exchange left in the peritoneal cavity (dwell) during the daytime.

Purpose

- This section provides principles, practices, and control methods to reduce infection and related safety risks in the dialysis setting based on evidence-based recommendations.

Risk Factors

- Dialysis patients are usually immunocompromised hosts because of alternations in immune function associated with dialysis chronic renal failure, and/or underlying co-morbid conditions (e.g., diabetes, hypertension, cardiovascular disease).
- Infection is second only to cardiovascular disease in having an impact on the morbidity and mortality of the patient with ESRD.
- Dialysis patients require vascular or peritoneal access, which bypasses the normal protective defenses.
- Dialysis supplies and equipment may become contaminated with microorganisms and/or endotoxins.

Strategies for Prevention

- Assessment
  - Patients should be assessed for airborne communicable diseases before being transported to dialysis services settings so that

appropriate Barrier Precautions can be used. (Refer to Section 2 - Isolation and Precautions)

- Refer to Sections 3 and 4 for General Prevention and Control Measures (e.g., handwashing and hand hygiene, Standard Precautions, aseptic technique, care of invasive devices, optimal cleaning, disinfection, and sterilization).
- Refer to Sections 2 and 3 for General Prevention and Control Measures (e.g., handwashing and hand hygiene, Standard Precautions, aseptic technique, care of invasive devices, optimal cleaning, disinfection, and sterilization).
- Refer to Section 5 for Employee Health considerations.
- Refer to Section 2 - Environmental Maintenance and Construction/Renovation.
- Setting Specific Measures
  - Asepsis

    Handwashing is essential when performing any procedure related to HD or CAPD.

    Clean nonsterile gloves and clean technique should be used during preparation and cannulation of access sites.

    Sterile gloves, surgical masks, and sterile technique should be used during initiation of central venous catheters and during dressing changes.

    Sterile gloves, surgical masks, and sterile technique should be used during initiation of CAPD treatment.

    Clean non-sterile gloves and clean technique should be used during dressing changes.
  - Equipment

    Policies and procedures for cleaning, disinfection, and dialyzer reuse and maintenance should be developed in accordance with the American Association of Medical Instrumentation (AAMI) recommendations.

Routine cultures (e.g., quarterly) should be done as recommended by AAMI to check the integrity of the reverse osmosis and other components of water purification system.

Water quality and treatment should meet AAMI and local standards.

Machine surfaces, monitors, blood pumps, and other related dialysis equipment should be thoroughly cleaned with an appropriate disinfectant.

Syringes and needles should be sterile and designated for single use.

Reusable patient care items and supplies should be cleaned and disinfected or sterilized as recommended by the manufacturer.

If sterile single-use items are reprocessed, there should be a policy and protocol to monitor this practice.

There should be a policy and procedure to recall items (e.g., dialysate) if necessary.

- Physical Plant - Refer to the American Institute of Architects (AIA) guidelines for design and construction of hospital and healthcare facilities (2001) for detailed information.

Dialysis centers may be in freestanding leased or owned facilities.

Treatment may be in an open area, but should be separate from administration and waiting rooms.

Individual treatment areas should have at least 80 square feet of space and at least a 4-foot space between beds and/or lounge chairs.

Handwashing sinks should be located near or in nursing stations and treatment areas.

The facility should have separate clean and soiled workrooms (utility rooms) and storage areas (e.g., linen, supplies, waste).

If a dialyzer is reused, a reprocessing room is required, sized to perform the reprocessing procedures and properly ventilated.

If a nourishment center (pantry or kitchen) is provided, it should have a sink, refrigerator, storage cabinets, and appropriate equipment.

Medication areas should have a sink, refrigerator, cabinets, controlled storage, and counter working space.

- Water treatment, distribution, and storage

  Water used for the production of dialysis fluid should be treated to remove chemical contaminants.

  Reverse osmosis or deionization water treatment systems are designed to remove electrolytes, bacteria, and bacterial endotoxins from dialysis water and are used in 99% of U.S. dialysis centers.

  A variety of filters are used to control bacterial contamination and remove organic chemicals and chlorine from the water (e.g., particulate, absolute, carbon, and ultra filters).

  Systems should be free of rough joints, dead-end spaces, and unused branches that could serve as reservoirs of bacteria that can persistently contaminate the system.

  There should be continuous flow of water through all distribution piping with a minimum flow velocity of 1.5 feet per second.

  Storage tanks serve as additional sources of contamination and should not be used unless they are frequently drained and adequately disinfected. An ultra filter should be used distal to the storage tank.

- Housekeeping

  Housekeeping services may be performed by employees or contracted personnel.

  All personnel performing housekeeping should be trained regarding the facility bloodborne pathogen exposure plan and cleaning and disinfection procedures.

  Waste management should comply with all applicable federal, state, and local regulations.

- Immunizations

  Hepatitis B vaccine should be available to patients and employees.

  Patients and employees should also be evaluated for immunization against influenza and pneumococcus.

  Patients with HBV and/or HCV should be evaluated for hepatitis A vaccine.

  Dialysis patients may have varied and possibly sub-optimal responses to vaccines.

- Disposable gloves should be worn when caring for the patient or touching the patient's equipment at the dialysis station; remove gloves and wash hands between each patient or station.
- Items taken into the dialysis station should be disposed of, dedicated for use only on a single patient, or cleaned and disinfected before being taken to a common clean area or used on another patient.
- Nondisposable items that cannot be cleaned and disinfected (e.g., adhesive take, cloth-covered blood pressure cuffs) should be dedicated for use only on a single patient.
- Unused medications (including multiple-dose vials containing diluents) or supplies (e.g., syringes, alcohol swabs) taken to the

patient's station should be used only for that patient and should not be returned to a common clean area or used on other patients.

- When multiple-dose medication vials are used (including vials containing diluents), prepare individual patient doses in a clean (centralized) area away from dialysis stations and deliver separately to each patient. Do no carry multiple-dose medication vials from station to station.
- Common medication carts should not be used to deliver medication to patients. Do not carry medication vials, syringes, alcohol swabs, or supplies in pockets. If trays are used to deliver medications to individual patients, they should be cleaned between patients.
- Clean areas should be clearly designated for the preparation, handling, and storage of medications and unused supplies and equipment. Clean areas should be clearly separated from contaminated areas where used supplies and equipment are handled. Do not handle and store medications or clean supplies in the same or an adjacent area to where used equipment or blood samples are handled.
- External venous and arterial pressure transducer filters/protectors should be used for each patient treatment to prevent blood contamination of the dialysis machines' pressure monitors. Change filters/protectors between each patient treatment, and do not reuse them. Internal transducer filters do not need to be changed routinely between patients.
- The dialysis station (e.g., chairs, beds, tables, machines) should be cleaned and disinfected between patients.
- Give special attention to cleaning control panels on the dialysis machines and other surfaces that are frequently touched and potentially contaminated with patients' blood.

- Discard all fluid and clean and disinfect all surfaces and containers associated with the prime waste (including buckets attached to the machines).
- For dialyzers and blood tubing that will be reprocessed, cap dialyzer ports and clamp tubing. Place all used dialyzers and tubing in leakproof containers for transport from station or reprocessing or disposal area.
- Routine testing for HBV and HCV infections is recommended in dialysis patients

    All patients on admission: HBsAg, Anti-HBc (total), Anti-HBs, Anti-HCV, ALT; results of HBV testing should be known before patient begins dialysis.

        HBV-susceptible: Monthly HBsAg

        Anti-HBs positive: Annual Anti HBs

        Anti-HBs and Anti-HBc positive: no additional testing needed

        Anti-HCV negative: monthly ALT, semi-annual Anti-HCV

- Hepatitis B Vaccination

    Susceptible patients should be immunized for hepatitis B [dose and vaccine frequency – see package insert].

    Test for anti-HBs one to two months after last dose.

        If anti-HBs is < 10 mlU/mL, consider patient susceptible, revaccinate with an additional three doses, and retest for anti-HBs.

        If anti-HBs > 10 mlU/mL, consider patient immune, and retest annually.

        Give booster dose of vaccine if anti-HBs declines to < 10 mlU/mL and continue to retest annually.

- Management of HBsAg-Positive Patients

    Follow infection control practices for hemodialysis units for all patients.

    Dialyze HBsAg-positive patients in a separate room using separate machines, equipment, instruments, and supplies.

    Staff members caring for HBsAg-positive patients should not care for HBV-susceptible patients at the same time (e.g., during the same shift or during patient changeover).

    HbsAg positive patients should not participate in dialyzer reprocessing programs.

➤ IC Program Aspects for Dialysis Settings

- Dialysis centers are often located outside of hospital settings. Collaboration between dialysis personnel and ICPs is important in maintaining an effective IC program in dialysis settings.
- Surveillance

    Classification of microorganism-related outcomes

        Bacteremia or peritonitis due to *Staphylococcus aureus* (outbreaks of both MSSA and MRSA reported in the literature) or other pathogens.

        Bacteremia or sepsis due to Gram-negative bacilli and/or endotoxins (i.e., toxins produced by Gram-negative bacilli).

        Bacteremia or peritonitis due to opportunistic microorganisms (e.g., *Candida sp.* and *Aspergillus sp.*).

    Patients and providers should be aware of the signs and symptoms of Gram-negative sepsis and pyrogenic reactions. Common symptoms of pyrogenic reactions are shaking, chills, fever, and hypotension. Symptoms can occur one to five hours after the initiation of dialysis and generally abate within a few hours after dialysis is discontinued.

Surveillance should include monitoring of water cultures. Total viable bacterial counts should not exceed 200 colony-forming units (cfu) per milliliter of water. Nontuberculous mycobacteria are relatively resistant to disinfection and may survive and multiply in water.

Surveillance should be a collaborative effort of the dialysis team, infection control, and other clinicians providing care to dialysis patients.

The scope of surveillance should be targeted for specific processes (e.g., monitoring of compliance with aseptic technique) or outcomes (e.g., access site infections or bloodstream infections).

Surveillance should be concurrently performed and designed for early detection of clusters and/or outbreaks of infections in the dialysis population.

Case finding may include review of culture reports, assessments, and review of patient admissions and emergency room visits. CDC definitions of infection should be used to identify nosocomial bacteremia and site infections.

The local health department should be notified of significant clusters/outbreaks and reportable communicable diseases in dialysis patients.

➤ Education

- Caregivers should be provided age/condition specific education regarding infection risks and strategies to reduce risks and prevent infection.
- Caregivers should be able to demonstrate understanding and skills.
- Patients should be instructed regarding the signs/symptoms of dialysis related infections and what actions to take when they are recognized.

References/Resources

- Association for Professionals in Infection Control and Epidemiology. APIC Text of Infection Control and Epidemiology. 2000, chapter 42, 1-18.
- Centers for Disease Control and Prevention, Healthcare Infection Control Practices Advisory Committee (HICPAC). Draft Guideline for Environmental Infection Control in Healthcare Facilities, 2001. Federal Register [final document pending]
- Centers for Disease Control and Prevention, Recommendations for Preventing Transmission of Infections Among Chronic hemodialysis Patients, MMWR, Recommendations and Reports, Vol. 50, No. RR-5, April 27, 2001, pp. 1-43.
- Garcia-Houchins S. Dialysis. In: Olmsted RN, editor. APIC infection control and applied epidemiology: principles and practice. St. Louis, MO: Mosby; 1996. p 89-1–89-9.
- Favero M, Alter M, Bland LA. Dialysis-associated infections. In: Bennett JV, Brachman PS, Sanford JP, editors. Hospital epidemiology and infection control. Galveston: Williams and Wilkins; 1996. p 693–698.
- Recommended IC Practices for HD Units at a Glance (from MMWR RR-5, pp 20-21).

Home Care Settings

Overview

- Home care services have grown over the past two decades. Additionally, more high-technology practices previously performed only in traditional healthcare settings are now performed in the home. Although basic infection control principles should be used in this setting, there are unique aspects to providing care in the home that impact the strategies for prevention of infections. These unique aspects relate to the setting itself (e.g., space, air handling, availability of equipment) and the shift for primary responsibility for care to family members and the patient/client with the formal home care provider acting in a more consultative role.
- The Division of Healthcare Quality Promotion of the CDC has not developed guidelines for infection control in home care settings. However, the following recommendations have been suggested in the literature.

Purpose

- Infection control strategies in home care services can be applied in order to reduce the risk of infections from healthcare delivery associated infections (e.g., vascular device infections) as well as targeting the reduction of community acquired infections in the home setting.

Risk Factors

- ➤ Inadequate knowledge or skills of informal healthcare providers related to asepsis (e.g., handwashing, disinfection, food handling, etc.).
- ➤ Inadequate facilities (e.g., sinks, laundry facilities, ventilations, etc.).
- ➤ Healthcare delivery devices used (e.g., urinary catheters, intravascular catheters, ventilators, etc.).
- ➤ Immunocompromised status of the home care patient/client.
- ➤ Construction in the home can expose home care patients/clients to airborne spores.

Strategies for Prevention

- ➤ Assessment
  - ▪ Patient and family caregivers should be assessed for their ability to perform care activities.
  - ▪ Patients should be assessed for the presence of infection upon admission to the home care setting.
- ➤ Refer to Sections 2 and 3 for General Prevention and Control Measures (e.g., handwashing and hand hygiene, Standard Precautions, aseptic technique, care of invasive devices, optimal cleaning, disinfection, and sterilization).
- ➤ Refer to Section 5 for Employee Health considerations.
- ➤ Refer to Section 2 - Environmental Maintenance and Construction/ Renovation. Although the guidelines do not apply to home care settings, the risk factors and general principles of risk reduction may be adapted for the home setting.
- ➤ Setting Specific Measures
  - ▪ An assessment of patient/client infection risks, setting specific issues, and the home caregiver knowledge/skills needs.

- A care plan should be developed with the home caregiver and patient/client to address and resolve issues identified in the assessment.
- Hygienic Practices

    Caregivers and patients/clients should practice handwashing following toileting, wound care, etc.

    Soap, instant hand sanitizers, disposable tissue, and paper towels should be readily available for use.

    Clean aseptic technique should be sufficient for most home care procedures.

    Intravascular devices and therapy

        Sterile aseptic technique should be used for intravascular line insertion and maintenance. (Refer to Section 4 - Vascular Device Related Infections).

    Urinary catheterization

        Clean aseptic technique should be used for intermittent urinary catheterization.

        Sterile aseptic technique should be used to insert chronic indwelling and suprapubic catheters.

        Catheters should be changed only when there are signs of damage, obstruction, or concretions.

    Respiratory care

        Suctioning (oral, nasal, trach tube) should be performed using clean aseptic technique.

        Freshly obtained tap water may be used for suctioning. Boiled water allowed to cool may also be used.

        White vinegar solution can be used as equipment disinfection.

        Boiled tap water or sterile water should be used for final rinsing of disinfected equipment.

Equipment should be allowed to dry before storing in a clean, dry place.

- Isolation is rarely indicated in the home setting. Caregivers should use barrier precautions. (Refer to Section 2)

  If a home care patient/client has an active airborne disease (e.g., Tuberculosis), caregivers should use appropriated respiratory protection. For the home caregiver, use of a surgical mask is sufficient. Formal home care providers should follow precautions outlined in Section 2.

- Environmental considerations

  Home setting should be kept clean and free from dust.

  Waste should be disposed of routinely. Sharps used in the home care setting should be disposed of in puncture-resistant containers.

  The home care provider may dispose of containers.

  If the informal caregiver disposes of the container, local sanitation rules should be followed.

  Precautions to reduce dust should be taken during home construction and renovation. (Refer to Section 2 - Construction and Renovation for general principles)

- Home care provider bag

  The bag can be placed on any clean surface.

  The bag should be placed out of reach of children and pets.

  The inside of the bag is considered clean.

  Reusable items should be cleaned and disinfected before being returned to the bag.

- Food preparation:

  Hands should be washed before food preparation, serving, and feeding.

Foods should be prepared, stored, and handled appropriately. (Refer to Section 2 - Food Handling)

Patients/clients should be educated regarding the risks of foodborne illness before preparing/handling food.

Enteral feeding bags should be rinsed after each feeding with fresh tap water or boiled and cooled tap water.

- IC Program
  - There should be interdisciplinary involvement between nursing, therapists, physicians, support personnel, and informal caregivers/patients/clients.
  - Surveillance

    Participants and staff should be evaluated for signs and symptoms of infections.

    Communicable disease reporting should be performed according to local and state regulations.
  - Nosocomial infection surveillance should be performed; draft home care definitions for infection may be applied. (Refer to Section 2)
- Educational of caregivers and patients/clients
  - Caregivers should be provided age/condition specific education regarding infection risks and strategies to reduce risks and prevent infection.
  - Caregivers should be able to demonstrate understanding and skills.
  - Staff and informal caregivers should be oriented to infection control principles and practices.
  - Standard Precautions and hygienic practices should be taught to caregivers and patients/clients.

References/Resources

- American Association for Respiratory Care. Guidelines for disinfection of respiratory care equipment used in the home. Respiratory Care 1988; 33:801-808.
- Association for Professionals in Infection Control and Epidemiology. APIC Text of Infection Control and Epidemiology. 2000, chapter 35,44,85-92,120.
- CDC. Caring for Someone with AIDS-Information for Friends, Relatives, Household Members and Others Who Care for a Person with aids at Home. www.cdc.gov
- Embry FC, Chinnes LF. Draft definitions for surveillance of infections in home healthcare. Am J Infect Control 2000, 28:449-53.
- Graham DR, Keldermans MM, Klemm LW, Semenza NJ, Shafer ML. Infectious complications among patients receiving home intravenous therapy with peripheral, central or peripherally placed central venous catheters. American Journal of Medicine 1991: 3B: 95S-100S.
- Simmons B, Trusler M, Roccaforte J, Smith P, Scott R. Infection control in home healthcare settings. Infection Control and Hospital Epidemiology 1990; 11:362 - 370.
- Valenti WM. Infection control, human immunodeficiency virus, and home healthcare: 1. Infection risk to the patient. American Journal of Infection Control 1994; 22:371-2.

Immunocompromised Patients

Overview

- Immunocompromised patients are often infected by their own flora (i.e., endogenous microorganisms). They may also be colonized and/or infected by cross-transmission from other people or contaminated equipment. Infections in the immunocompromised patient may be life threatening as defects in the body's immune system predispose them to infections. Patients are at increased risk for acquisition of bacteremia, pneumonia, tuberculosis, urinary tract infections, soft tissue infections, as well as opportunistic organisms (e.g., *Candida sp.* and *Aspergillus sp.*). Handwashing, adherence to aseptic technique, use of barrier precautions, and elimination of environmental reservoirs are important infection control strategies.

Purpose

- Recognition of the compromised patient, identifying and correcting risk factors and reducing infection sources can decrease the potential for infection.

Risk Factors

- Absolute granulocyte counts < 500 cells/mm^3
- HIV-related illness (i.e., AIDS)
- Bone marrow/organ transplant
- Hematologic malignancy
- Cancer
- Chemotherapy
- Elderly status

- Neonatal status
- Major surgery, burns, tissue trauma
- Poorly controlled diabetes
- Chronic malnutrition

Strategies for Prevention

- Patient assessment
  - Patients should have a nutritional assessment and a care plan to improve nutritional status.
- Refer to Sections 2 and 3 for General Prevention and Control Measures (e.g., handwashing and hand hygiene, Standard Precautions, aseptic technique, care of invasive devices, optimal cleaning, disinfection, and sterilization).
- Refer to Section 5 for Employee Health considerations.
- Refer to Section 2 - Environmental Maintenance and Construction/Renovation. Although the guidelines do not apply to home care settings, the risk factors and general principles of risk reduction may be adapted for the home setting.
- Population specific measures
  - Patients should avoid eating raw foods (e.g., eggs, fruits, vegetables) and unpasteurized milk or cheeses.
  - Sterile water should be used for respiratory therapy procedures and wound irrigation.
  - Household members/visitors should be instructed to use thorough handwashing and sanitary practices.
  - Patients should avoid contact with persons having upper respiratory tract infections.
  - Neutropenic patients should wear surgical masks when leaving their own room/dwelling.

- Patients should avoid cleaning litter boxes, birdcages, or aquariums.
- In the inpatient setting, patient-specific equipment should be used when possible (e.g., thermometer, blood pressure cuff, and stethoscope).
- Patients should be assessed for allergy/sensitivity to latex. Latex-free alternative should be provided to these patients.
- Isolation and precautions should be applied to immunocompromised patients following the same guidelines as for the general patient population as there are no conclusive data to support protective or reverse isolation.
- Flowers (fresh and dried) and ornamental plants should be excluded from patient rooms and areas where immunocompromised patients may be located.
- Use of carpeting should be avoided in patient care areas where the incidence of spills is likely.
- In the inpatient setting, use of high-efficiency particulate air (HEPA) filtration may be indicated for highly immunocompromised persons such as bone marrow transplant patients, burn patients, and patients with prolonged granulocytopenia.

➤ IC Program

- Immunocompromised persons are often treated across settings including home, outpatient, and inpatient heightening the importance of integrating infection control program aspects between all settings and formal/informal caregivers and the patient.

- Surveillance

  Immunocompromised persons are at higher risk for infection and closer monitoring for clusters and outbreaks may be indicated.

  Immunocompromised persons may have increased numbers of invasive devices that should be considered in surveillance activities.

References/Resources

- Center for Disease Control and Prevention, Healthcare Infection Control Practices Advisory Committee (HICPAC). Draft Guideline for Environmental Infection Control in Healthcare Facilities, 2001. 2001 Federal Register [final document pending]
- Mooney BR, Revers SA, Larson E. Infection control and bone marrow transplantation. Am J Infect Control 1993; 21:131-138.
- Naussef WM, Maki DG. A study of the value of simple protective isolation in patients with granulocytopenia. N Engl J Med 1981; 304:448-453.
- Rise GF, Tomascak V. Prevention of infection in the immunocompromised host. Am J Infect Control 1998:26:594-602.
- USPHS/ISDA Prevention of Opportunistic Infections Working Group. USPHS/ISDA guidelines for the prevention of opportunistic infections in persons infected with human immunodeficiency virus: disease-specific recommendations. Clin Infect Dis 1995; 21(Suppl): 32 - 43.

Long-Term Care Facilities

Overview

- The U.S. population aged 65–85 years is increasing rapidly and persons aged >85 years have doubled in recent years. Currently, about 20% of the latter group resides in Long-term care Facilities (LTCFs). One of every four persons >65 years can expect to spend part of his/her life in this type of setting and currently, about 1.5 million reside in LTCFs.
- With increased chronic illness and co-morbidities in the LTCF population, residents' risk of healthcare associated infections is similar to that of hospitalized patients.

Purpose

- Although the basic principles of infection control apply to LTCF settings, these settings have unique requirements due to the patient populations served and the residential nature of the LTCF.

Risk Factors

- Patient/Resident characteristics
  - Age-related decline in immunologic function, specifically cell-mediated immunity and antibody humoral system response
  - Local host defense problems (e.g., thinning of skin, urinary retention, decreased mucociliary clearance of airways, ineffective cough).
  - Presence of underlying chronic diseases (e.g., diabetes, COPD, malignancy.)
  - Decreased mental status

- Multiple medications
- Indwelling devices (e.g. urinary catheters)
- Gastric achlorhydria
- Incontinence – fecal and/or urinary
- Immobility and/or limited ambulation
- Pressure ulcers
- Close contact of residents as roommates and in communal areas

➤ Common healthcare associated infection in LTCFs
- UTIs vs. asymptomatic bacteriuria
- Respiratory tract infections
    - Pneumonia
    - Influenza
    - Tuberculosis
- Skin and soft-tissue infections
- GI infections
- Bacteremia
- Conjunctivitis

➤ Common cluster/epidemic infections
- Antibiotic-resistant bacteria
- Scabies infestations
- Influenza
- TB
- Viral gastroenteritis
- Bacterial gastroenteritis
- *Clostridium difficile*–associated diarrhea

Strategies for Prevention

- Refer to Sections 2 and 3 for General Prevention and Control Measures (e.g., handwashing and hand hygiene, Standard Precautions, aseptic technique, care of invasive devices, optimal cleaning, disinfection, and sterilization).
- Refer to Section 5 for Employee Health considerations.
- Refer to Section 2 - Environmental Maintenance and Construction/ Renovation. Although the guidelines do not apply to home care settings, the risk factors and general principles of risk reduction may be adapted for the home setting.
- Setting specific measures - An effective IC program is the most practical and resourceful prevention strategy. The following elements include a **partial** selection from the SHEA Long-Term Care Committee and APIC Guidelines Committee on infection prevention and control in the long-term care facility.
  - A-Good evidence to support the recommendation
  - B-Moderate evidence to support the recommendation
  - C-Poor evidence to support the recommendation
  - Categories reflecting the quality of evidence for the recommendation

    I-Evidence from at least one properly randomized, controlled trial.

    II-Evidence from at least one well-designed clinical trial without randomization, from cohort or case-controlled analytic studies (preferably from more than one center), from multiple time-series studies, or from dramatic results in uncontrolled experiments.

    III-Evidence from opinions of respected authorities, based on clinical experience, descriptive studies, or reports of expert committees.

➤ Regulations

- LTCFs are governed by federal, state, and voluntary agency guidelines.
- Skilled nursing facilities are required by the Omnibus Budget Reconciliation Act of 1987 to have an IC program.
- The CMS, formerly HCFA, has published requirements for LTCFs accepting Medicare or Medicaid residents. These requirements address the need for an IC program, surveillance, isolation, employee health, and handwashing.
- LTCFs should comply with federal and state OSHA guidelines. Exposure control plans are required to protect employees from bloodborne pathogens and TB.
- LTCFs accredited by JCAHO should comply with applicable JCAHO standards.
- LTCFs should comply with applicable federal, state, and local regulations for waste management and food handling and preparation.

➤ Infection Control Program

- An active, effective, facility-wide infection control program should be established in the LTCF to help prevent the development and spread of infectious diseases *(BIII)*.
- *Comment:* LTCF infection control programs developed in response to studies of LTCF infections and regulations. The elements of a program generally include the following:

  Surveillance based on systematic data collection to identify infections in residents.

  A system for detection, investigation, and control of institutional outbreaks of infectious diseases.

  An isolation and precautions system to reduce the risk of transmission of infectious agents.

Infection control policies and procedures. Continuing education in infection prevention and control.

A resident health program.

An employee health program.

A system for antibiotic review and control.

Disease reporting to public health authorities.

- The infection control program should be in compliance with federal, state, and local regulations.

➤ Infection Control Administrative Structure

- Oversight of the infection control program should include participation of the ICP, administration, nursing staff, and physician staff. *(BIII)*
- Management of the IC program involves establishing policies and procedures for investigating, controlling, and preventing infection transmission in the facility. Other functions include review of infection control data, approval of policies and procedures, monitoring program activities, and recommending policy to the facility administration. *(BIII)*
- *Comment:* Those responsible for infection control program oversight should meet on a regular basis and as needed for emergent situations and should keep written minutes of all meetings. The minutes should reflect problem identification and follow-up action.

➤ Infection Control Practitioner (ICP)

- One person, the ICP, should be assigned the responsibility of directing infection control activities in the LTCF. The ICP should be someone familiar with LTCF resident-care problems. *(BIII)*
- The ICP should have a written job description of infection control duties. *(BIII)*

- The ICP is responsible for implementing, monitoring, and evaluating the infection control program for the LTCF. *(BIII)*
- The ICP requires the support of administration to function effectively. *(BIII)*
- The ICP should be guaranteed sufficient time to direct the infection control program. *(BIII)*
- The ICP (or another appropriate individual, such as the medical director) should have written authority to institute infection control measures (such as isolation or visitor restrictions) in emergency situations. *(BIII)*
- *Comment:* The ICP should have a sufficient infection control knowledge base to carry out responsibilities appropriately. A background in infectious diseases, microbiology, geriatrics, and educational methods is advisable. Management and teaching skills also are helpful. Continuing education is essential for the ICP. The ICP should know the federal, state, and local regulations dealing with infection control in the LTCF. Communication is an important part of infection control. The ICP should communicate with relevant facility committees and personnel. The ICP should communicate openly with hospital ICPs about residents transferred into or out of the LTCF, to ensure appropriate isolation and collection of surveillance information.

➤ Surveillance

- The LTCF should have a system for ongoing collection of data on infections in the institution. *(BIII)*
- A documented surveillance procedure should be used, including written definitions of infections. *(BIII)*
- *Comment:* Concurrent surveillance is preferable to retrospective surveillance. The frequency of surveillance for nosocomial infections should be based on factors such as acuity level of the

resident population. Surveillance, generally at least once a week is needed to collect timely data. Surveillance data should be collected primarily from communication with staff; this may be during walking rounds in the LTCF. Medical progress notes in the chart, laboratory or radiology reports, nursing notes, treatment records, medication records, physical assessment environmental observations, and follow-up information from transfers to acute care hospitals provide clues to the presence of infections.

- The ICP should review surveillance data frequently and recommend infection control measures, as appropriate, in response to identified problems. *(BIII)*
- *Comment:* Analysis of surveillance data should include at least the following elements on each infection to detect clusters and trends: type of infection, data of onset, location in the facility, appropriate culture information, and risk factors. An infection surveillance report form facilitates recording of data on residents with nosocomial infections.
- Infection rates should be calculated periodically, recorded, analyzed, and reported to the administration and staff. *(BIII)*
- *Comment:* Infection rates usually are calculated monthly, quarterly, and annually. Nosocomial infection rates are calculated preferably as nosocomial infections per days of risk (e.g., resident days, catheter days). A standard infection report form facilitates reporting of surveillance information. Tables, graphs, and charts may be used to facilitate education of personnel.
- Surveillance data should be used for planning infection control effort, detecting epidemics, directing continuing education, and identifying individual resident problems for interventions. *(BIII)*

- **Outbreak Control**
  - Surveillance data should be used to detect and prevent outbreaks in the LTCF. *(BIII)*
  - The facility should define authority for intervention during an outbreak. *(BIII)*
  - A TB control program should focus on detection of cases in residents, period screening of employees, and isolation or transfer of residents with known or suspected TB disease. *(BIII)*
- **The Facility**
  - Handwashing facilities that are conveniently located with adequate supplies should be available for residents and staff. *(BIII)*
  - Clean and dirty utility areas should be functionally separate and designated. *(BIII)*
  - Appropriate ventilation and air filtration should be addressed by the LTCF. *(BIII)*
  - Housekeeping in the facility should be performed on a routine and consistent basis to provide for a safe and sanitary environment. *(BIII)*

    Measures should be instituted to correct unsafe and unsanitary practices. *(BIII)*

    Areas in the LTCF with unique infection control concerns (e.g., laundry, kitchen, physical therapy) should have appropriate policies and procedures developed. *(BIII)*

    Policies and procedures for disposal of infectious medical waste (including waste categorization, packaging, collection, transport, and disposal) should be developed in accordance with federal, state, and local regulations. *(BIII)*

➤ Isolation and Precautions

- Isolation and precautions policies and procedures should be developed, evaluated, and updated. Compliance (e.g., with handwashing) should be monitored. *(BIII)*
- Any isolation and precautions system used should include wearing of masks, eye protection, and gowns when contamination or splashing with blood or body fluids is likely. *(BIII)*
- Used needles and syringes should not be manually recapped, broken, or bent. They should be disposed of, as with all sharps, in a puncture-resistant, leak-proof container. *(BIII)*
- Gloves are indicated for contact with blood or body fluids, contaminated items, mucous membranes, or non-intact skin. *(BIII)*
- Policies should be developed to deal with spills and personnel exposure to blood or body fluids. Employees should know how to respond to an exposure. *(BIII)*
- The facility should have infection control policies dealing with acceptance and transfer of residents with infectious diseases. *(BIII)*

➤ Asepsis and Handwashing

- Handwashing should be encouraged. Hands should be washed after contact with body fluids, after removing gloves, when soiled, and when otherwise indicated. *(AII)*
- A handwashing policy and procedure should be developed by the LTCF. *(BIII)*
- Policies and procedures for disinfection and sterilization should be developed. *(BIII)*

➤ Resident Care

- Resident rooms should have an accessible sink, with soap, water, towels, and toilet facilities. *(BIII)*
- A resident skincare program should be developed to maintain the skin as a barrier to infection. *(BIII)*

- A program to prevent UTIs should address catheter use, catheter insertion, closed drainage systems, irrigation of catheters, maintenance of urinary flow, and indications for changing the catheter. *(BIII)*
- *Comment:* If leg bags are used, the LTCF should develop policies and procedures for aseptic connection, cleaning, and storage of leg bags. Intermittent catheterization is an alternative to an indwelling catheter.
- A program to minimize the risk of pneumonia in the LTCF should address immunizations, reducing the potential for aspiration following feeding, minimizing atelectasis, and caring for respiratory therapy equipment. *(BIII)*
- Policies and procedures should be developed for prevention of infections associated with nasogastric and gastrostomy feeding tubes, including preparation, storage, refrigeration, and administration of feeding solutions. *(BIII)*
- Policies and procedures should be developed for prevention of IV infections, if IV devices are used. *(BIII)*

➤ **Resident Health Program**

- Each resident should have an initial history (including important past and present infectious diseases), immunization status evaluation, recent physical examination, and intradermal (Mantoux) tuberculin skin test. *(BIII)*
- *Comment:* A recent chest radiograph is advisable if the skin test is positive.
- All newly admitted residents should receive TB screening by the intradermal (Mantoux) tuberculin method unless a physician's statement is obtained that the resident had a past positive reaction to tuberculin. When new or active TB is suggested by a positive skin-test result and/or by symptoms, a chest radiograph and medical evaluation should be obtained. *(BIII)*

- Follow-up skin testing for TB should be performed periodically or after discovery of a new case of TB in a resident or staff member. The intradermal Mantoux method should be used. *(BIII)*
- Each resident should receive tetanus and diphtheria vaccine every 10 years (or when clinically indicated). This should be recorded in the resident's chart. *(AII)*
- Each resident should receive the pneumococcal vaccine if indicated. This should be recorded in the resident's chart. *(BIII)*
- Each resident should receive the influenza vaccine annually in the fall, unless medically contraindicated. This should be recorded in the resident's chart. *(AII)*
- Policies and procedures addressing visitors should be developed to deal with introduction of community infections (such as influenza) into the LTCF. *(BIII)*

➤ **Employee Health Program**

- All new employees should have a baseline health assessment, including immunization status and history of relevant past or present infectious diseases. *(BIII)*
- All new employees should receive TB screening by the intradermal (Mantoux) method unless a physician's statement is obtained that the employee had a positive reaction to tuberculin. When new or active TB is suggested by a positive skin-test result and/or symptoms, a chest radiograph and medical evaluation should be obtained. *(BIII)*
- Follow-up skin testing for TB should be performed periodically or after discovery of a new case of TB in a resident or staff member. Skin test-negative personnel should undergo repeat skin testing at regular intervals as determined by a risk assessment. The intradermal Mantoux method should be used. *(BIII)*

- All employees should have current immunizations, with documentation in the employee's (health) record, including tetanus and diphtheria vaccination every 10 years. *(BIII)*
- Employees with blood or body fluid contact should be offered HBV vaccination. Administration of the vaccine or refusal should be documented in the employee's health record. *(AII)*
- Employees should be offered the influenza vaccine annually in the fall. *(AII)*
- Each employee should be taught basic hygiene and handwashing and to consider blood and all body fluids as potentially infectious. *(BIII)*
- Employees with signs or symptoms of communicable disease (e.g., cough, rash, and diarrhea) should not have contact with the residents or their food. *(BIII)*
- All employees should be educated to report any significant infectious illnesses to the staff member responsible for employee health. *(BIII)*
- The LTCF should develop protocols for managing employee illnesses and exposures (such as HBV, HIV, TB scabies). *(BIII)*
- *Comment:* An employee absentee policy that discourages the employee from working while ill should be developed.

➤ Education

- Infection control education should be provided at the initiation of employment and regularly thereafter. Training should include all staff; especially those providing direct resident care. *(BIII)*
- All programs should be documented with the date, topic, names of attendees, and evaluations. *(C)*
- *Comment:* Program topics and frequency should be based on assessment and relevant to infection prevention and control.

➤ **Policies and Procedures**

- Infection control policies and procedures should be approved, reviewed, and revised on a regular basis. *(BIII)*
- Employees should be made aware of infection control policies and procedures. *(BIII)*
- *Comment:* The ICP should develop a system for monitoring staff compliance with infection control policies and procedures.

➤ **Antibiotic Resistance and Monitoring**

- The ICP should monitor antibiotic susceptibility results from cultures to detect clinically significant antibiotic-resistant bacteria (such as MRSA or VRE) in the institution. Changes in antibiotic-susceptibility trends should be communicated to appropriate individuals and committees. *(BIII)*
- The LTCF should have a policy dealing with resistant bacteria. *(BIII)*
- Infection control programs in LTCFs should be encouraged to include a component of antimicrobial utilization review. *(BIII)*
- *Comment:* The LTCF should encourage prudent antimicrobial prescribing. In selected LTCFs, a more intensive antimicrobial utilization review program may be developed, including review of antibiotic appropriateness.

➤ **Miscellaneous Aspects**

- There should be a system for reporting notifiable disease to proper public health officials.
- The ICP should communicate with the director of the QM program. *(BIII)*

The ICP may be involved with the infection control implications of new products and the safety program as needed. *(C)*

The ICP may be involved with other activities relevant to infection control, as compatible with program goals and time constraints. *(C)*

References/Resources

- Association for Professionals in Infection Control and Epidemiology. APIC Text of Infection Control and Epidemiology. 2000, chapters 35, 46.
- Bartley J Ed. Guidelines for Prevention and Control of Antimicrobial Resistant Organisms (ARO) – Focus on: MRSA and VRE. 2002. Michigan Society for Infection Control. www.MSIC-online.org
- Bonilla HF, Zervos MA, and Lyons MJ, et al. Colonization with vancomycin-resistant Enterococcus faecium: Comparison of a long-term care unit with an acute care hospital. Infect Control Hosp Epidemiol 1997; 18:333–339.
- Joint Commission on Accreditation of Healthcare Organizations. Long-term care standards. Chicago: JCAHO; 2000.
- Nicolle LE. Asymptomatic bacteriuria in the elderly. Infect Dis Clin North Am 1997; 11:647–662.
- Smith PW, Rushnak PG. Infection prevention and control in the long-term care facility. Am J Infect Control 1997; 25(6):488–512.

Neonates

Overview

- Neonates are a special population with the potential for increased risk of infection. Several factors affect risk including method of acquisition, maternal complications, and infant host factors.
- Improved technologies coupled with interventional procedures have allowed survival of immature neonates not possible a few years ago. Additionally, improved prenatal care has allowed proactive approaches to decrease complications and undesirable outcomes.

Purpose

- Both basic and specialized infection control strategies can help reduce infections in neonates.

Risk Factors

- Method of acquisition may affect risk:
  - Transplacental *(in utero)* transmission.
  - Intrapartum as a result of direct contact with maternal genital tract, blood, or stool.
  - Postnatal as a result of contact with mother, other newborns in the nursery, personnel, visitors, or inanimate objects.
  - Infections in the first few days of life; usually due to organisms acquired from the maternal genital tract that have colonized in the newborn's gastrointestinal or respiratory tract, skin, or mucous membranes.
  - Later infections occurring during nursery stay as a result of organisms acquired from sources in the nursery (e.g., other infants).

- Maternal complications that affect risk of neonatal infections:
  - Low birth weight and premature delivery.
  - Premature rupture of membranes; especially if more than 24 hours before delivery (increases the exposure of the fetus to potential pathogens from the maternal genital tract).
  - Fetal monitoring devices (e.g., scalp electrodes and skin abrasions from traumatic delivery); may provide portals of entry for potential pathogens from maternal genital tract.
  - C-section delivery; may be associated with an increased incidence of respiratory distress syndrome and consequent risk of infection.
- Neonatal host factors that affect risk of infection:
  - Absence of normal (protective) flora at birth; facilitates colonization with potential pathogens.
  - Prematurity, low birth weight, congenital anomalies and perinatal anoxia; associated with prolonged hospital stay, increased invasive device utilization, and higher risk of nosocomial infection.
  - Impaired barrier function (e.g., skin, lungs).
  - Immature immune system (e.g., poor antibody production).
  - Breast milk; considered to be protective by favoring growth of "normal flora" and providing specific IgA antibody, macrophages, lymphocytes, and antibacterial substances (e.g., lactoferrin, lysozyme).
- Microorganisms of nosocomial importance in the neonate:
  - *S. aureus:* Newborn colonization is common but disease is rare; outbreaks of MRSA may occur in the NICU; personnel may become carriers; most infections are superficial and cutaneous; less commonly bacteremia, pneumonia, and other serious infections.
  - Coagulase-negative staphylococci: Normal inhabitants of the skin and nose; rarely cause disease in healthy term newborns; colonize prosthetic material, especially intravascular catheters, ventricular

drains and shunts, and endotracheal tubes; low birth weight, prolonged stay in the NICU, parenteral lipids, and central venous catheters are risk factors; the most frequent manifestation is indolent bacteremia without focal findings.

- Enterococci: A cause of late-onset bacteremia, meningitis, pneumonia, and soft-tissue abscesses in the NICU; bowel resection and central venous catheters increase risk of infection; relatively resistant to antibiotics.
- Aerobic Gram-negative bacilli (e.g., *E. coli, Klebsiella, Citrobacter, Enterobacter)*: Part of the newborn's stool flora acquired from the mother or the NICU; important causes of bacteremia, meningitis, pneumonia, and UIT.
- *Pseudomonas sp.*: Found in water or moist environment; may cause sepsis, pneumonia, and UTIs; the major cause of nosocomial neonatal endophthalmitis.
- *Candida sp.*: Intrauterine infection is rare; acquired frequently at birth; *C. albicans* most common; manifestation varies from superficial skin infection to disseminated infection involving lungs, central nervous system, and other organs; risk factors for disseminated infection include low birth weight, antibiotic therapy, parenteral nutrition (particularly lipids), abdominal surgery, prolonged NICU stay (longer than four weeks).
- *Malassezia sp.*: May cause fungemia in infants receiving lipids; colonizes on skin and intravascular catheters.
- RSV: Outbreaks are common in NICU; pneumonia is more common in premature infants; newborn may acquire infection from mother, family, hospital staff, or other infants in the nursery; may be transmitted by fomites.
- Rotavirus infection: Endemic in many NICUs; majority of infected infants are asymptomatic; premature infants have less severe disease possibly because of immaturity of the GI tract;

endemic nursery strains may be less virulent than those from the community.

- Hepatitis A: Excretion is prolonged in the newborn; infected infants usually are asymptomatic; outbreaks may be recognized only when staff or parents become ill.

Strategies for Prevention and Control

- Refer to Sections 2 and 3 for General Prevention and Control Measures (e.g., handwashing and hand hygiene, Standard Precautions, aseptic technique, care of invasive devices, optimal cleaning, disinfection, and sterilization).
- Refer to Section 5 for Employee Health considerations.
- Refer to Section 2 - Environmental Maintenance and Construction/Renovation. Although the guidelines do not apply to home care settings, the risk factors and general principles of risk reduction may be adapted for the home setting.
- Setting/Population specific considerations
  - Recognize transmission of selected infectious agents from mother to the newborn and screen mother and treat as appropriate.

    Cytomegalovirus

    In utero transmission occurs in 1–3% of all pregnancies; most infections are asymptomatic in the newborn; may occur with primary maternal infection or reactivation; primary maternal infection associated with a transmission rate of 4%, with 10–20% of infected infants being symptomatic; infection after reactivation is rarely symptomatic.

    Intrapartum and postnatal transmission via breast milk are more common than *in utero* infections; usually asymptomatic; severe disease may occur in very low birth weight infants.

Herpes simplex virus

Transmission increased with maternal primary genital infection (~40% vs. ~5% with recurrent infection); lack of maternal antibody and high viral shedding found in primary infection are thought to facilitate transmission in this setting.

Transmission is usually intrapartum; increased risk with prolonged rupture of membranes, premature delivery, maternal cervical lesions at delivery, and use of scalp electrodes.

Transplacental transmission is less common but can be associated with severe infections (e.g., hydronencephaly, microcephaly, ocular malformations, and intracranial calcifications); postnatal transmission may also result in severe disease (e.g., encephalitis, disseminated disease).

Varicella-zoster virus

Congenital varicella syndrome (e.g., limb hypoplasia, cutaneous scarring, ocular defects, mental retardation) occurs in ~2% of newborns of mothers with varicella in the first or early second trimester.

Severe disseminated neonatal varicella (e.g., vesicular skin/mucosal lesions, pneumonia, hepatitis, meningoencephalitis) due to lack of antibody in the newborn may occur if maternal varicella develops from five days before to two days after delivery; maternal infection >5 days before delivery or postnatal transmission usually is associated with mild disease in the newborn.

Rubella

In utero transmission during first trimester is efficient (~80%) and is associated with severe congenital disease (e.g., cardiac malformations, deafness, cataracts, microphthalmia, hepatosplenomegaly, petechiae, retinopathy, radiographic bone abnormalities) in infected fetus in 85% of cases.

Second-trimester transmission risk is 39% with a lower risk of congenital defects (primarily hearing loss).

Third-trimester transmission risk is high particularly during the last month (up to 100%), but symptomatic disease in the newborn is rare.

Hepatitis B virus (HBV)

Transmission is primarily intrapartum; highest risk associated with mothers with positive hepatitis B early antigen (HBe) but no anti-HBe antibody (rate is 80–90%), or with acute hepatitis in the third trimester (rate is 60–70%).

In utero transmission is rare and occurs mostly during acute maternal infection.

Most infected newborns are asymptomatic, but are at high risk (75–100%) of becoming chronic carriers of HBV.

Hepatitis B vaccine and Hepatitis B Immune Globulin (HBIG) should be administered within 12 hours of birth to babies born to mothers with positive HbsAg.

Human immunodeficiency virus (HIV)

Intrapartum or postnatal transmission via breast milk accounts for 70% of cases *in utero* transmission.

Overall risk of transmission without antiretroviral therapy in the mother is 14–39%; reduced to 8% by use of zidovudine initiated during pregnancy.

Advanced maternal disease and high maternal viral titers increase risk of transmission.

Initially asymptomatic in newborn; later complications such as failure to thrive, pneumonitis, and opportunistic infections.

Parvovirus B19

Transmission occurs during primary acute maternal infection; the rate is unclear.

Overall rate of fetal loss is 4–9%; highest with infection during first 20 weeks of gestation.

Associated with hydrops fetalis and anemia in the newborn.

Enteroviruses (e.g., Echovirus, Coxsackie virus)

Transmission intrapartum is most common; often associated with mild febrile illness, rash, or aseptic meningitis.

Disease at birth may be associated with severe hepatitis, myocarditis, and meningoencephalitis, suggestive of transplacental transmission.

Toxoplasmosis

Transmission occurs during primary maternal infection.

First trimester transmission rate is 10–15%, but associated with high risk of severe disease (e.g., hydrocephalus, chorioretinitis, jaundice, deafness).

Second trimester transmission rate is 30%, associated with 40% asymptomatic infection.

Third trimester transmission rate is 60%, but most infections are asymptomatic.

Pregnant women should avoid contact with cat feces and litter.

Syphilis

Transmission occurs primarily *in utero*; occasionally by passage through birth canal.

Transmission rate varies: maternal primary or secondary syphilis is 70–100%; tertiary syphilis is 30%.

Most infected infants develop symptoms in infancy (e.g., hepatosplenomegaly, jaundice, lymphadenopathy, pneumonia, meningoencephalitis, hepatitis, anemia) or early childhood (e.g., dental and bone abnormalities, interstitial keratitis, deafness).

Chlamydia trachomatis

Transmission is intrapartum (rate is 50%).

Conjunctivitis in 25–50% of infected newborns; mild pneumonia at 1–4 months of age in 5–20% of infected newborns.

Gonorrhea

Transmission is intrapartum.

Commonly associated with conjunctivitis, which may progress to corneal damage and endophthalmitis.

Newborns should receive silver nitrate drops, erythromycin, or tetracycline ointment in eyes immediately after birth.

Group B streptococcus

Transmission is usually peripartum (shortly before or intrapartum); rate is 50%.

Only 1–2% of colonized newborns develop disease.

Postnatal transmission from mother, family, or nursery sources also may occur.

Associated with respiratory distress, hypoperfusion, coagulopathy, bacteremia, and meningitis (the leading cause of neonatal sepsis and meningitis in most centers in North America and Europe).

Listeriosis

Transmission may occur *in utero*; transplacental transmission may result in disseminated abscesses and/or granulomas in multiple internal organs (granulomatosis infantiseptica).

Intrapartum or postpartum infection may also occur and is associated with central nervous system infection (e.g., meningitis) after three days of age.

Tuberculosis

Transmission may occur *in utero* with miliary TB, intrapartum via aspiration of endometrial organisms, and postnatal secondary to pulmonary TB.

Fever, hepatomegaly, lymphadenopathy, splenomegaly, pneumonia, failure to thrive, and biliary obstruction may occur.

- Normal newborn nursery

Most nursery-acquired infections are superficial infections of the skin, mucous membranes, and eyes.

Outbreaks are commonly due to true pathogens (e.g., *S. aureus*, group A streptococci, respiratory viruses, GI pathogens).

- Neonatal intensive care units (NICU)

Skin and mucous membrane infections are common.

Bacteremia (usually related to central venous catheters), respiratory tract infections, and GI tract infections occur frequently.

Common pathogens include *S. aureus*, coagulase-negative staphylococci, Gram-negative bacilli, *Candida*, and respiratory tract viruses.

Twenty-five percent (25%) of newborns with bacteremia have meningitis; signs and symptoms are similar.

Risk of early onset (7 days or less after birth) sepsis is increased with prematurity, low birth weight, premature rupture of membranes, maternal fever, chorioamnionitis, bacteremia, and UTI; common causes include group B streptococci, *E. coli*, and *Listeria* species.

Late-onset sepsis (longer than seven days after birth) acquired in the NICU is associated with low birth weight, central venous lines, parenteral hyperalimentation (particularly lipids), and surgery; often due to coagulase-negative *Staphylococcus, S. aureus*, enterococci, or aerobic Gram-negative bacilli.

Early-onset pneumonia is usually related to intrapartum infection and early-onset sepsis, particularly group B streptococci; nosocomial pneumonia often due to Gram-negative bacilli, *S. aureus, S. epidermidis*, or viruses; ureoplasma of maternal origin may cause severe pneumonia in very low birth weight babies; endotracheal intubation is a major risk factor; definite diagnosis is often difficult.

Necrotizing enterocolitis (NEC) results from injury to the immature GI tract; associated with ischemia, GI bacteria, and oral feeding, providing substrate for bacterial growth and/or toxin production. Diagnosis requires the following conditions (CDC, 1988):

Two of the following, without other recognized cause: vomiting, abdominal distention, or prefeeding residuals *and* persistent blood in the stools on microscopic or gross examination *and* any of the following radiographic abnormalities: pneumoperitoneum, pneumatosis intestínalis, or unchanged "rigid" loops of the small bowel.

- IC Program
  - Surveillance

    Normal newborns usually have a very short length of stay and routine surveillance is not indicated.

    High-risk neonates in Neonatal Intensive Care Units are at higher risk for infection and closer monitoring for clusters and outbreaks is indicated.

    High-risk neonates have increased numbers of invasive devices that should be considered in surveillance activities.

References/Resources

- American Academy of Pediatrics www.aap.org
- American Academy of Pediatrics. 1999 Red Book: Elk Grove Village, IL: American Academy of Pediatrics.
- Armstrong D. Listeria monocytogenes. In: Mandell GL, Bennett JE, Dolin R, Eds. Principles and practice of infectious diseases. New York: Churchill Livingstone; 1995. p 1880–1885.
- Association for Professionals in Infection Control and Epidemiology. APIC Text of Infection Control and Epidemiology. 2000, chapters 36,48,49,50
- Connor EM, Sperling RS, Gelber R, et al. Reduction of maternal–infant transmission of human immunodeficiency virus type I with zidovudine treatment. N Engl J Med 1994; 331:1173–1180.
- Moore DL. Infections in neonates. In: Olmsted RN, editor. Infection control and applied epidemiology: principles and practice. St. Louis, MO: Mosby; 1996. P. 47-1–47-18.

- Pelke S, Ching D, Easa D, Melish ME. Gowning does not affect colonization or infection rates in a neonatal intensive care unit. Arch Pediatr Adolesc Med 1994; 148:1016-20.
- Tramont EC. Treponema pallidum (syphilis). In Mandell GL, Bennett JE, Dolin R, editors. Principles and practice of infectious diseases. New York: Churchill Livingstone; 1995. P. 2117–2133.

Obstetrics

Overview

➤ The majority of obstetric (OB) patients have intact host defense mechanisms and have not had prolonged exposure to systemic antimicrobial therapy nor prolonged hospitalization prior to delivery. In addition, most do not require extensive invasive diagnostic and monitoring procedures. Therefore most OB patients are not generally at high risk for infection prior to delivery. High-risk OB patients are more likely to require multiple prepartum hospitalizations and exposure to invasive devices such as indwelling urinary catheters, intravascular devices, and intrauterine pressure and fetal monitoring placing them and their fetus at increased risk of infection.

Purpose

➤ During prepartum and intrapartum care, both the health and well-being of the mother and the neonate must be considered and infection control prevention strategies implemented to reduce associated infection risks for both mother and neonate.

Risk Factors

➤ Prepartum

- Maternal infection prepartum (e.g., Hepatitis B, Varicella, Listeria, Group B Strep, HIV, Chlamydia, *Herpes simplex*) (Refer to Section 5 - Pregnant Employee and Section 4 – Neonates)
- Lack of prenatal care
- Malnutrition
- Anemia
- Prolonged prepartum hospitalization

- Prolonged rupture of membranes (PROM) (usually > 24 hours prior to delivery), which is associated with perinatal infection, preterm delivery, and related complications.
- Use of internal pressure catheter for monitoring contractions or for amnioinflusion, which is associated with increased risk of Intraamniotic fluid infection.
- Use of internal fetal electrodes for fetal heart rate monitoring.
- Vaginal examinations.
- Use of baths and whirlpools.
- Intraamniotic infection syndrome (IAIS) risk estimated at 1% to 2% of term deliveries and up to 25% for preterm deliveries. Risk factors include:

  PROM

  Intrauterine trauma

➤ Delivery

- Endometritis-For vaginal deliveries, risk estimated to be between 0.9% and 3.9% of deliveries; for Caesarian Section (C/S), risk estimated from 5% for elective procedures and up to 85% for nonelective procedures with large teaching centers caring for indigent patients at the highest end. Risk factors include:

  Placement in vagina of intrauterine forceps or physicians hands at time of delivery.

  Retained placenta.

- Surgical site infection

  Episiotomy infections occur in about 0.09 to 0.3 per 100 procedures and are usually mild.

  C/S incision infections occur in about 4% of deliveries.

    Superficial site infection

Deep site infection

Organ/Space infection

- Postpartum
  - Maternal infection risks:

    Septic pelvic thrombophlebitis estimated to occur in one out of every 2000 deliveries. Risk factors include:

      C/S after prolonged labor

      PROM

      Traumatic delivery

      Anemia

      Malnourishment

      Other systemic disease

    Breast infection risk estimated at 1% to 3%; risk factors include:

    Inadequate emptying of breasts

    Improper positioning of infant

    Inadequate nipple care

    Urinary tract infection occur frequently in postpartum women; risk factors include:

      Bladder catheterization at delivery

      History of UTI

      C/S

      Forceps delivery or vacuum extraction

      Epidural anesthesia

- Neonatal infection risk factors:

  Contact of neonates with their infected mothers. (Refer to Section 4-Neonates)

  Neonate ingestion of contaminated breast milk.

  Other risk factors. (Refer to Section 4 – Neonates)

Strategies for Prevention

- ➤ Assessment
  - Screening and treatment for maternal infections should be done early in prepartum care.
  - Screening and counseling should be provided for maternal nutrition, infection risks, and general health and safety throughout the prepartum period.
- ➤ Refer to Sections 2 and 3 for General Prevention and Control Measures (e.g., handwashing and hand hygiene, Standard Precautions, aseptic technique, care of invasive devices, optimal cleaning, disinfection, and sterilization).
- ➤ Refer to Section 5 for Employee Health considerations.
- ➤ Refer to Section 2 - Environmental Maintenance and Construction/Renovation.
- ➤ Although the guidelines do not apply to home care settings, the risk factors and general principles of risk reduction may be adapted for the home setting.
- ➤ Population specific strategies
  - Prepartum

    Clinical guidelines for management of the patient with PROM should be developed although the literature does not provide any conclusive evidence for strategies that reduce infection.

Aseptic technique should be used including use of sterile solutions, appropriate disinfection and sterilization of transducer domes and maintenance of a closed system for internal pressure catheters and fetal electrodes.

The number of vaginal examinations should be limited to those clinically necessary and personnel should wash hands and don clean gloves before performing examinations.

Digital examination of the cervix should be avoided until active labor occurs or until the decision has been made to induce labor.

Bladder catheterization should be avoided whenever possible.

Shaving of perineal (pubic) hair has not been shown to decrease risk of infection and in fact has been associated with increased infection risks; if better visualization is needed, clipping of hair is recommended.

Baths and whirlpools should be drained, cleaned, and disinfected according to manufacturer's guidelines. Refer to Section 4 - Rehabilitation Services for details on maintaining whirlpools and tubs.

- Delivery

Vaginal delivery

There is no supportive literature to require family members attending vaginal delivery to don scrub attire versus wearing a clean gown over street clothing.

Caesarean delivery (C/S)

All standards for surgical services should be used in the C/S suites. (Refer to Section 4-Surgical Services)

Studies have demonstrated that short-course prophylaxis significantly decrease endometritis after nonelective C/S (e.g., C/S after ROM or prolonged labor).

Meticulous surgical technique to reduce contamination of peritoneal cavity with amniotic fluid (Refer to Section 3 – Surgical Site Infections).

- Postpartum

  Breast milk strategies should include:

  Mothers handwashing before touching nipples.

  Mothers cleansing of nipples with water and drying before expressing milk.

  Mothers discarding the first 5-10 mL of milk.

  Storage of breast milk at 34-40°F.

  Storage of breast milk for no longer than 48 hours, unless frozen.

  Rapid thawing of frozen milk and discarding of unused thawed milk after 24 hours.

  Sterile transfer of milk between containers.

  Change of syringe and tubing every 12 hours for continuous infusion of breast milk.

  Thorough cleaning and disinfection of breast pumps between use if individual breast pumps cannot be used.

  Mothers with vesicular HSV lesions on the breasts, active TB, Primary CMV, Hepatitis B, and HIV and HTLV I/II should discuss potential contraindications for breast-feeding with their physicians.

➤ IC Program aspects

- Interdisciplinary involvement in the IC program should include nursing, physicians, therapists, and other support personnel.

- Surveillance

  Data collection for endometritis and surgical site infections should include post discharge methods due to the shortness of maternal/newborn length of stay (average two days for vaginal delivery and four days for C/S for uncomplicated deliveries) (Refer to Section 1 – Acute Care Nosocomial Surveillance).

  A single case of Group A Beta hemolytic streptococci (GAS), also known as puerperal fever/sepsis or childbed fever, should be considered a sentinel event and an outbreak investigation and control plan initiated due to the potential for transmission to other patients in labor and delivery. (Refer to Section 1 - Outbreak Investigation)

  Postpartum fevers in C/S patients are common and often not associated with infection.

  Infections in neonates resulting from passage through the birth canal are considered to be nosocomial.

  An infection known or proved to have been acquired transplacentally (e.g., cytomegalovirus, rubella) and that becomes evident at or before 48 hours after birth is not considered to be nosocomial.

➤ Education

- Staff should be provided age/condition specific education regarding infection risks and strategies to reduce risks and prevent infection.
- Staff should be able to demonstrate understanding and skills.
- Mothers should be taught techniques and importance of perineal care especially after voiding and defecation.
- Mothers should be taught techniques to reduce nipple trauma and mastitis.
- Mothers and family members should be taught techniques for preventing breast milk contamination.

References/Resources

- The American College of obstetricians and Gynecologists. Evaluation of Cesarean Delivery. 2000.
- The American College of obstetricians and Gynecologists. Guidelines for Perinatal Care, Fourth Ed. 1997.
- The American College of Obstetricians and Gynecologists. Precis: Obstetrics, Second Ed. 2000.
- The American College of obstetricians and Gynecologists. www.acog.org
- Association for Professionals in Infection Control and Epidemiology. APIC Text of Infection Control and Epidemiology. 2000, chapter 49.
- Infectious Diseases Society for Obstetrics and Gynecology. In: Mead PB, Hager WD, Eds. Infection Protocols for Obstetrics and Gynecology. Montaval NJ: Medical Economics; 1992
- Mead PB. Prevention and control of nosocomial infection in obstetrics and gynecology. In: Wentzel RP, Ed. Prevention and Control of Nosocomial Infection. 3rd Ed, revised. Baltimore: Williams and Wilkins; 1997.

Pediatrics

Overview

- Pediatric patients may be cared for in ambulatory or inpatient settings. Children cared for may be well or seriously ill. Pediatric settings are designed to provide comfort to the child as well as provide a safe environment for treatment. Infection risks and prevention strategies will depend upon the extent of illness and the child's age group.

Purpose

- Pediatric settings pose special risks that require unique infection control strategies in addition to basic strategies.

Risk Factors

- Risk of infection varies for children depending on their age group.
  - Age-specific personal hygiene

    Immunologic maturation

    Physiologic factors
- Age-related anatomic and functional characteristics place infants and younger children at higher risk for many infections in comparison to older children (adolescents) and adults.
- Behavior of younger children, including frequent soiling of hands, drooling, runny noses, and mouthing behaviors, contribute to increase risk of infection.
- Young children have close contact with their caregivers(s) and with other children in day care centers, schools, and during play, which also increases the risk of infection transmission.

- Children with chronic health conditions and/or compromised immune systems have more contact with both inpatient and outpatient healthcare settings, increasing their risk for healthcare associated infection.
- Infections of special importance
  - Respiratory syncytial virus (RSV) can cause upper respiratory illness in persons of any age.

    RSV is the most important cause of bronchiolitis and pneumonia in infants and young children.

    During peak RSV season, many infected infants and children may be hospitalized.

    A number of staff and family members may also be infected.
  - Streptococcus group and *Staphylococcus aureus*
  - Infections (e.g., impetigo) are transmitted by direct contact with contaminated items and secretions.
  - Tuberculosis (TB)

    Cough is usually absent in children; however, communicability is still possible.
  - Cystic fibrosis (CF) patients

    CF patients are at increased risk for pulmonary infections.

    Common organisms associated with CF pulmonary infections or colonization include *S. aureus*, *P. aeruginosa*, and *P. cepacia*.
- Latex allergy/sensitivity

    Children with conditions such as spina bifida or history of multiple surgeries are at increased risk for latex allergy.

Strategies for Prevention and Control

- Refer to Sections 2 and 3 for General Prevention and Control Measures (e.g., handwashing and hand hygiene, Standard Precautions, aseptic technique, care of invasive devices, optimal cleaning, disinfection, and sterilization).
- Refer to Section 5 for Employee Health considerations.
- Refer to Section 2 - Environmental Maintenance and Construction/ Renovation. Although the guidelines do not apply to home care settings, the risk factors and general principles of risk reduction may be adapted for the home setting.
- Population specific measures
  - Prevention of RSV transmission. The following strategies are recommended to reduce cross-contamination during peak season:

    Lab screening (rapid test) for RSV upon admission of pediatric patients.

    Cohorting of infected patients/staff.

    Excluding visitors with respiratory infections in the healthcare setting.

    Restricting staff with respiratory infections.

    Strict adherence to handwashing and environmental sanitation.
  - Prevention of Streptococcus group and *Staphylococcus aureus* transmission.

    Handwashing and general asepsis are means of prevention.
  - Tuberculosis (TB)

    Children with asymptomatic primary TB are considered noncontagious; special preventive measures are not necessary.

In children with active TB, a cough is usually absent and cultures are often negative, however, children with active TB should still be isolated using the same precautions as for adults; visitors should wear surgical masks and employees should wear facility-approved respirators.

- Cystic fibrosis (CF) patients

  Meticulous handwashing, environmental sanitation, equipment reprocessing are recommended to reduce cross-transmission of organisms via hands, environmental surfaces, and respiratory equipment.

- Children with latex allergy/sensitivity

  Children with conditions such as spina bifida or history of multiple surgeries should be assessed for latex allergy.

  Latex-free supplies should be available for caring for these individuals.

- Ambulatory care pediatric settings

  Forty percent (40%) of pediatric visits are attributed to infectious diseases; the waiting area may contribute to transmission of infection between children as well as to adult caregivers.

  Consideration should be given to triaging children with communicable diseases to examination rooms as soon as possible to minimize risk of infection transmission.

  Children of all ages should be assessed at each outpatient or inpatient visit for immunization status.

  Children should be immunized according to the recommendations set forth by the Advisory Committee on Immunization Practices (ACIP), the American Academy of Pediatrics (AAP), and the American Academy of Family Physicians (AAFP); Refer to Section 2 – Immunizations.

The local health department should be informed of reportable communicable diseases including sexually transmitted diseases; in some situations, these cases may require referral to social services.

The parents and/or caregivers should be educated regarding risks of infection transmission and preventive strategies including handwashing, food handling, and sanitation.

Caregivers of children with special medical conditions (e.g., with central lines or requiring respiratory treatments) will require additional training to provide care and assess for symptoms of infection.

- Intensive care pediatric settings.

  Risk of nosocomial infection is affected by underlying disease and immune status.

  Use of invasive devices (e.g., vascular catheters, ventilatory devices) and use of antimicrobial agents contribute to higher risk for nosocomial infection.

- Pediatric general care units

  Playrooms and sharing of toys may add to transmission of infection; stuffed animals are not appropriate for shared toys.

  There should be a procedure for routine cleaning of toys and surfaces in the playroom; toys should be washable.

- Day care centers (Refer to Section 4 - Day care Centers)

References/Resources

- American Academy of Pediatrics. Policy Statement: recommendations for preventive pediatric healthcare (RE9939). Pediatrics 2000, 105(3):645.
- American Academy of Pediatrics. 2000 Red Book: Elk Grove Village, IL: American Academy of Pediatrics.

- Churchill RB, Pickering LK. Infection control challenges in child-care centers. In: Rutala WA, Weber DJ, Eds. Infectious disease clinics of North America. Philadelphia: WB Saunders; 1997. P 347–366.
- Association for Professionals in Infection Control and Epidemiology. APIC Text of Infection Control and Epidemiology. 2000, chapters 40, 50.
- Heymann SJ, Brewer TF, Wilson ME, Colditz GA, et al. Pediatric Tuberculosis: what needs to be done to decrease morbidity and mortality. Pediatrics 2000; 106:1-7 available at www.pediatrics.org/cgi/content/full/106/1/e1
- McPherson M, Arang P, Fox H, Lauver C, et al. A new definition of children with special healthcare needs. Pediatrics 1998,102(1): 137-39.

Rehabilitation Services

Overview

- Rehabilitation therapies may be provided in inpatient and outpatient settings. Rehabilitation services include collaborative efforts of nursing, physical therapy, occupational therapy, speech therapy, recreation therapy, informal caregivers, and the client/patient.

Purpose

- Patients may be at higher risk for urinary tract infections, soft tissue infections, aspiration pneumonia, scabies, and airborne diseases due to setting and treatment factors. There are no standard infection control guidelines for rehabilitation services, however, basic infection control principles for prevention and control should be followed in order to reduce infection transmission risks.

Risk Factors

- Patients/clients may have one or more factors or disabilities that increase infection risks (e.g., urinary catheters, incontinence, immobility, chronic disease).
- Treatment modalities/devices are shared amongst patients/clients.
- Use of pools, whirlpools, and aquatic therapy are common and may increase the risk of infection due to contamination by organic matter (e.g., feces, urine, and wound drainage).
- Patients/clients frequently participate in food preparation as part of their treatment plan.

- Admissions to acute and long-term care facilities are common and may expose patients/clients to colonization with antibiotic resistant organisms.
- Long-term use of antibiotics is common.

Strategies for Prevention and Control

- Assessment
  - Patients/clients should be assessed for signs/symptoms of infection prior to participation in activities.
- Refer to Sections 2 and 3 for General Prevention and Control Measures (e.g., handwashing and hand hygiene, Standard Precautions, aseptic technique, care of invasive devices, optimal cleaning, disinfection, and sterilization).
- Refer to Section 5 for Employee Health considerations.
- Refer to Section 2 - Environmental Maintenance and Construction/ Renovation. Although the guidelines do not apply to home care settings, the risk factors and general principles of risk reduction may be adapted for the home setting.
- Setting Specific Measures
  - Policies for participant and caregivers' medical evaluation and follow-up post infectious illness should be established.
  - Policies for providing care to sick patients/clients should be established including criteria for exclusion for communicable illnesses.
  - Hygienic practices

    Caregivers and patients/clients should practice handwashing following toileting, wound care, etc.

    There should be an adequate numbers of sinks at accommodating heights of children and wheelchairs.

Soap, instant hand sanitizers, disposable tissue, and paper towels should be readily available for use.

- Environmental considerations

  Occupational therapy manipulatives and other shared equipment such as walkers, parallel bars, eating surfaces should be washable and cleaned according to an established schedule or when visibly soiled.

  Bathrooms and commodes should be cleaned routinely and when there is visible soiling or contamination.

- Food Preparation:

  Hands should be washed before food preparation, serving, and feeding

  Vinyl gloves should be worn when handling ready to eat and unwrapped food.

  Food brought in from home should be labeled with client name and date and appropriately stored.

  Unused food should be disposed of within 24 hours.

  Foods should be prepared, stored, and handled appropriately. (Refer to Section 2 - Food Handling)

  Patients/clients should be educated regarding the risks of foodborne illness before preparing/handling food.

- Equipment/personal items

  Each participant should have a separate area for storing personal belongings.

  Orthotics used to assist with activities of daily living may need to be molded for body parts having impaired skin integrity resulting in contamination.

    Barriers should be used between patients/clients skin and the orthotic device to reduce contamination risks.

Orthotic devices should be cleaned and disinfected routinely and when visibly soiled.

Pharyngeal/laryngeal visualization and pharyngeal thermal stimulation equipment.

These items should be single-use whenever possible.

Multi-use devices should be cleaned and disinfected with appropriate disinfection after each use. (Refer to Section 2 - Disinfection and Sterilization)

Needles used for sensation testing and surface electrodes should be disposable and disposed of appropriately after each use. (Refer to Section 2 - Environmental Maintenance)

- Pools, aquatic therapy, and whirlpools

  Appropriate levels of chlorine/bromine disinfectant equivalent to 1.2 - 2 ppm free chlorine at a pH of 7.5-7.8 should be maintained and monitored.

  If gross contamination occurs or monitoring indicates, water should be drained and shock disinfection performed by raising chlorine levels to 10 ppm or more per manufacturer instructions. To avoid injury, pools should not be used until chlorine levels return to 1.5-2.0 ppm.

- Hubbard tanks and whirlpools should be cleaned and disinfected between each patient use; manufacturers' instructions should be followed for disinfection surfaces and agitator jets.

➤ IC Program

- There should be interdisciplinary involvement between nursing, therapists, physicians, support personnel, and informal caregivers/ patients.
- Surveillance

  Participants and staff should be evaluated for signs and symptoms of infections.

Communicable disease reporting should be performed according to local and state regulations.

Nosocomial infection surveillance should be performed; long-term care definitions for infection may be applied. (Refer to Section 1)

- Educational of caregivers
  - Caregivers should be provided age/condition specific education regarding infection risks and strategies to reduce risks and prevent infection.
  - Caregivers should be able to demonstrate understanding and skills.
  - Staff, students, volunteers, and family members who provide care should be oriented to the centers infection control policies and procedures.
  - Standard Precautions should be taught to caregivers and patients/clients.

References/Resources

- Association for Professionals in Infection Control and Epidemiology. APIC Text of Infection Control and Epidemiology. 2000, chapters 34,35,46,69.
- Cagle PE. Infection control in special areas, physical therapy. In: Safety and Infection Control. Springhouse, PA: Springhouse Corp. Pp. 249-255.

Surgical Services

Overview

- Surgical Site Infection (SSI) prevention methods must be consistent across the continuum, regardless of healthcare venue. It has been estimated that approximately 75% of all operative procedures in the U.S. are performed in ambulatory, same-day, or outpatient settings. (Also Refer to Sections 2 and 3)

Purpose

- Invasive surgical procedures increase risk of infection transmission. Infection control in surgical services is focused primarily on surgical team technique, operating room air handling, and patient intrinsic risk.

Definitions

- **Intraoperative area** - may include the operating room suite or a procedure room where invasive surgical procedures occur. The intraoperative area of an operating room suite includes the semirestricted (area surrounding the operating room suite) and the restricted (the operating room suite) areas. Intraoperative care begins when the patient enters the invasive procedure area and/or the operating room suite.
- **P/P** - policy / procedure
- **Preoperative area**- may be a holding area for invasive procedures and/or the preoperative area of the operating room. Some preoperative care may be performed in other areas including a central testing area, the inpatient room, or a clinic exam/treatment

room. Preoperative care of the patient begins prior to the start of the surgery.

- **Perioperative** - includes preoperative, intra-operative, and postoperative areas or settings.
- **Postoperative area** - may include the operating room suite, the procedure room, a recovery room/postoperative area, a patient room, or a clinic/treatment room. Postoperative care of the patient begins immediately after the surgical procedure has been completed and/or when the incision is being closed.

Risk Factors

- Patient characteristics
  - Age
  - Nutritional status
  - Diabetes
  - Smoking
  - Obesity
  - Coexistent infections at a remote body site
  - Colonization with microorganisms
  - Altered immune response
  - Length of preoperative stay
- Operative associated characteristics
  - Duration of surgical scrub
  - Skin antisepsis
  - Preoperative shaving
  - Preoperative skin prep
  - Duration of operation
  - Antimicrobial prophylaxis

- Operating room ventilation
- Inadequate sterilization of instruments
- Foreign material in the surgical site
- Surgical drains
- Surgical technique
- Poor hemostasis
- Failure to obliterate dead space
- Tissue trauma
- Insertion of indwelling urinary catheter

Strategies for Prevention and Control

- Assessment
  - Signs and symptoms of upper respiratory infection in the patient should be referred to anesthesia and/or surgeon.
  - Latex allergy status should be determined preoperatively and appropriate personnel should be notified; patients with known or suspected latex allergy must be properly identified per P/P.
  - Surgical patients should be assessed for signs and symptoms of tuberculosis (TB) and other infectious agents that may be spread via airborne, droplet, and/or contact route; P/P should reflect transportation and isolation precautions for such patient.
- Refer to Sections 2 and 3 for General Prevention and Control Measures (e.g., handwashing and hand hygiene, Standard Precautions, aseptic technique, care of invasive devices, optimal cleaning, disinfection, and sterilization).
- Refer to Section 5 for Employee Health considerations.

- Refer to Section 2 - Environmental Maintenance and Construction/ Renovation. Although the guidelines do not apply to home care settings, the risk factors and general principles of risk reduction may be adapted for the home setting.
- Setting specific considerations
  - Preoperative preparation of the patient

    The patient should be provided a clean gown and a cap to cover the hair prior to entering the intraoperative area for the purpose of asepsis.

    The patient should ingest nothing by mouth (NPO) six to eight hours prior to surgical procedure to reduce risk of vomiting, help maintain asepsis, and reduce the risk of aspiration pneumonia.

    Prescribed enema(s) or douche should be performed prior to entrance into the perioperative area whenever possible; ambulatory patients and those admitted the day of surgery should be instructed to self-administer the enema(s) or douche at home.

    Urinary catheterization should be done only if clinically necessary. (Refer to Section 3 – Urinary Tract Infections)
  - Antimicrobial prophylaxis

    Antimicrobial prophylaxis, when ordered, should be provided as directed by the Pharmacy and Therapeutics Formulary or equivalent; prophylaxis should not routinely exceed 24 hours.

    A prescribed antibiotic should be administered by appropriate personnel (e.g., anesthesia) prior to initiation of the surgical procedure, preferably within 60 minutes of incision.
  - Operative Garb

    Proper attire should be worn in compliance with facility policies and procedures. (Refer to Section 2 – Scrubs and Surgical Apparel)

Shoe covers are optional, but recommended when shoes have been worn outside the healthcare facility; shoe covers should be changed whenever visibly soiled or wet; shoe covers must be removed when leaving perioperative area.

Surgical masks should be discarded after use and whenever visibly soiled or wet; masks should not be worn on top of head or around the neck.

Personnel within the surgical field should wear protective eyewear and whenever performing tasks where there is potential for splash; facial shields may be worn over the surgical masks.

Personnel and patients should wear laser-safe eye protection with appropriate wavelength and optical density whenever laser is used.

Fluid resistant gowns and/or fluid resistant boots/footwear should be worn whenever there is a possibility of contamination from large amounts of blood (e.g., massive bleeding trauma cases).

All personnel within the sterile field should wear sterile gowns; gowns must be disposable or reprocessed using manufacturer's guidelines.

- Gloves, surgical scrub, and hand hygiene

  Sterile gloves should be worn when performing sterile procedures and discarded after use or when damaged/torn.

  Double gloving is permitted; both gloves must be discarded after use or when damaged or torn; peeling of layered gloves is not accepted practice.

  Petroleum products should never be used with latex gloves.

  Policies and procedures should address jewelry, nails, nail polish, artificial nails, appliqués, etc. (Refer to Section 2 - Handwashing and Hand Hygiene)

For surgical scrub recommendations, refer to Section 2 - Asepsis and Section 3 - Surgical Site Infections.

- Anesthesia

  A bacterial filter must be placed on the expiration side of the breathing circuit of the ventilation unit.

  The soda lime used in anesthesia is changed after the case; soda lime requirements - top layer is discarded, bottom layer is placed on top, and new layer is placed on bottom.

  Endotracheal tube, filter, and circuit used for anesthesia are discarded after use on the patient.

  Oxygen should be administered using a disposable mask/nasal canula and discarded after each patient use.

  Suction catheters must be used in a manner that prevents infection to the patient and personnel (follow aseptic technique for suctioning through endotracheal tube); a closed circuit catheter is preferred; discard catheter after each use.

  Laryngoscope blades should be decontaminated with an enzymatic solution immediately after patient use; the blades must be high-level disinfected or sterilized after cleaning.

  Anesthesia machines, carts, and monitors not in contact with the patient should be disinfected when contaminated or at least daily; follow manufacturer's guidelines and P/P.

  Ventilators should be dismantled and cleaned according to manufacturer's guidelines; filters should be used on patient circuit to prevent exposure to the ventilator unit; develop P/P.

- Intraoperative techniques

  Aseptic technique and maintenance of the sterile field must be used for all invasive procedures.

  Transferring and positioning of the patient onto the procedure table should be performed using a method to preserve skin integrity, maintain safety, prevent microbial contamination, and provide adequate exposure of the surgical site.

Drainage tubes and catheters should be connected to proper collection containers.

A vomiting patient should be placed on his/her side, to prevent aspiration; severe vomiting should be treated to prevent harm to incision.

Surgical supplies should be opened only when there is reasonable certainty of use during the procedure; facility specific policies and procedures should address reuse.

Counts should be maintained for all sponges, sharps, and/or instruments used during the surgical procedure due to the risk of physical damage to the patient; incorrect counts are handled and reported per procedure.

The pneumatic tourniquet should be used in a manner that prevents damage to the skin and provides protection from fluids; the tourniquet must be disinfected when contaminated with blood or other potentially infectious material or at the end of the surgical case.

Pulse oximetry sensor probes should be placed on clean, dry, intact skin only.

Perfusion equipment that is in direct contact with mucous membranes, blood, or body fluids should be disposable or be cleaned, and high-level disinfected or sterilized after each patient use.

Blood bag(s) should be handled in a manner to prevent contamination to blood and/or blood bag.

- Disinfection and sterilization of equipment.

  Decontamination of instruments should begin immediately after completion of the surgical procedure; an enzymatic solution is preferred.

Sharp instruments should be handled using a non-contact method to prevent injury from blood and/or body fluids; disposable sharps must be discarded into approved sharps disposal containers.

Perfusion machines, carts, and monitors not in contact with the patient should be disinfected when contaminated or at least daily; follow manufacturer's guidelines and facilities procedures.

Equipment/instrumentation with fluid tank may pose risk as microorganism reservoir and should be approved by Infection Control; must have P/P for disinfecting and maintaining the equipment.

Creutzfeldt-Jakob disease (CJD)
(Refer to Section 2 - Disinfection and Sterilization)

- Pathology

  Tissue should be collected and transferred using aseptic technique; tissue should be transplanted immediately, whenever possible; tissue not used immediately should be processed and/or stored in a controlled, safe environment per facility policies and procedures.

  Refrigerators used for tissue storage should be monitored according to hospital policy; an alarm system may be required for temperature control.

  Blood and blood products should be obtained and administered following guidelines and facility specific policies and procedures.

  Follow Standard Precautions in handling blood/tissue/specimens and other potentially infectious material when obtaining, transporting, and preparing specimens for transport.

  Culture specimen(s) should be transported immediately to the laboratory in order to prevent contamination, overgrowth, or degradation.

Tissues for histology should be carefully placed in preservative as soon as practical per procedure.

Amputated limbs should be placed in impervious wrappers, double-bagged, and delivered to appropriate area per P/P.

Release of surgical specimens and/or items contaminated with blood or other potentially infectious materials is discouraged. It is important to develop specific policies and procedures and it is recommended that an affidavit be signed prior to release.

- Environment

  Handwashing sinks should be equipped with foot, knee, or electronically activated levers whenever possible.

  Sinks used for the disposal of liquid wastes should be available in soiled utility rooms; if a separate room is not available, these sinks must be designated with appropriate signage.

  Storage of clean and sterile supplies must be in an area kept dry and free of dust.

  Items should be removed from external shipping cartons before entry into the perioperative area whenever possible; external shipping cartons must not be used for storage; corrugated cardboard should be avoided in the intraoperative area.

  Ventilation in patient care areas and work areas must be adequate for the task(s) performed; air grills must be kept dust free and maintained in good working condition.

  The ventilation system within the operating room should provide a minimum of 15 exchanges of filtered (95%) air per hour, with three fresh air changes, all under positive pressure.

  Air should be introduced at the ceiling and exhausted near the floor.

  The relative humidity of air should be 30% - 60% and air temperature should be controlled at 68°F - 73°F (20°C - 23°C);

refer to specific P/P regarding temperature requirements for specialized surgical procedures.

Smoke and plume generated during electro-surgery and laser surgery should be controlled and/or removed whenever possible; evacuation systems are recommended to prevent the potential hazard(s) from inhalation of smoke and associated byproducts.

Sharps disposal container(s) should be available and easily accessible in all areas where sharps are used.

The size of the sharps container should provide adequate space for all types of sharps used during the procedure.

The sharps container should allow entry of contaminated items by a non-touch method in order to maintain asepsis.

Environmental cultures should only performed if approved and/or directed by the ICP.

Traffic in the semi-restricted and restricted areas should be minimized in order to prevent air turbulence, which can increase airborne contamination.

The number and movement of persons should be kept to a minimum while surgery is in progress.

Doors to the operating room should remain closed whenever possible; opening during surgery is discouraged (signage may be required).

Housekeeping services should be defined through a "statement of services" provided by the department and/or contracted with support services in the building.

Disinfectants used in the surgical area must be EPA-registered and approved by ICP.

Patient surgical tables, thermia pads, and/or pans should be cleaned and disinfected daily after the surgical case.

Floors should be cleaned daily and when soiled, using a wet-vacuum; if the wet-vacuum system is not available, a two-bucket wet mop system should be used.

At the conclusion of the day's routine schedule, operating rooms, scrub areas, hallways, and substerile areas must be terminally cleaned.

Waste handling and disposal should follow state and local regulations. Disposable equipment containing large amounts of blood and/or body fluid requires special biohazard containers and/or double bagging to prevent leakage.

A regularly scheduled inspection of the area should be performed collaboratively with Facilities, Housekeeping, Surgical Services, and ICPs.

Medication, specimen, and food refrigerators should be maintained and monitored according to appropriate guidelines.

➤ IC Program aspects

- An interdisciplinary and collaborative team approach is recommended in order to provide consistent care to reduce adverse patient outcomes, prevent infection, and improve patient safety outcomes.
- Products and medical devices should meet infection control/safety standards and sterilization parameters when applicable; an interdisciplinary surgical product evaluation committee should include ICP representation.
- Surveillance

  Postsurgical patients are susceptible to infections following surgery including postoperative wound infections, pneumonia, intravascular device associated infections, and catheter associated urinary tract infections and facilities performing surgical procedures should assess and select procedures for surveillance activities. (Refer to Section 2 - Acute Care Surveillance)

Surgical patients often have short lengths of stay, or procedures may be performed on an ambulatory basis, therefore post discharge surveillance data collection should be considered. (Refer to Section 2)

- Education
  - Policies and procedures (P/P), education, training, and competencies should be written and revised to reflect current scientific-based evidence and strategies related to infection prevention and related healthcare worker/patient safety in the perioperative setting.
  - Patients should be instructed regarding preoperative preparation (e.g., bathing) and postoperative wound care.

References/Resources

- American Institute of Architects, Guidelines for design and construction of hospital and healthcare facilities, 2001 edition, The American Institute of Architects, Washington, D.C.; 2001.
- Association for Professionals in Infection Control and Epidemiology. APIC Text of Infection Control and Epidemiology. 2000, chapter 53 pp.1-11.
- Association of Operating Room Nurses. Recommended practices for surgical attire. Standards and recommended practices. Denver: AORN; 1995. p. 141-142.
- Belkin NL. APIC State-of-the-art report: Use of scrubs and related apparel in healthcare facilities. Am J Infect Control 1997; 25:401-404.

- Centers for Disease Control and Prevention, Healthcare Infection Control Practices Advisory Committee (HICPAC). Draft guideline for environmental infection control in healthcare facilities, 2001. 2001, Federal Register.
- Department of Labor and Department of Health and Human Services (US), Occupational Safety and Health Administration. Instruction CPL 2 - 2/69. Enforcement procedures for the Occupational Exposure to Bloodborne Pathogen Standard. 29 CFR 1910.1030 m.4.c (1) (b) Nov. 27, 2001.
- Shojania KG, Duncan BW, McDonald KM, et al., Eds. Making Healthcare Safer: A Critical Analysis of Patient Safety Practices. AHRQ Publication No. 01-E058, Rockville, MD: Agency for Healthcare Research and Quality. July 2001.

Travelers

Overview

- Thousands of Americans travel abroad each year. In the past, local health departments often provided travel immunizations, but many have discontinued this practice. However, they may be able to provide information and phone numbers for local travel clinics. While travel agencies may downplay the importance of travel immunizations and counseling, travelers may enter a country without immunization and/or appropriate counseling for personal health and safety. Tourists should have information to make informed decisions about issues including food/water selection and risks of certain travel activities. Fortunately, there are many excellent reference sources (published and electronic) available to professionals and the general public regarding healthy travel.

Purpose

- ICPs may be requested to provide References/Resources and resources for travelers.

Risk Factors

- Immunizations are not available for all travel-related health and infection risks.
- Some countries allow an exemption from vaccination due to age and/or on medical grounds; this may leave the traveler unprotected.
- Under the International Health Regulations adopted by the World Health Organization, a country may, under certain conditions,

require an International Certificate of Vaccination against yellow fever from international travelers; the unprepared traveler may encounter difficulty.

- Time for effective development of antibody postimmunization may be insufficient and/or simultaneous administration of certain vaccines may be contraindicated.
- If certain vaccines (e.g., MMR and varicella) are given with immune globulin (IG, formerly called immune serum globulin, and immunoglobulin) preparations, antibody response can be diminished.
- Preventative therapy/prophylaxis is not available for all agents; resistance is emerging (e.g., malaria).
- Existing personal/health conditions may increase risk for the traveler.
- Lack of knowledge or means for safety and health precautions will increase risk of illness.
- Recommendations may rapidly change at destination due to outbreaks or other events (e.g., natural disasters).

Strategies for Prevention and Control

- A travel itinerary should be defined to identify special needs dependent on trip destination including:
  - Time/season of travel.
  - Endemic/epidemic diseases/infectious agents.
- Travelers should prepare by:
  - Obtaining a current medical history including:

    Present medical therapies.

    Allergies.

Chronic diseases or current significant health issues (e.g., pregnancy or contraindications to certain vaccine).

Immunization history.

- Obtaining information needed for trip regarding:

  Location of nearby US government offices—consulates, embassies.

  Contact local health department for location of local Travel Clinics.

  How to obtain medical assistance while traveling.

  Jet lag effects.

  Malarial precautions.

  Food precautions.

  Water precautions and safe practices.

  Traveler's diarrhea – signs and treatment.

  Insect and other hazardous wildlife protection.

  Climate (e.g., altitude sickness, sun exposure, cold exposure) and appropriate gear.

- Obtaining needed supplies/medications:

  A traveler's medical kit.

  Adequate supply of current medications.

  Additional items such as hand sanitizer, water filters/purification tablets, etc.

- Reviewing current information and alerts at www.cdc.gov/travel.
- If conditions at destination changes, (e.g., outbreak or natural disaster) travelers should be advised either to contact the CDC Fax Information Service (request document number 000005) or to consult the CDC Travelers' Health Website for the most up-to-date information.

References/Resources

- Association for Professionals in Infection Control and Epidemiology. APIC Text of Infection Control and Epidemiology. 2000, chapter 122 pp.1-2.
- Centers for Disease Control www.cdc.gov/travel
- CDC Information for International Travel (published biannually by the U.S. Department of Health and Human Services, (also known as the yellow book) available at CDC travel website
- Dupont H, Steffen R. Textbook of Travel Medicine and Health. Malden, MA: Blackwell Science, Inc.; 1997
- International Society of Travel Medicine www.istm.org
- National Center for Infectious Diseases at www.cdc.gov/ncidod/index.htm
- Summary of Health Information for International Travel (also known as the Blue Sheet; updated biweekly) is available both from the Centers for Disease Control and Prevention (CDC) website at www.cdc.gov/travel/blusheet.htm and from the CDC Fax Information Service by telephoning 1-888-CDC-FAXX (232 - 3299) and requesting document number 220022

Section V

EMPLOYEE/ OCCUPATIONAL HEALTH

Overview and Work Restrictions

Overview

- Healthcare organizations provide a safe environment of care for clients and healthcare workers (HCWs). The infection control professional (ICP) has a vital role within each organization to help identify infectious risks to patients and HCWs, assess potential outcomes, implement preventative policies and procedures, and evaluate the effectiveness of control measures.
- Factors to consider when selecting what is appropriate for a particular facility include the characteristics of the patient/client/resident population and worker pool, the type of healthcare setting, the geographic location, and diseases endemic in the communities served.
- Familiarity with this section will assist the ICP in updating the organization's program to keep current with changing trends. Tables on multiple subjects are designed in a quick reference format.
- The prevention strategies addressed include immunizations for vaccine-preventable diseases (Refer to Section 2 – Immunizations for HCWs, Adults and Children, Isolation and Precautions), management of healthcare personnel exposure to infected persons, including postexposure prophylaxis (Refer to Section 5 – Exposure Management), and work restrictions for exposed or infected healthcare personnel in this chapter.

Purpose

- The transmission of infections between patients and HCWs can be accomplished by utilizing IC components of a healthcare organization's occupational health program to promote a safe environment of care for the HCW and clients served. This section includes recommendations considered prudent by consensus of the Hospital Infection Control Practices Advisory Committee (HICPAC). [N.B., "Hospital" has been replaced with "Healthcare" in subsequent HICPAC guidelines]

- The ICP should facilitate a thorough review of the recommended practices and adapt only those applicable to the given healthcare organization.

Risk Factors

- HCWs have the potential for exposure to infectious materials, including body substances, contaminated medical supplies and equipment, contaminated environmental surfaces, or contaminated air. (Refer also to Section 5 – Exposure Management)
- These personnel may include but are not limited to emergency medical service personnel, dental personnel, laboratory personnel, autopsy personnel, nurses, nursing assistants, physicians, technicians, therapists, pharmacists, students and trainees, contractual staff not employed by the healthcare facility, and persons not directly involved in patient care but potentially exposed to infectious agents (e.g., clerical, dietary, housekeeping, maintenance, and volunteer personnel).
- In general, HCWs in or outside healthcare settings who have contact with patients, body fluids, or specimens have a higher risk of acquiring or transmitting infections than do other healthcare personnel who have only brief casual contact with patients and their environment (e.g., beds, furniture, bathrooms, food trays, medical equipment).

Strategies for Prevention

- Program elements necessary to attain the IC goals of an employee/occupational health service:
  - Coordination with other departments.
  - Medical evaluations.
  - Health and safety education.
  - Immunization programs.
  - Management of job-related illnesses and exposures to infectious diseases, including policies for work restrictions for infected or exposed personnel.
  - Counseling services for personnel on infection risks related to employment or special conditions.
  - Maintenance and confidentiality of personnel health records.

References/Resources

- Association for Professionals in Infection Control and Epidemiology. APIC Text of Infection Control and Epidemiology. 2000, chapters 79-84.
- Centers for Disease Control and Prevention. HICPAC guideline for infection control in healthcare personnel. Am J Infect Control 1998; 26(3): 289–354.
- Centers for Disease Control and Prevention. Public Health Service guidelines for immunization of healthcare workers. MMWR 1997; 46(RR-18):23.

Guidelines for Work Restrictions and Management of Infetious Illnesses

Disease	Work Restriction	Duration	Category*
Conjunctivitis	Restrict from patient contact and contact with patient's environment.	Until discharge ceases.	II
Cytomegalovirus	No restriction.	NA	II
Diarrheal diseases Acute stage (diarrhea with other symptoms)	Restrict from patient contact, contact with the patient's environment, or food handling.	Until symptoms resolve.	IB
Convalescent stage, *Salmonella spp.*	Restrict from care of high-risk patients.	Until symptoms resolve; consult with local and state health authorities regarding need for negative stool cultures.	IB
Diphtheria	Exclude from duty.	Until antimicrobial therapy complete and two cultures obtained ≥ 24 hours apart are neg.	IB
Enteroviral infections	Restrict from care of infants, neonates, and immunocompromised patients and their environments.	Until symptoms resolve.	II

Guidelines for Work Restrictions and Management of Infetious Illnesses

Disease	Work Restriction	Duration	Category*
Hepatitis A	Restrict from patient contact, contact with patient's environment, and food handling.	Until seven days after onset of jaundice.	IB
Hepatitis B HCW with acute or chronic hep. B surface antigemia who do not perform exposure-prone procedures.	No restriction,* refer to state regulations; Standard Precautions should always be observed.	NA	II
Personnel with acute or chronic hepatitis Be antigemia who perform exposure-prone procedures.	Do not perform exposure-prone invasive procedures until counsel from expert review panel; panel should review and recommend procedures the worker can perform, taking into account specific procedure and skill/technique of worker; refer to state regulations.	Until hepatitis Be antigen is negative.	II
Hepatitis C	No recommendation.	NA	Unresolved

Guidelines for Work Restrictions and Management of Infetious Illnesses

Disease	Work Restriction	Duration	Category*
Herpes simplex Genital	No restriction.	NA	1A
Hands (herpetic whitlow)	Restrict from patient contact and contact with patient's environment.	Until lesions heal.	II
Orofacial	Evaluate for need to restrict from care of high-risk patients.	NA	II
HIV	Do not perform exposure-prone invasive procedures until counsel from an expert review panel, etc. (as stated above for Hepatitis B)	NA	II
Measles Active	Exclude from duty.	Until seven days after the rash appears.	IA
Postexposure (susceptible personnel)	Exclude from duty.	From fifth day after first exposure through 21st day after last exposure and/or four days after rash appears.	IB

Guidelines for Work Restrictions and Management of Infetious Illnesses

Disease	Work Restriction	Duration	Category*
Meningococcal infections	Exclude from duty.	Until 24 hours after start of effective therapy.	IA
Mumps			
Active	Exclude from duty.	Until nine days after onset of parotitis.	IB
Postexposure (susceptible personnel)	Exclude form duty.	Until nine days after onset of parotitis.	IB
Pediculosis (lice)	Restrict from patient contact.	Until treated and observed to be free of adult and immature lice.	IB
Pertussis			
Active	Exclude from duty.	From beginning of catarrhal stage thru third wk after onset of paroxysms or until five days after start of effective antimicrobials.	IB
Postexposure (asymptomatic HCW)	No restriction; prophylaxis recommended.	NA	II

Guidelines for Work Restrictions and Management of Infetious Illnesses

Disease	Work Restriction	Duration	Category*
Postexposure (symptomatic HCW)	Exclude from duty.	Until five days after start of effective antimicrobials.	IB
Rubella Active	Exclude from duty.	Until five days after rash appears.	IA
Postexposure (susceptible personnel)	Exclude form duty.	From seventh day after first exposure through 21st day after last exposure.	IB
Scabies	Restrict from patient contact.	Until cleared by medical evaluation.	IB
Staphylococcus aureus Active, draining skin lesions	Restrict from contact w/ patients and their environment or food handling.	Until lesions have resolved.	IB
Carrier state	No restriction, unless personnel are epidemiologically linked to transmission of the organism.	NA	IB

Guidelines for Work Restrictions and Management of Infetious Illnesses

Disease	Work Restriction	Duration	Category*
Streptococcal infection, Group A	Restrict patient care, contact with patient's environ., or food handling.	Until 24 hours after adequate treatment started.	IB
Tuberculosis Active pulmonary disease	Exclude from duty	Until proven noninfectious.	IA
PPD converter	No restriction.	NA	IA
Varicella-zoster (**chickenpox**) Active disease	Exclude from duty.	Until all lesions dry and crust.	IA
Postexposure (susceptible personnel)	Exclude from duty.	From 10th day after first exposure through 21st day (28th day if VZIG given) after last exposure or, if varicella occurs, until all lesions dry and crust.	IA

Guidelines for Work Restrictions and Management of Infetious Illnesses

Disease	Work Restriction	Duration	Category*
Varicella-zoster **(shingles)**			
Localized in healthy person	Cover lesions; restrict from care of high-risk patients.¶	Until all lesions dry and crust.	II
Generalized or localized in immunosuppressed person	Restrict from patient contact.	Until all lesions dry and crust.	IB
Postexposure (susceptible personnel)	Restrict from patient contact.	From 10th day after first exposure through 21st day (28th day if VZIG) after last exposure or, if varicella occurs, until all lesions dry and crusted.	IA
Viral respiratory infections, acute febrile	Consider excluding from the care of high-risk patients§ or contact with their environment during community outbreak of RSV and influenza.	Until acute symptoms resolve.	IB

* Unless epidemiologically linked to transmission of infection.

¶ Those susceptible to varicella and who are at increased risk of complications of varicella, such as neonates and immunocompromised persons of any age.

§ High-risk patients as defined by the ACIP for complications of influenza.

* Recommendation Categories

IA: Strongly recommended for all hospitals and strongly supported by well-designed, experimental, or epidemiologic studies.

IB: Strongly recommended for all hospitals and reviewed as effective by experts in the field and a consensus of Hospital Infection Control Practices Advisory Committee members on the basis of strong rationale and suggestive evidence, even though definitive scientific studies have not been done.

II: Suggested for implementation in many hospitals. Recommendations may be supported by suggestive clinical or epidemiologic studies, a strong theoretic rationale, or definitive studies applicable to some but not all hospitals.

No recommendation; unresolved issue: Practices for which insufficient evidence or consensus regarding efficacy exists.

Exposure Management

Overview

- Healthcare workers may be exposed to a variety of infectious agents in the course of their employment. The risk of acquisition of microorganisms varies and is related to several factors including: worker training and skill level; Standard Precautions protocol including appropriate use of PPE and handwashing; isolation protocol; type of agent; nature and duration of exposure; physiological factors; postexposure management; facility design.
- Common infectious agents encountered in the healthcare setting include bloodborne pathogens (HIV, HBV, HCV), tuberculosis, chickenpox, and influenza.

Purpose

- Infectious work-related exposures occur in healthcare settings. Each facility should develop, implement, and educate employees regarding specific exposure management procedures in order to reduce infection and adverse outcomes.

Definitions

- **Bloodborne pathogen exposure** - event places HCW at risk for HBV, HCV, or HIV infection; defined as a percutaneous injury (e.g., a needlestick or cut with a sharp object) or contact of mucous membrane or non-intact skin (e.g., exposed skin that is chapped, abraded, or afflicted with dermatitis) with blood, tissue, or OPIM.
- **Healthcare workers** - persons (e.g., employees, students, contractors, attending clinicians, public-safety workers, or volunteers) whose activities involve contact with patients or with

blood or other body fluids from patients in a health-care, laboratory, or public-safety setting.

- **PEP** - Postexposure prophylaxis that varies based upon agent type and source, exposure parameters, and evaluation of exposed HCW by physician; PEP may include a combination of antiretroviral agents, antibiotics (e.g., for TB), passive immune globulin (e.g., HBIG), and/or vaccine (e.g., chickenpox or influenza).

Risk Factors

- The risk of acquiring an infectious agent is related to:
  - Worker training and skill level (Refer to Section 1).

    Provide education about infectious agents and prevention strategies at orientation, when there is a change in policy/procedure, and annually.

    Return demonstration competencies, e.g., phlebotomy and IV procedures, cleaning, and reprocessing of reusable equipment, and wound and dressing changes.

    Management oversight as appropriate.
  - Observance of Standard Precautions including appropriate use of PPE and handwashing.

    Selection and use of PPE including facial protection, gowns, and gloves.

    Handwashing/hand hygiene.

    Respirator fit testing and fit checks.
  - Isolation and other precaution protocols. (Refer to Section 2)

    Evaluation of patients for appropriate use of transmission based precautions.

Education of patient/family re: cooperation and involvement, e.g., leaving room, PPE and handwashing, rationale for protocol.

Appropriate management of shared equipment.

- Type of agent. (Refer to Section 2 – Communicable Disease Reporting)
  - Bloodborne pathogens including HIV, HBV, HCV, syphilis—found in blood/body fluids; exposure from needlestick or other contaminated sharp, splash to mucous membranes, contact with non-intact skin.
  - TB bacilli inhaled in the form of droplet nuclei.
  - Influenza spread through respiratory secretions.
  - Chickenpox spread through contact with respiratory secretions or vesicle fluid.
- Nature and duration of exposure. (Refer to Section 1 – Communicable Disease Reporting-Common Communicable Disease table and Section 5 – Overview and Work Restrictions)
  - Type of encounter with agent, e.g., sharp device vs. intact skin vs. mucous membranes; organism "load"; inhalation of droplets, airborne agents, aerosols, or plumes; self-inoculation from contaminated hands.
  - Time exposed to agent, e.g., entering patient's room for vitals check vs. prolonged care.
  - Number or frequency exposure events.
- Physiological factors. (Refer to Sections 2, 3, and 4)
  - Immunity to agent
  - Skin integrity and personal hygiene
  - Health status and immunocompetence
  - Medications, smoking and/or substance abuse

- Chronic illnesses/co-morbidities
- Pregnancy

➤ Postexposure management

- Availability of first aid treatment
- Promptness of assessment
- Availability of prophylaxis
- Thoroughness and accuracy of recordkeeping for trends; using information to improve equipment or devices and procedures.

➤ Facility design and upkeep (Refer to Sections 2, 3, and 4)

- Location of handwashing stations and related supplies, alcohol based hand rinses, PPE.
- Ventilation as appropriate (negative, positive, air changes per hour, duct design, and exhaust).
- Maintenance of water systems (Legionella).
- Maintenance of surfaces (damage, porosity).
- Housekeeping protocol including agents and frequency of cleaning.

Strategies for Prevention

➤ Wound care/management

- First aid and routine wound/splash cleansing.
- Notify appropriate supervisor or personnel:

  Assess for medical needs.

  Assess for counseling needs: risks and precautions.
- Provide tetanus immunization (Td) if five years or longer since last vaccination.
- Document exposure facts.

- Source person serological evaluation and prophylaxis.
  - If exposed HCW is unsure whether he or she wishes to be tested for HIV, a blood sample may be drawn to store for 90 days to allow the HCW time to decide.
  - Test for HBsAg, HCV, antibody.
  - Test for HIV antibody after obtaining informed consent.
  - Rapid testing should be available to initiate prophylactic treatment, if indicated.
  - If source is unknown, assess for likelihood of presence of bloodborne viral infection.
  - Hepatitis B evaluation/prophylaxis following significant/percutaneous exposure.

    Exposed Person Serological Evaluation

    Baseline: HBsAg, HBs antibody/ALT/AST (SGPT/SGOT); HBs antibody optional if exposed person is known to have adequate titers within the last 24 months.

    Follow-up: HBsAg, HBs antibody/ALT/AST/HBC antibody in three and six months.

    Prophylaxis (See table later in this section).
  - Hepatitis C evaluation/prophylaxis following significant/percutaneous exposure

    Exposed Person Serological Evaluation

    Baseline: anti-HCV, ALT/AST.

    Follow-up: anti-HCV, ALT/AST at three and six months.

    Prophylaxis: None recommended.
    - Human Immunodeficiency Virus (HIV) evaluation/prophylaxis following significant/percutaneous exposure (See tables later in this section).

RECOMMENDATIONS FOR POSTEXPOSURE HEPATITIS B PROPHYLAXIS

	Treatment When Source Is Found to Be:		
* Exposed Person status	HBsAg † Positive	HBsAg † Negative	Unknown or Untested
Unvaccinated	HBIG § × 1 plus HBV vaccine series	HBV vaccine series	HBV vaccine series
Previously vaccinated			
Known responder**	No Treatment	No Treatment	No Treatment
Known nonresponder ††	HBIG × 2 §§ or HBIG § × 1 and reinitiate vaccine series.	No treatment	If known high risk*** treat as if source were HBsAg positive.
Response unknown	Test exposed for anti-HBs: 1. If adequate, no treatment. 2. If inadequate, HBIG × vaccine booster.	No treatment	Test exposed for anti-HBs: 1. If adequate, no treatment. 2. If inadequate, vaccine booster and recheck titer in one to two mos.

* Persons who have previously been infected with HBV are immune to reinfection and do not require postexposure prophylaxis.

† Hepatitis B surface antigen.

§ Hepatitis B immune globulin; dose is 0.06 mL/kg intramuscularly.

¶ Hepatitis B vaccine.

** A responder is a person with adequate levels of serum antibody to HBsAg (i.e., anti-HBs > 10 mIU/mL).

†† A nonresponder is a person with inadequate response to vaccination (i.e., serum anti-HBs < 10 mIU/mL).

§§ The option of giving 1 dose of HBIG and reinitiating the vaccine series is preferred for nonresponders who have not completed a 2nd 3-dose vaccine series. For persons who completed a second vaccine series but failed to respond, two doses of HBIG are preferred.Antibody to HBsAg.*

Recommended HIV postexposure prophylaxis for percutaneous injuries					
Infection status of source					
* Exposure type	HIV-pos Class 1*	HIV-pos Class 2*	Unknown status§	Unknown source§	HIV-neg
Less severe¶	Recommend basic 2 - drug PEP	Recommend expanded 3-drug PEP	Generally, no PEP warranted; consider basic 2 - drug PEP** for source with HIV risk factors††	Generally, no PEP warranted; consider basic 2 - drug PEP** in settings where exposure to HIV-infected persons is likely	No PEP warranted
More severe§§	Recommend expanded 3-drug PEP	Recommend expanded 3-drug PEP	Generally, no PEP warranted; consider basic 2 - drug PEP** for source with HIV risk factors††	Generally, no PEP warranted; consider basic 2 - drug PEP** in settings where exposure to HIV-infected persons is likely	No PEP warranted

Recommended HIV postexposure prophylaxis for percutaneous injuries—legend for facing chart

HIV-Positive, Class 1 – asymptomatic HIV infection or known low viral load (e.g., <1,500 RNA copies/mL). HIV-Pos., Class 2 – symptomatic HIV infection, AIDS, acute seroconversion, or known high viral load. If drug resistance is a concern, obtain expert consultation. Initiation of PEP should not be delayed pending expert consultation, and, because expert consultation alone cannot substitute for face-to-face counseling, resources should be available to provide immediate evaluation and follow-up care for all exposures.

† Source of unknown HIV status (e.g., deceased source person with no samples available for HIV testing).

§ Unknown source (e.g., needle from sharps disposal container).

¶ Less severe (e.g., solid needle/superficial injury).

** The designation "consider PEP" indicates that PEP is optional and should be based on an individualized decision between the exposed person and the treating clinician.

†† If PEP is offered and taken and the source is later determined to be HIV- negative, PEP should be discontinued.

§§ More severe (e.g., large-bore hollow needle, deep puncture, visible blood on device or needle from artery/vein).

Recommended HIV postexposure prophylaxis for percutaneous injuries

Infection status of source					
* Exposure type	HIV-pos Class 1*	HIV-pos Class 2*	Unknown status§	Unknown source§	HIV-neg
Small volume**	Consider basic 2 - drug PEP††	Recommend basic 2 - drug PEP	Generally, no PEP warranted; consider basic 2 - drug PEP†† for source with HIV risk factors§§	Generally, no PEP warranted; consider basic 2 - drug PEP†† in settings where exposure to HIV-infected persons is likely	No PEP warranted
Large volume¶¶	Recommend basic 2 - drug PEP	Recommend expanded 3-drug PEP	Generally, no PEP warranted; consider basic 2 - drug PEP†† for source with HIV risk factors§§	Generally, no PEP warranted; consider basic 2 - drug PEP†† in settings where exposure to HIV-infected persons is likely	No PEP warranted

* For skin exposures, follow-up is indicated only if there is evidence of compromised skin integrity (e.g., dermatitis, abrasion, or open wound).

† HIV-Positive, Class 1 — asymptomatic HIV infection or known low viral load (e. g., < 1,500 RNA copies/mL). HIV-Positive, Class 2 — symptomatic HIV infection, AIDS, acute seroconversion, or known high viral load. If drug resistance is a concern, obtain expert consultation. Initiation of postexposure prophylaxis (PEP) should not be delayed pending expert consultation, and, because expert consultation alone cannot substitute for face-to-face counseling, resources should be available to provide immediate evaluation and follow-up care for all exposures.

§ Source of unknown HIV status (e. g., deceased source person with no samples available for HIV testing).

¶ Unknown source (e.g., splash from inappropriately disposed blood).

** Small volume (i.e., a few drops).

†† The designation, “consider PEP,” indicates that PEP is optional and should be based on an individualized decision between the exposed person and the treating clinician.

¶¶ Large volume (i.e., major blood splash).

§§ If PEP is offered and taken and the source is later determined to be HIV-negative, PEP should be discontinued.

Situations for which expert* consultation for HIV postexposure prophylaxis is advised

- Delayed (i.e., later than 24–36 hours) exposure report:
  - The interval after which there is no benefit from postexposure prophylaxis (PEP) is undefined.
- Unknown source (e.g., needle in sharps disposal container or laundry):
  - Decide use of PEP on a case-by-case basis.
  - Consider the severity of the exposure and the epidemiologic likelihood of HIV exposure.
  - Do not test needles or other sharp instruments for HIV.
- Known or suspected pregnancy in the exposed person:
  - Does not preclude the use of optimal PEP regimens.
  - Do not deny PEP solely on the basis of pregnancy.
- Resistance of the source virus to antiretroviral agents:
  - Influence of drug resistance on transmission risk is unknown.
  - Selection of drugs to which the source person's virus is unlikely to be resistant is recommended; if the source person's virus is known or suspected to be resistant to >1 of the drugs considered for the PEP regimen.
  - Resistance testing of the source person's virus at the time of the exposure is not recommended.
- Toxicity of the initial PEP regimen:
  - Adverse symptoms, such as nausea and diarrhea are common with PEP.
  - Symptoms often can be managed without changing the PEP regimen by prescribing antimotility and/or antiemetic agents.
  - Modification of dose intervals (i.e., administering a lower dose of drug more frequently throughout the day, as recommended by the manufacturer), in other situations, might help alleviate symptoms.

*** Local experts and/or the National Clinicians' Postexposure Prophylaxis Hotline (PEPline 1-888-448-4911)**

- Tuberculosis (TB) exposure management:
  - As soon as possible after an exposure to TB (i.e., exposure to a person with pulmonary or laryngeal TB for whom proper isolation precautions were not implemented), PPD testing should be performed on personnel who are known to have negative PPD-test results.
  - The PPD test should be repeated 12 weeks after the exposure if the initial postexposure PPD-test result is negative.
  - PPD tests or chest radiographs should not be performed on personnel with previous positive PPD-test results, unless they have symptoms suggestive of active TB.
  - Preventive therapy should be offered to the following personnel, regardless of age, who have conversion of their PPD test: (a) recent converters, (b) close contacts of persons with active TB, (c) those with medical conditions that increase their risk for active TB, (d) those with HIV infection, (e) injecting-drug users.
- Chickenpox. (Refer to Section 5 and the CDC Guideline for infection control in healthcare personnel, 1998; see reference for citation)
- Influenza. (Refer to Section 5 and the CDC Guideline for infection control in healthcare personnel, 1998; see reference for citation)

References/Resources

- Association for Professionals in Infection Control and Epidemiology. APIC Text of Infection Control and Epidemiology. 2000, chapters 79-84.
- Centers for Disease Control and Prevention, Guideline for infection control in healthcare personnel, 1998. Am J of Inf Control, 1998:26; 289-354.

- Centers for Disease Control and Prevention. Management of possible sexual, injecting-drug–use, or other nonoccupational exposure to HIV, including considerations related to antiretroviral therapy: Public Health Service statement. MMWR 1998; 47 (no. RR-17).
- Centers for Disease Control and Prevention. Public Health Service Guidelines for immunization of healthcare workers. MMWR 1997; 46(RR-18):23.
- Centers for Disease Control and Prevention. Public Health Service Guidelines for the management of healthcare worker exposure to HIV and recommendations for postexposure prophylaxis. MMWR 1998;47(RR-7):1–33.
- Centers for Disease Control and Prevention. Updated U.S. Public Health Service Guidelines for the Management of Occupational Exposures to HBV, HCV, and HIV and Recommendations for Postexposure Prophylaxis. MMWR 2001; 50(RR-11).
- Food and Drug Administration - Report unusual or severe toxicity to antiretroviral agents. Phone: (800) 332 - 1088 Address: Med Watch, HF-2, FDA, 5600 Fishers Lane, Rockville, MD 20857 or www.fda.gov/medwatch
- Hepatitis Hotline: (888) 443-7232 or www.cdc.gov/hepatitis
- HIV Antiretroviral Pregnancy Registry. Phone:(800) 258-4263 Fax: (800) 800-1052 Address: 1410 Commonwealth Drive, Suite 215, Wilmington, NC 28405; www.glaxowellcome.com/preg_reg/antiretroviral
- HIV/AIDS Treatment Information Service www.hivatis.org
- National Clinicians' Postexposure Prophylaxis Hotline (PEPline) Phone: (888) 448-4911 or www.ucsf.edu/hivcntr
- Needlestick! Website for clinicians www.needlestick.mednet.ucla.edu

- Popejoy SL. Occupational blood exposure. In: Olmsted RN, editor. Infection control and applied epidemiology: principles and practice. St. Louis, MO: Mosby; 1996. p 23-1–23-6.
- Reporting to CDC: Occupationally acquired HIV infections and failures of PEP. Phone: (800) 893-0485

Immunocompromised Employees

Overview

- The immunocompromised healthcare worker (IHCW) is an individual with decreased cellular or humoral immunity. The person may have one or more defects in the body's normal defense mechanisms that predispose them to infections.

Purpose

- Immunocompromised employees may be at increased risk for infection.

Risk Factors

- All organisms may be opportunistic in that they gain advantage of a failure in host defense mechanisms. The greater the compromise to these defenses, the less virulent the organism may be to cause an infection. Consequently, those with major immune defects are subject to a larger number and greater variety of infections.
- Infectious or chemical agents that may cause immunosuppression include, but are not limited to, human immunodeficiency virus (HIV), hematologic malignancies such as leukemia and lymphoma, chemotherapeutic agents, high-dose systemic steroids and anti-rejection drugs for transplant patients.

Strategies for Prevention and Control

- Develop a program that includes participation by Employee/ Occupational Health, Infectious Disease/Epidemiology, Infection Control, Risk Management, Human Resources, Medical Legal Affairs, Psychiatry, and/or others as indicated.

- Establish a Healthcare Worker Advisory Group (HCWAG) to be responsible for providing assistance to the IHCW.
  - The HCWAG could be a set group or an ad hoc assembly based upon circumstances.
  - Guidance to seek appropriate medical care and periodic evaluation of health status, counseling on the advisability of continuing to work in the healthcare setting, and information on safer sex and partner notification may be provided by the HCWAG.
  - IHCWs should inform their physician and/or healthcare facility when there is a significant risk of compromised patient care.
  - The HCWAG may also be responsible for advising HCWs with bloodborne pathogens under what circumstances, if any, that the IHCW may perform invasive procedures.
  - The HCWAG may arrange counseling regarding job employee's modification or reassignment and any issues related to the Americans with Disabilities Act; career counseling and job retraining should be promoted.
- IHCWs should receive counseling as to their responsibilities to reduce infection-related risks to self and others.
- Confidentiality must be maintained in accordance with institutional policy and legal statues; if job modification is required, information must be limited to those who have a legal right to know.
- Education to all healthcare workers, including volunteers and students, should include encouragement to provide health information including immunocompromising conditions to Employee/Occupational Health.

References/Resources

- Association for Professionals in Infection Control and Epidemiology. APIC Text of Infection Control and Epidemiology. 2000, chapters 31,33, 37,79,105,110.

- Centers for Disease Control and Prevention, Guideline for Infection Control in Healthcare Personnel 1998. 1998 Am J Infect Control: 26; 289-354.
- Centers for Disease Control and Prevention, Healthcare Infection Control Practices Advisory Committee (HICPAC). Draft guideline for environmental infection control in healthcare facilities, 2001. 2001, Federal Register.
- Phillips KA, Lowe RA, Kahn JG, Lurie P, et al. The cost-effectiveness of HIV testing of physicians and dentists in the United States. JAMA 1994; 271:851–858.
- Robert LM, Chamberland ME, Cleveland JL, Marcus R, et al. Investigation of patients of healthcare workers infected with HIV. Centers for Disease Control and Prevention Database. Ann Intern Med 1995; 122:653–657.

Pregnant Employees

Overview

- Exposure to certain infectious agents may cause congenital syndromes in the fetus when the primary infection is acquired during pregnancy. Therefore, all healthcare workers of childbearing age should be educated on potential adverse effects on the fetus of specific infectious agents. Restriction of the pregnant healthcare worker from patient care may be required for certain infectious agents. Obtaining immunization history of non-pregnant women of childbearing age as well as consistent use of Standard Precautions can prevent or minimize exposure to most infectious diseases.

Purpose

- Provision of education, principles, and control methods to women of childbearing age and the pregnant healthcare worker will decrease anxiety and potentially increase compliance to control measures.

Risk Factors:

- Airborne Disease
  - Tuberculosis-congenital tuberculosis is extremely rare and is only associated with mothers who have an active diseases process.
  - Varicella-Zoster
  - Rubeola, Rubella, Mumps
- Non Airborne Diseases
  - Risks of congenital transmission after exposure due to maternal contact with infectious agents while not using PPE.

    Cytomegalovirus (CMV)

Transmitted by direct contact, person-to-person with virus containing secretions. Sexual transmission most frequent. May also passed from mother to baby before, during, or after birth.

Patient to HCW transmission very rare.

Hepatitis B

Transmitted through blood or body fluids such as wound exudates, semen, cervical secretions, and saliva.

Mother-to-infant transmission during the perinatal period in infants born to HBs Ag-positive mothers.

Chronic HBV infection with persistence of Hepatitis B surface antigen (indicates infectious state) occurs in as many as 90% of infants who become infected during perinatal transmission.

Nonimmunized healthcare worker exposure occurs primarily via sharps injuries.

Hepatitis C

Perinatal transmission most likely occurs, but the risks and consequences have not been defined.

Herpes Simplex

HSV-1 usually involves face and skin above the waist. HSV-2 usually involves the genitalia and skin below the waist. However either type can be found in either site.

Occupational acquision is unlikely.

Transmission occurs through direct contact.

Herpes simplex in the genital area can be transmitted as the infant passes through the birth canal.

HIV (Human-Immunodeficiency Virus)

HIV transmission has been documented from blood, semen, cervical secretions, and human milk.

Predominant modes of transmission are through sexual contact, percutaneous or mucous membrane exposure to blood or contaminated needles or sharps, and mothers-to-infant transmission before or around the time of birth.

Parvovirus B19 (Erythema Infectiosum, Fifth Disease)

Transmission occurs through respiratory secretions and blood.

Transmission to hospital personnel has been infrequently reported.

Parvovirus B19 infection that occurs during pregnancy can cause fetal hydrops or death.

Risk of fetal death <10% in the first half of pregnancy and negligible in the second half.

Congenital anomalies among newborns associated with B19 infection has not been reported.

Syphilis

Open lesions of primary or secondary syphilis may contain many infectious bacteria.

Infants born with congenital syphilis have highly-infectious secretions.

HCWs who have had close, unprotected contact with an infant with congenital syphilis prior to antibiotic therapy are at risk of developing lesions and may require prophylaxis.

Congenital syphilis can be contracted from an infected mother via transplacental transmission at any time during pregnancy or birth.

In women with untreated early syphilis, 40% of pregnancies result in spontaneous abortion, stillbirth or perinatal deaths.

Strategies for Prevention and Control

- Strict adherence to Standard Precautions with all patients and transmission-based precautions as indicated prevents acquisition of infection in most cases.
- A thorough immunization and communicable disease history should be obtained upon employment; update annually.
- Susceptible non-pregnant women of childbearing age, should be immunized against the following diseases: Rubeola, Rubella, Hepatitis B, Mumps, Diphtheria, Tetanus and Varicella-Zoster. Obtain serologic screening if beneficial.
- If exposure occurs, education and reassurance of the employee with involvement from her own healthcare provider are important aspects of management.
- TB
  - In the event of TB exposure, PPD skin testing on pregnant women is not contraindicated and is recommended.
  - Pregnant women demonstrating a positive skin test, after exposure without pulmonary disease, may need preventative therapy with INH during pregnancy (depending on certain risk factors). If there are no risk factors, prophylactic therapy can be delayed until after delivery.
  - Fit testing for N-95 respirators should be documented; changes in pregnancy weight may affect fit and fit testing should be repeated.
- Varicella
  - Non-immune pregnant employees should not care for patients with suspected or confirmed herpes zoster or chickenpox.
  - In the event of varicella exposure, serologic susceptibility should be obtained if HCW has not been immunized.
  - Varicella vaccine is contraindicated in pregnancy. Education and communication with HCW obstetrician is warranted.

- Rubeola, rubella, mumps
  - Non-immune pregnant personnel should not care for patients with suspected or confirmed infections.
- Hepatitis B (HBV)
  - Hepatitis B Immune Globulin (HBIG) and HBV vaccine is not contraindicated in pregnancy if an exposure to HBV occurs.
- Hepatitis C
  - In the event of Hepatitis C exposure, baseline and follow-up testing for anti-HCV should be performed.
  - Education and communication with HCW obstetrician is warranted.
- Human Immunodeficiency Virus (HIV)
  - Pregnancy testing should be offered if status unknown.
  - The risk of infection should be evaluated and need for Postexposure Prophylaxis (PEP) as with any other HIV exposure. (Refer to Section 5 - Exposure Management)
  - The decision to use any antiviral drug during pregnancy should involved HCWs healthcare provider regarding potential benefits and risk to self and fetus.
  - Efavirenz (EFV) should not be used during pregnancy; all prophylactic regimens must be considered for teratogenic effects.
  - HIV-antibody testing for at least six months postexposure (e.g., at baseline, six weeks, three months, and six months) should be performed.

- Parvovirus B19
  - Pregnant women should be educated about the potential risks of Parvovirus B19 infection to the fetus and the importance of adherence to precautions.
  - Routine exclusion of pregnant employees caring for patients with Parvovirus is not necessary.
- Syphilis
  - Prophylactic antibiotic therapy may be indicated for HCW who have had close, unprotected contact with an infant with congenital syphilis.

References/Resources

- Association for Professionals in Infection Control and Epidemiology. APIC Text of Infection Control and Epidemiology. 2000, chapter 81, 1-9.
- Center for Disease Control and Prevention, Guideline for Infection Control in Healthcare Personnel. Federal Register October 1998.
- Centers for Disease Control and Prevention, Updated U.S. Public Health Service Guidelines for the Management of Occupational Exposures to HBV, HCV, and HIV and Recommendations for Postexposure Prophylaxis. 2001, MMWR 50 (RR-11).
- Immunization of Healthcare Workers: Recommendations of the Advisory Committee on Immunization Practices (ACIP) and the Hospital Infection Control Practice Advisory Committee (HICPAC).
- 1997 MMWR 46(RR-18), 1-42. www.cdc.gov/mmwr/mmwrpvol.html

Section VI

LABORATORY

Laboratory Testing

Overview

- The medical laboratory provides support to infection control by supplying information that is evaluated in conjunction with clinical components of the patient's condition.
- Laboratories may also be asked to assist in environmental, equipment, cluster, or outbreak investigation.
- Laboratories are configured in a variety of designs providing services appropriate to the patient population mix. Testing may be performed at the bedside, in an onsite testing facility, and/or be sent to a reference, regional, or other laboratory.
- Regardless of service facilities, there are numerous elements to consider, including how to interpret and apply test results. The microbiology section of the laboratory encompasses the major portion of this service although immunology, chemistry, hematology, urinalysis, blood bank, and coagulation may contribute to the clinical picture.
- An understanding and application of epidemiology, common healthcare associated infections, and specialized populations and settings for provision of healthcare must be considered in conjunction with laboratory results.

Purpose

- The ICP should have access to fundamental information related to understanding and interpreting laboratory results.
- A detailed exploration is beyond the scope of this handbook. However, References/Resources and resources for supplementary information are supplied.

Risk Factors

- Pathogenic bacteria, fungi, and viruses
- Opportunistic bacteria, fungi, and viruses
- Parasites

Strategies for Prevention and Control

- An understanding of host-factors and agent properties coupled with knowledge of human-microbial interactions are foundational in infection control. Agent, reservoir, means of transmission, and host comprise the chain of infection (Refer to Section 1 – Infection Control and Epidemiology); laboratory testing is focused on identifying the agent in order to initiative appropriate prevention or control measures.
- Microbiology
  - Study of bacteria, fungi (molds and yeasts), parasites, viruses, and algae (rare in healthcare).
  - Differentiation of normal or commensual flora, transient microorganisms, colonization, and infection.
  - Virulence or pathogenicity.
  - Distinguish between contamination and representation.
  - Classification schemes.
  - Detection techniques.
  - Specimen collection.
  - Preliminary and final results.
  - Turn-around times.
  - Treatment evaluation.
  - Laboratory biosafety.

- Bacteria
  - Air tolerance.

    Aerobic – require oxygen.

    Anaerobic – oxygen intolerant.

    Microaerophilic – tolerate low oxygen.

    Special gas blends – required to recover certain bacteria in the laboratory.

  - Gram-stain classification.

    Based upon cell wall structure.

    Used for most bacteria.

    Gram positive – retain crystal violet dye in gram stain.

      Examples: *Staphylococcus sp., Streptococcus sp., Bacillus sp., Corynebacterium sp., Clostridium sp.*

    Gram negative – don't retain crystal violet.

      Examples: Haemophilus influenzae, *E. coli, Enterobacter sp., Pseudomonas sp., Serratia sp., Acinetobacter sp., Klebsiella sp., Citrobacter sp., Neisseria sp., Moraxella sp. and Bacteroides sp.*

    Morphological shape under microscope:

      Cocci – spheres

      Bacilli – rod or stick form

      Coccobacilli – very short bacilli

      Spirochete – curled or corkscrew

    Configuration under microscope

      Pairs or diplo – kidney bean *(Neisseria sp.)* or spear-head *(S. pneumoniae)*

      Chains - like a string of beads *(Streptococcus pyogenes)*

      Clusters, tetrads, or clumps *(Staphylococcus sp.)*

- Acid-fast stain classification

  For mycobacteria (*M. tuberculosis, M. intracellular-avium* complex or MAC).

  Cell wall high lipid content do not take up gram-stain dyes well.

  Ziehl-Neelson or Kinyoun methods using a special dye (carbol-fuchsin) that resists removal by acid or alcohol rinse, thus, the term "acid-fast bacilli" (AFB).

  Fluorochrome stains using auramine with or without rhodamine dye.

  Caveat: Nonviable organisms may stain positive.

  Caveat: Presence of mycobacteria on direct examination of stained specimens does not establish the diagnosis of tuberculosis as atypical mycobacteria and some other microorganisms will stain as AFB.

> Microorganism identification

- Bacteria

  Dependent on incubation; growth on agar or other media offers preliminary ID; growing availability of rapid screening tests.

  Many grow within 24–72 hour; others take longer.

  Once grown on media, bacteria can be further identified using a variety of chemical or enzymatic tests.

  Some bacteria require special environmental conditions to grow; if suspected, special requests must be made (i.e., anaerobes, fungi, mycobacterium, mycoplasma, viruses).

- Viruses

  Most laboratories do not have the appropriate equipment and resources to culture viruses; if cultures are ordered, specimens require "holding" in a special transport media until transport to a referral lab can occur.

Living cell cultures can be used for isolation of some pathogenic viruses.

Viral growth in cells can be detected in several ways, including changes in the cell morphology or structure and cell death.

Some viruses grow slowly in the laboratory and may take up to four weeks to detect.

Common viruses such as herpes simplex can be grown in one to two weeks.

- Antimicrobial susceptibility testing

  Disk diffusion - placing antibiotic disks on agar plates inoculated with bacteria and measuring zones of clearance (Kirby-Bauer).

  MIC - minimum inhibitory concentration of bacterial growth in liquid media containing serially diluted concentration of an antibiotic (e.g., microwell titer).

  Results are commonly reported as (S) sensitive/susceptible or (R) resistant.

  Determination of MIC provides concentration of an antibiotic required to inhibit growth of specific bacteria *in vitro*.

  Interpretation based on the comparison of the results with predetermined nationally accepted standard values or cutoffs (NCCLS) for specific antibiotics and bacteria.

  Some bacteria have predictable antibiotic patterns and therefore do not routinely undergo antibiotic susceptibility testing (e.g., Group A Streptococcus, Pasteurella multocida).

  Caveat: A positive culture may indicate true disease, contamination, or colonization without disease. Factors such as type of bacteria, source of specimen, and host characteristics should always be considered when interpreting culture results.

- Serological testing
  - Often used for detection of antibodies against specific microorganisms, particularly viruses.
  - IgM antibody may be detected early during the course of infection, but may also be associated with false-positive results due to nonspecific stimulation of the immune system.
  - IgG antibody is produced later during the course of infection; a fourfold or greater rise in IgG titers between acute (early during the illness) and convalescent (two to four weeks later) serum samples supports recent infection.
  - Examples of infections diagnosed serologically: Hepatitis A, B, and C; cytomegalovirus; Epstein-Barr virus, and HIV.
- Toxin assays
  - Most common is performed on stool specimens for diagnosis of *Clostridium difficile*–associated diarrhea; detects presence of bacterial toxin by examining for pathologic changes in certain types of cells.
  - Antigen assays

    Detection of antigens of pathogens in certain body fluids, for early diagnosis or when cultures may show no growth.

    Examples: cryptococcal antigen in serum or cerebrospinal fluid (CSF); *L. pneumophila* antigen in urine; *S. pneumoniae, H. influenzae, N. meningitidis,* and Group B *Streptococcus* antigen in CSF.

    Caveat: A negative antigen assay result, particularly as regards CSF bacterial antigens, does not rule out infection.
- Molecular Biology
  - Nucleic acid probes.

    Often used to directly detect either the single-stranded DNA or RNA of a specific species or genera of potential pathogens in clinical specimen; variety of methods (e.g., chemiluminescence or radioactivity).

Advantages include direct detection of pathogens that are difficult to grow or are present in low numbers in clinical specimens (e.g., *Legionella sp.*), and culture confirmation of isolates that grow too slowly on agar media for timely identification (e.g., *M. tuberculosis*).

Probe-based tests may be routinely used in many laboratories for rapid detection of *C. trachomatis* and *N. gonorrhea* in clinical specimens.

- Polymerase chain reaction (PCR)

  Used for difficult-to-grow or detect pathogens in clinical specimens by *in vitro* amplification of their nucleic acid.

  Potentially capable of detecting even minute number of organisms in clinical specimens (e.g., herpes simplex in the CSF and HIV in blood).

- Plasmid profile analysis

  Involves the extraction of plasmid DNA followed by the separation of plasmid molecules by agarose gel electrophoresis.

  Has been successfully used for isolation of plasmid DNA from a variety of bacteria (e.g., *Enterobacteriaceae* and *Staphylococcus sp.*).

- Restriction endonuclease analysis

  Used to cleave double-stranded DNA of plasmids or chromosomes.

  Differentiation of one bacterial isolate from another in the same species group (e.g., *S. aureus, Enterococcus sp., C. difficile, K. pneumoniae*).

- Pulse field gel electrophoresis

Allows analysis of bacterial DNA fragments representing the entire bacterial chromosome by agarose gel electrophoresis (e.g., *E. coli, P. aeruginosa, S. aureus, Legionella sp., Acinetobacter sp.*, multidrug-resistant enterococci).

- Ribotyping

  Allows fingerprinting of ribosomal RNA.

  Restriction endonuclease analysis of ribosomal RNA used to distinguish bacterial isolates in the same species group (e.g., *Staphylococcus sp., Enterobacter cloacae, Acinetobacter sp.*).

➤ Human Immunodeficiency Virus (HIV) testing

- HIV viral load testing.
- The two most common methods for measuring HIV load in the plasma are by using branched DNA (bDNA) and PCR technologies.
- PCR which targets a specific region of a nucleic acid sequence and makes a large number of copies of that sequence before measuring the quantity.
- bDNA technique does not alter the number of molecules in the sample; instead, it attaches probes and bDNA to each HIV RNA molecule to increase the molecule's size, followed by a chemiluminescent substrate that emits light.
- The light signal, which is directly proportional to the HIV RNA load, is then measured (assay by Chiron Corp.) and the HIV RNA level is calculated.
- Currently, bDNA is the most reproducible method for measuring viral load, which may help predict HIV-related disease progression.

HEPATITIS TESTING

Interpretation of viral hepatitis tests

Test	Abbreviation	Interpretation
Hepatitis A virus	HAV	
IgM antibody to HAV	Anti-HAV IgM	Signifies acute infection; present < 6 months after acute infection.
IgG antibody to HAV	Anti-HAV IgM	Represents past infection when IgM without anti-HAV.
Hepatitis B virus	HBV	
Hepatitis B surface antigen	HBsAg	Indicates ongoing infection and infectivity.
Hepatitis B e antigen	HBeAg	Correlates with ongoing infection and high infectivity.
Hepatitis B DNA	HBV DNA	Correlates with infectivity.
Antibody to surface antigen	Anti-HBs	Indicates past HBV infection or vaccination and immunity.
Antibody to core antigen	Anti-HBc	Represents distant or acute infection; not associated with vaccination; may be false pos.
IgM antibody to core antigen	Anti-HBc IgM	Indicates acute HBV infection.
Hepatitis C virus	HCV	
Antibody to hepatitis C	Anti-HCV	Usually indicates prior exposure to HCV, ongoing infection and infectivity; may be false positive.
HCV RNA	HCV RNA	Correlates with viral replication and infectivity.

HEPATITIS TESTING

Interpretation of viral hepatitis tests

Test	Abbreviation	Interpretation
Hepatitis D virus	HDV	
Delta antigen	HDAg	Found in early acute delta infection (requires presence of HBV).
Antibody HDV	Anti-HDV	Indicates current or past HDV infection; high titers associated with chronic infection).
HDV RNA	HDV RNA	Represents viral replication.
Hepatitis E virus Antibody to HEV	HEV Anti-HEV	Indicates present or past HEV infection.
IgM antibody to HEV	IgM anti-HEV	Represents recent HEV infection.
HEV RNA	HEV RNA	Associated with viral replication and infectivity.

CEREBROSPINAL FLUID (CSF) TESTING

Common findings in cerebrospinal fluid lab tests for meningitis

Aspect	Normal	Bacterial	Viral	Fungal
Color	Clear	Cloudy	Clear, hazy	Clear, hazy
White blood cells (Wbc)/mm	0–8	400–100,000	5–500	40–400
Protein mg/dL	12–60	80–500	30–150	40–150
Glucose mg/dL	40-70	<35	Normal to low	Normal to low
Percent on Differential	PMNs* 0–6% Monocytes 94–100%	PMNs >90%	Monocytes >50%	Monocytes >50%

* PMNs = polymorphonucleocytes

References/Resources

- American Academy of Pediatrics. 2000 Red Book: report of the committee on infectious diseases. 24th ed. Elk Grove Village, Ill: American Academy of Pediatrics; 1997.
- Association for Professionals in Infection Control and Epidemiology. APIC Text of Infection Control and Epidemiology. 2000, chapter 63,67,70,93.
- Chin J, Ed. Control of communicable diseases manual, 17th Ed. Washington, DC: American Public Health Association. 2000.
- Centers for Disease Control and Prevention. Guidelines for preventing transmission of tuberculosis in healthcare facilities, 1993. MMWR 1994;43(RR-17).

- Centers for Disease Control and Prevention, Healthcare Infection Control Practices Advisory Committee (HICPAC). Draft Guideline for Environmental Infection Control in Healthcare Facilities, 2001. 2001, Federal Register.
- Greene JN, Stratton CW. Role of the microbiology lab in hospital epidemiology and infection control. In Mayhall CG, Ed. Infection control and hospital epidemiology. Baltimore: Williams and Wilkins; 1996. p 1126–1137.
- Mellors J, et al. Quantitation of HIV-1 plasma predicts outcome after seroconversion. Ann Intern Med 1995; 122:573–579.
- Murray PR, editor. Manual of Clinical Microbiology. 7th Ed. Washington, DC: American Society for Microbiology, 1999.
- Thomas DL. Hepatitis viruses. In: Mayhall CG, editor. Hospital epidemiology and infection control. Baltimore: Williams and Wilkins; 1996. p 446–465.
- Tietze NW, editor. Clinical guide to laboratory tests. 3rd ed. Philadelphia: WB Saunders; 1995.
- U.S. Department of Health and Human Services, Centers for Disease Control and Prevention, and National Institutes of Health, Biosafety in Microbiological and Biomedical Laboratories, 4th ed., Washington, DC: U.S. Government Printing Office, 1999.

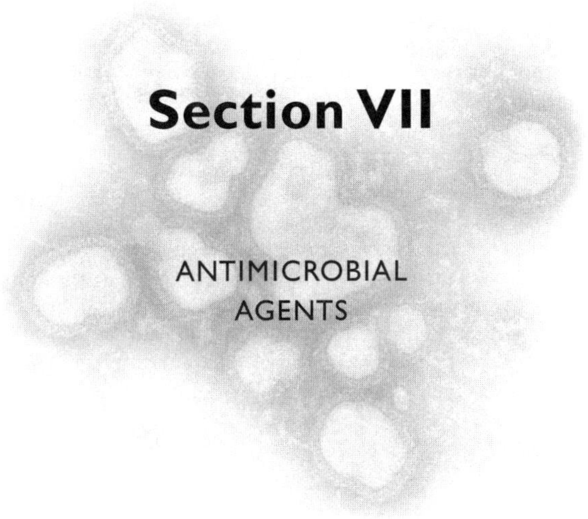

Section VII

ANTIMICROBIAL AGENTS

Antimicrobial Utilization

Overview

- This section is adapted from The Michigan Society for Infection Control (MSIC) "*Guidelines for Prevention and Control of Antimicrobial Resistant Organisms-2000.*" Copies of this booklet can be obtained from MSIC—see references at the end of this section.
- Prudent utilization of antimicrobials (primarily antibiotics) is critical to prevent the emergence and/or reduce the prevalence of antimicrobial resistant organisms. Methicillin-resistant Staphylococcus aureus (MRSA) first emerged in England in 1960, soon after methicillin was introduced for the treatment of penicillin-resistant staphylococci. MRSA was first reported in the U.S. in 1968 and is now endemic in many regions of the country.
- There has been a rapid increase in the incidence of infection and colonization with Vancomycin Resistant Enterococci (VRE) since the late 1980s. In the late 1990s, there were reports of Vancomycin Intermediate Susceptibility (VISA). There is also increasing antimicrobial resistance of many gram-negative bacilli including *E. coli, Enterobacter, Klebsiella, Serratia, Acinetobacter, Pseudomonas* and others and *M. tuberculosis*. Increasing resistance is associated with previous antimicrobial use, underlying disease, and invasive procedures.

Purpose

- The Infection Control Professional (ICP) is encouraged to take a leadership role in efforts within the healthcare setting to assure this stewardship.

- Collaboration with pharmacy, medical and nursing staff, and administration is critical. Each organization is encouraged to develop goals with process and outcome measures to optimize antimicrobial use within the patient populations or clients it serves.

Risk Factors

- Previous antimicrobial use
- Underlying disease
- Invasive procedures

Strategies for Prevention

- Community programs should include:
  - Education for providers and consumers regarding the completion of treatment regimens and inappropriate use of antimicrobials.
- Healthcare facilities should consider the following when developing facility specific policies and procedures:
  - Limitation of the antimicrobial formulary.
  - Implementation of therapeutic guidelines including criteria for appropriateness.
  - Restriction of antimicrobial ordering for selected agents to infectious disease physicians.
  - Implementation of an antimicrobial order form.
  - Institution of automatic stop orders.
  - Limited susceptibility reporting to selected agents (e.g., first generation cephalosporins).
  - Antimicrobial surveillance program and inclusion of antimicrobial use/outcomes in peer review activities.

- Implementation of critical pathways/guidelines/protocol to provide decision support for antimicrobial selection.
- Antimicrobial rotation or "cycling."
- Promotion of vaccines to reduce risk of diseases that might lead to secondary bacterial infections and subsequent resistance (e.g., *S. pneumoniae*, influenzae).
- Careful consideration for the implementation of isolation for resistant organisms versus adherence to Standard Precautions.

References

- APIC 1997 Guidelines Committee - Position Statement. The Use of Antimicrobial Household Products. APIC News November/December 1997, p 13.
- Association for Professionals in Infection Control and Epidemiology. Conference Proceedings: Global Consensus Conference on Infection Control Issues Related to Antimicrobial Resistance. March 1999. Washington, DC:
- Association for Professionals in Infection Control and Epidemiology. APIC Text of Infection Control and Epidemiology. 2000, chapter 61.
- Bartley J Ed. Guidelines for Prevention and Control of Antimicrobial Resistant Organisms (ARO) – Focus on: MRSA and VRE. 2002. Michigan Society for Infection Control. www.MSIC-online.org
- Nicolle LE, Dyck B, Thompson G, et al. Regional dissemination and control of epidemic methicillin-resistant Staphylococcus aureus. Infect Control Hosp Epidemiol 1999; 20:202-5.
- Rahal K, Wang F, Schindler J, et al. Reports on surveillance of antimicrobial resistance in individual countries. Clin Infect Dis 1997; 24(Suppl 1):S169-75.

- Roman RS, Smith J, Walker M, et al. Rapid geographic spread of a methicillin-resistant Staphylococcus aureus strain. Clin Infect Dis 1997; 25:698-705.
- Rutala WA, Stiegel MM, Sarubbi FA, et al. Susceptibility of antibiotic-susceptible and antibiotic-resistant hospital bacteria to disinfectants. Infect Control Hosp Epidemiol 1997; 18:417-21.
- Shlaes DM, Gerding DN, John JF Jr, et al. Society for Healthcare Epidemiology of America and Infectious Diseases Society of America Joint Committee on the Prevention of Antimicrobial Resistance: guidelines for the prevention of antimicrobial resistance in hospitals. Infect Control Hosp Epidemiol 1997; 18:275-91.
- Sieradzki K, Roberts RB, Haber SW, Tomasz A. The development of vancomycin resistance in a patient with methicillin-resistant Staphylococcus aureus infection. N Engl J Med 1999; 340:517-23.
- Smith TL, Pearson ML, Wilcox KR, et al. Emergence of vancomycin resistance in Staphylococcus aureus. N Engl J Med 1999; 340:493-501.
- Struelens MJ. The epidemiology of antimicrobial resistance in hospital acquired infections: problems and possible solutions. Br Med J 1998; 317:652-4.

RESISTENCE ORGANISM FLOWCHART

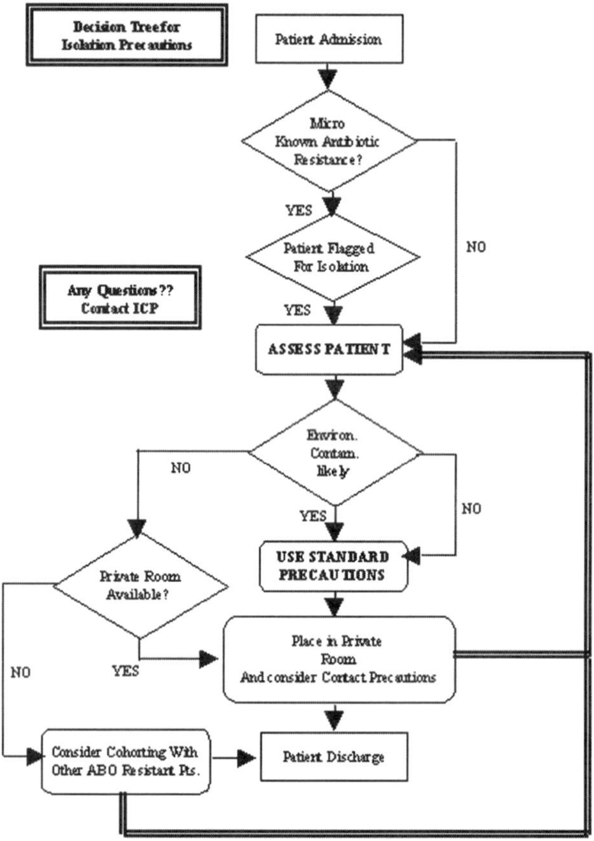

SPECTRUM OF ACTIVITY OF SELECTED ANTIMICROBIAL AGENTS

Antimicrobial Agent (*Trade Name*)	Major *InVitro* Activity*	NOT Commonly Recommended For
Acyclovir (*Zovirax®*)	Herpes simplex, varicella-zoster	Cytomegalovirus, all other viruses
Amikacin (*Amikin®*)	Many AGNB† (including *Pseudomonas spp.*, *Enterobacter spp.*)	Anaerobes, Gram-positive bacteria
Amoxicillin-clavulanate (*Augmentin®*)	Similar to ampicillin, plus some ampicillin-resistant *Escherichia coli*, anaerobes, oxacillin-sensitive *Staphylococcus spp.*, *H. influenzae*, *Moraxella catarrhalis*	MRSA‡, MRSE¶, *Pseudomonas spp.*, *Enterobacter spp.*
Amphotericin B (*Fungizone®*)	Many *Candida albicans*, non-*albicans* *Candida spp.*, *Aspergillus spp.*, *Cryptococcus neoformans*, *Torulopsis glabrata*, Mucorales fungi	*Candida lusitanea*, *Pseudallescheria boydii*
Ampicillin/ amoxicillin (*Omnipen®*/ *Amoxil®*)	*Streptococcus spp.*, *Enterococcus spp.*, some *E. coli*, *H. influenzae* (β-lactamase negative), and *Salmonella spp.*, *Listeria monochjnytogenes*	*Pseudomonas spp.*, β-lactamase-positive AGNB and *H. influenzae*, *Staphylococcus spp.*, *M. catarrhalis*

SPECTRUM OF ACTIVITY OF SELECTED ANTIMICROBIAL AGENTS

Antimicrobial Agent (*Trade Name*)	Major *InVitro* Activity*	NOT Commonly Recommended For
Ampicillin-sulbactam (*Unasyn®*)	*Streptococcus spp.*, *Enterococcus spp.*, oxacillin-sensitive *S. aureus*, *H. influenzae*, most *E. coli* and *Klebsiella spp.*, *anaerobes*, *M. catarrhalis*	MRSA, MRSE, *Pseudomonas aeruginosa*, *Enterobacter spp.*, *Neisseria gonorrhea*
Aztreonam (*Azactam®*)	Many AGNB, including *E. coli*, *Klebsiella spp.*, *P. aeruginosa*, *M. catarrhalis*, *H. influenzae*	Gram-positive bacteria, anaerobes
Capsofungin (*Cancidas*)	Aspergillus spp., Candida spp.	Cryptococcus spp.
Cefazolin (*Ancef®*)	*Streptococcus spp.*, oxacillin-sensitive *Staphylococcus spp.*, *E. coli*, *Klebsiella spp.*	MRSA, MRSE, *Pseudomonas spp.*, *Enterobacter spp.*, *Enterococcus spp.*, *Bacteroides fragilis*

SPECTRUM OF ACTIVITY OF SELECTED ANTIMICROBIAL AGENTS

Antimicrobial Agent *(Trade Name)*	Major *InVitro* Activity*	NOT Commonly Recommended For
Cefepime *(Maxipime®)*	*Streptococcus spp.*, oxacillin-sensitive *S. aureus*, many AGNB (incl. *Pseudomonas spp.*, ceftazidime-resistant *Klebsiella spp., and Enterobacter spp.)*	MRSA, MRSE, *Enterobacter spp.*, *anaerobes*
Cefprozil *(Cefzil®)*	Similar to cefuroxime	Similar to cefuroxime
Cefpodoxime proxetil *(Vantin®)*	*Streptococcus spp.*, *H. influenzae*, *M. catarrhalis*, *E. coli*, *K. pneumoniae*, *P. mirabilis*, *N. gonorrheae*	MRSA, MRSE, *Pseudomonas spp.*, *Enterococcus spp.*
Ceftibuten *(Cedax®)*	*Streptococcus spp.*, *H. influenzae*, *M. catarrhalis*	MSSA, MRSA, MRSE, *Pseudomonas spp.*, *Enterococcus spp.*
Ceftizoxime *(Cefizox®)*	Similar to cefazolin, plus some cefazolin-resistant AGNB, some anaerobes, *H. influenzae*, *Neisseria spp.*	MRSA, MRSE, *Pseudomonas spp.*, *Enterococcus spp.*, fully penicillin-resistant *Streptococcus pneumoniae*

SPECTRUM OF ACTIVITY OF SELECTED ANTIMICROBIAL AGENTS

Antimicrobial Agent *(Trade Name)*	Major *InVitro* Activity*	NOT Commonly Recommended For
Cefotaxime/ceftriaxone *(Claforan®/Rocephin®)*	Similar to cefazolin, plus some cefazolin-resistant AGNB, moderately penicillin-resistant *S. pneumoniae, H. influenzae, Neisseria spp.*	MRSA, MRSE, *Pseudomonas spp., Enterococcus spp.,* fully penicillin-resistant *S. pneumoniae,* anaerobes
Cefoxitin/cefotetan *(Mefoxin®/Cefotan®)*	Similar to cefazolin, plus some cefazolin-resistant AGNB, many anaerobes; less active than cefazolin against staphylococci	MRSA, MRSE, *Pseudomonas spp., Enterobacter spp., Enterococcus spp.*
Ceftazidime *(Fortaz®)*	Many AGNB (including *Pseudomonas spp.), H. influenzae, M. catarrhalis*	Staphylococci, anaerobes, *Enterococcus spp., Enterobacter spp.*
Cefuroxime *(Zinacef®)*	Similar to cefazolin, plus *H. influenzae, Neisseria spp., M. catarrhalis*	MRSA, MRSE, *Pseudomonas spp., Enterobacter spp., Enterococcus spp.*

SPECTRUM OF ACTIVITY OF SELECTED ANTIMICROBIAL AGENTS

Antimicrobial Agent *(Trade Name)*	**Major** ***InVitro*** **Activity***	**NOT Commonly Recommended For**
Chloramphenicol (*Chloromyctin®*)	Some Gram-positive bacteria (including *S. pneumoniae*), *H. influenzae*, *Neisseria meningitidis*, many anaerobes, *Rickettsia spp.*	*Staphylococcus spp.*, many AGNB
Ciprofloxacin/ofloxacin (*Cipro®/Floxin®*)	Many Gram-negative bacteria (including *Pseudomonas spp.*), *N. gonorrhea*, *Legionella spp.*	Many Gram-positive bacteria (including MRSA, MRSE, *S. pneumoniae*, *Enterococcus spp.*), anaerobes
Clarithromycin/ azithromycin (*Biaxin®/Zithromax®*)	Many Gram-positive bacteria, *H. influenzae*, *M. catarrhalis*, some atypical mycobacteria	MRSA, MRSE, many AGNB, anaerobes, *Enterococcus spp.*
Clindamycin (*Cleocin®*)	*Streptococcus spp.*, some *S. aureus*, many anaerobes	MRSA, MRSE, AGNB, *C. difficile*, *Enterococcus spp.*
Erythromycin (*Eryc®,E.E.S.®*)	Many Gram-positive bacteria, *Legionella spp.*, *Chlamydia spp.*, *Mycoplasma spp.*, *M. catarrhalis*	AGNB, MRSA, MRSE, *Enterococcus spp.*
Famciclovir (*Famvir®*)	Herpes simplex, varicella-zoster	Cytomegalovirus, all other viruses

SPECTRUM OF ACTIVITY OF SELECTED ANTIMICROBIAL AGENTS

Antimicrobial Agent *(Trade Name)*	Major *InVitro* Activity*	NOT Commonly Recommended For
Fluconazole *(Diflucan®)*	*Candida albicans, Cryptococcus neoformans*	*Aspergillus spp., C. krusei, T. glabrata,* Mucorales fungi
Foscarnet *(Foscavir®)*	*Herpes simplex*, varicella-zoster, cytomegalovirus	All other viruses
Ganciclovir *(Cytovene®)*	Herpes simplex, varicella-zoster, cytomegalovirus	Acyclovir-resistant viruses
Gatifloxacin *(Tequin)*	*S. pneumoniae, S. aureus, H. influenzae, M. catarrhalis*, anaerobes, and many AGNB	MRSA, MRSE
Gentamicin *(Garamycin®)*	Many AGNB, synergistic killing of many enterococci in combination with penicillin, ampicillin, or vancomycin	Anaerobes, Gram-positive bacteria
Imipenemcilastatin *(Primaxin®)*	Many Gram-positive bacteria (including oxacillin-sensitive *S. aureus*), AGNB (including *P. aeruginosa, Enterobacter spp.*), anaerobes	MRSA, MRSE, *Stenotrophomonas maltophilia, Enterococcus faecium, Pseudomonas cepacia*

SPECTRUM OF ACTIVITY OF SELECTED ANTIMICROBIAL AGENTS

Antimicrobial Agent (*Trade Name*)	Major *InVitro* Activity*	NOT Commonly Recommended For
Itraconazole (*Sporanox®*)	*Candida albicans*, *Cryptococcus neoformans*, *Histoplasma spp.*, *Blastomyces spp.*, *Aspergillus spp.*	Mucorales fungi, *Candida krusei*, *Torulopsis glabrata*
Ketoconazole (*Nizoral®*)	*Candida albicans*	*Aspergillus spp.*, non-albicans *Candida spp.*, *Torulopsis glabrata*, Mucorales fungi
Levofloxacin (*Levaquin®*)	Many AGNB incl. *Pseudomonas spp.*, *M. catarrhalis*, *H. influenzae*, *C. trachomatis*, *Legionella spp.*, *S. aureus*	MRSA, MRSE, *Enterococcus spp.* anaerobes
Linezolid (*Zyvox*)	Enterococci (including vancomycin-resistant strains) staphylococci (including MRSA and MRSE), streptococcis (including *S. pneumoniae*)	Gram-negative bacteria
Lomafloxacin (*Maxaquin®*)	Many AGNB incl. *Pseudomonas spp.*, *H. influenzae*, *M. catarrhalis*	MRSA, MRSE, *Enterococcus spp.* *S. pneumoniae*, anaerobes

SPECTRUM OF ACTIVITY OF SELECTED ANTIMICROBIAL AGENTS

Antimicrobial Agent *(Trade Name)*	Major *InVitro* Activity*	NOT Commonly Recommended For
Loracarbef *(Lorabid®)*	*Streptococcus spp.*, *S. aureus*, *H. influenzae*, *M. catarrhalis*	MRSA, MRSE, *Enterococcus spp.* *Pseudomonas spp.*
Meropenem *(Merrem)*	Many gram-positive bacteria (including oxacillin-sensitive *S. aureus*), AGNB (including *P. aeruginosa*, *Enterobacter spp.*), anerobes	MRSA, MRSE, *Stenotrophomonas maltophilia*, *Enterococcus faecium*
Metronidazole *(Flagyl®)*	Anaerobes (including *C. difficile)*, *Entamoeba histolytica*, *Giardia lamblia*	Aerobic Gram-positive bacteria, AGNB
Moxifloxacin *(Avelox)*	*S. pneumoniae*, *S. aureus*, *H. influenzae*, *M. catarrhalis*, anerobes and many AGNB	MRSA, MRSE
Nafcillin/oxacillin *(Unipen®)*	*Streptococcus spp.*, *many Staphylococcus spp.*	MRSA, MRSE, anerobes, AGNB, *Enterococcus spp.*
Penicillin G or V *(Bicillin®/PenVee K®)*	*Streptococcus spp.*, *Enterococcus spp.*, some anaerobes, *Pasteurella multocida*, *N. meningitidis*	*Staphylococcus spp.*, most AGNB, *B. fragilis*

SPECTRUM OF ACTIVITY OF SELECTED ANTIMICROBIAL AGENTS

Antimicrobial Agent *(Trade Name)*	**Major** ***InVitro*** **Activity***	**NOT Commonly Recommended For**
Piperacillin *(Pipracil®)*	Similar to Penicillin G, plus many AGNB (including P. aeruginosa), many anaerobes	Some AGNB (including some *E. coli, Klebsiella spp., Acinetobacter spp., and Enterobacter spp.), S. aureus, S. epidermidis*
Piperacillin-tazobactam *(Zosyn®)*	Same as piperacillin, plus oxacillin-sensitive S. aureus, anaerobes, and expanded AGNB (including E. coli) activity	MRSA, MRSE
Quinupristin/ dalfopristin *(Synercid®)*	*Enterococcus faecium* (including vancomycin-resistant strains), staphylococci (including MRSA and MRSE), streptococci (including *S. pneumoniae*)	*Enterococcus faecalis,* gram-negative bacteria
Rifampin *(Rifadin®)*	Many Gram-positive bacteria (including MRSA, MRSE), *H. influenzae* (for prophylaxis), *N. meningitidis* (for prophylaxis), *M. tuberculosis*, some atypical mycobacteria, *Legionella spp.*	Monotherapy for treatment of established infection, many AGNB

SPECTRUM OF ACTIVITY OF SELECTED ANTIMICROBIAL AGENTS

Antimicrobial Agent *(Trade Name)*	Major *InVitro* Activity*	NOT Commonly Recommended For
Tetracyclines (e.g., *Achromycin®*, *Minocin®*, *Vibramycin®*)	Some Gram-positive bacteria, *Chlamydia spp.*, *Mycoplasma spp.*, *Rickettsia spp.*, *Ehrlichia spp.*, *M. catarrhalis*	AGNB, MRSA (except minocycline), MRSE (except minocycline)
Ticarcillin-clavulanate *(Timentin®)*	Many Gram-positive bacteria (including oxacillin-sensitive *S. aureus*), AGNB (including *P. aeruginosa*) and anaerobes	*Enterococcus spp.*, MRSA, MRSE
Tobramycin *(Nebcin®)*	Similar to gentamicin, plus enhanced activity vs. *P. aeruginosa*	Similar to gentamicin
Trimethoprim-sulfamethoxazole *(Septra®, Bactrim®)*	Many Gram-positive bacteria (including some MRSA and MRSE), some AGNB (including *E. coli, Klebsiella spp.), L. pneumophila, M. catarrhalis, Pneumocystis carinii, Listeria monocytogenes, S. maltophilia*	*P. aeruginosa,* anaerobes, *Enterococcus spp.*
Trovafloxacin *(Trovan®)*	Many AGNB, incl. *Pseudomonas spp., S. aureus, Streptococcus spp., M. catarrhalis, N. gonorrheae, Legionella spp., Chlamydia spp.*, many anaerobes	MRSA, MRSE, *Enterococcus spp.*

SPECTRUM OF ACTIVITY OF SELECTED ANTIMICROBIAL AGENTS		
Antimicrobial Agent ***(Trade Name)***	**Major** ***InVitro*** **Activity***	**NOT Commonly Recommended For**
Valacyclovir *(Valtrex®)*	Similar to acyclovir	Similar to acyclovir
Valganciclovir *(Valcyte)*	Herpes simplex, varicella-zoster, cytomegalovirus	Acyclovir-resistant viruses
Vancomycin *(Vancocin®)*	Many aerobic Gram-positive bacteria (including MRSA, MRSE, *Enterococcus spp.*), *C. difficile*	Gram-negative bacteria (except *Flavobacterium meningosepticum*)

* Whenever possible, antibiotic selection should be based on *in vitro* susceptibility of the specific isolate.

† AGNB: aerobic Gram-negative bacilli.

‡ MRSA: Methicillin-resistant *S. aureus*.

¶ MRSE: Methicillin-resistant *Staphylococcus epidermidis*

Section VIII

APPENDICES

GLOSSARY

COMMON TERMS IN INFECTION CONTROL

Antibiogram
Record of resistance of microbe to various antibiotics; used to identify trends and patterns of resistance.

Antimicrobial prophylaxis
Use of antimicrobial agents before an infection has occurred, to prevent a subsequent infection.

Antimicrobial resistance
Loss of activity against microorganisms. The mechanism of resistance may be associated with enzymatic inactivation of the drug, altered permeability barriers, altered target protein in cell wall, or altered cytoplasm targets.

Bacteriostatic
Quality of inhibition of growth of bacteria.

Bench mark
Use of either internal or external information to compare a sample to a population; it is important to use the same methodology and that the sample adequately represents the population with respect to risk factors. Usually, the benchmark is considered the best result for the comparison based on valid research.

Body substance isolation
Isolation of all moist and potentially infectious body substances (blood, feces, urine, sputum, saliva, wound drainage, and other body fluids) from all patients, regardless of their presumed infection status, primarily through the use of gloves.

Baseline
Objective quantitative data collected to determine endemic infection rates or rates of risk factors in a population.

Case control study

A retrospective study that starts with the outcome (e.g., infection, disease) and looks back to identify the associated risk factors/causes.

Cleaning

Removal of all foreign material from objects (e.g., removal of dirt or grossly visible body fluids from endoscope surfaces).

Cluster

Events such as infections that occur closely together in a population.

Cohort

A group of patients exposed to a common factor(s) who are compared to an unexposed group to see what the effect of the factor is on the disease.

Cohorting

Grouping of patients/staff together who have had exposure to the same infection or who have the same infection and segregating from those who have not had the exposure or do not have the infection.

Colonization

Presence of microorganisms at a body site not associated with active invasion of the host.

Common source outbreak

Outbreak of infections attributed to the same single exposure source (e.g., contaminated food item).

Communicable

Capable of being transmitted from one person to another.

Concurrent

Occurring at the same time; in the case of surveillance, collecting data as close as possible to the time of exposure to a risk factor (e.g., indwelling catheter).

Congenital disease

Illness present at birth or shortly thereafter that results from intrauterine infection.

Contamination

The presence of microorganisms on inanimate objects (e.g., clothing, surgical instruments) or in substances (e.g., water, food, milk).

Continuous quality improvement

The base theory that quality can be improved on a continuous, never-ending basis.

Device days

The total number of days that a specific type of device is used in a population within a specific timeframe. Device days are used as a denominator in surveillance.

Disinfection

A process that eliminates many or all microorganisms except bacterial spores.

Empiric

Treatment by remedies that experience has proved to be useful.

Endemic

The usual or expected occurrence of disease.

Endogenous

Infections caused by the patient's own flora.

Epidemic

An excess over the expected incidence of disease within a geographic area during a specified time period.

Epidemiology

Study of the distribution and determinants of disease.

Exogenous

Infections that result from transmission of organisms from a source other than the patient.

Hypothesis

A supposition or "best guess" to account for known facts.

Immunosuppressive

Any chemical, pharmacological, physical, or immunologic agent that inhibits the immune response.

In utero (congenital) infection

Infection of the newborn acquired in utero and present at birth.

Incidence

Number of new cases of disease in a population over a period of time.

Incubation period

The time interval between initial contact with an infectious agent and the first appearance of symptoms associated with the infection and/or laboratory detection.

Infection

Condition in a host resulting from presence and invasion by microorganisms.

Index case

The first known case with a specific microorganism or disease; usually used as the first known case in a cluster or outbreak.

Inflammation

Condition resulting from tissue response to injury or stimulation by noninfectious agents (e.g., thermal burns, chemicals, toxins).

Intrapartum (natal) infection

Infection acquired during passage through the birth canal.

Isolation

Separation of infected/exposed persons from others for the period of communicability in order to reduce infection transmission risks.

Neonatal infection

Infection occurring in the first 28 days of life.

Outbreak

Synonymous with epidemic, but a term often preferred when dealing with the public; does not evoke the same fear response as the term epidemic.

Pathogenicity

The ability of microorganisms to induce disease.

Pandemic

An epidemic that involves large geographical areas or several continents.

Perinatal infection

Infection acquired during period from shortly before to shortly after birth.

Postnatal (postpartum) infection

Infection acquired after birth.

Propagated source outbreak

An outbreak which continues over time due to the person-to-person spread.

Proportion

A type of ratio in which the numerator must be included in the denominator. It is often expressed as a percentage.

Prospective study

Individuals are identified with a common risk factor and followed forward in time to identify potential outcomes (e.g., infection).

Reservoir

Place in which an infectious agent can survive but may or may not multiply.

Risk factor

A characteristic, behavior, or experience that increases the probability of developing a negative health outcome (e.g., infection).

Risk stratification

A method to allow comparisons of outcomes by grouping similar subgroups together within in samples and populations (e.g., Surgical Site Infection Risk Index).

Sanitation

A process resulting from reduction in the microbial population to a safe or relatively safe level on an inanimate object.

Sensitivity

Ability of a test to detect a disease if the disease is truly present.

Sentinel event

An unusual critical event that, when it occurs, should prompt immediate investigation.

Specificity

Ability of a test to not detect a disease when not present.

Standard Precautions

Precautions designed to reduce the risk of transmission of microorganisms from both recognized and unrecognized sources of infection in hospitals.

Sterilization

A process that completely eliminates or kills all microorganisms.

Surveillance
The process of data collection, collation, and analysis for the purposes of characterizing risk groups and identifying control strategies.

Susceptible
A person or animal not possessing sufficient resistance against a particular pathogenic agent to prevent contracting infection or disease when exposed to the agent.

Therapeutic
The science and art of healing.

Threshold
The level that must be exceed for an effect to be produced or action to be taken.

Transmission
Link in the chain of infection in which passing of infection to a host occurs; requires a susceptible host, means of transmission, infectious agent, resevoir, and means of escape.
(Refer to Section 1 – Infection Control and Epidemiology for a picture of the chain of infection)

Trend
A specific tendency or direction of findings as identfied during surveillance analysis.

Universal precautions
Method used to prevent the spread of infectious agents. All human blood and body fluids are treated as if known to be infectious. Now commonly referred to as Standard Precautions.
(Refer to Section 2 – Isolation and Precautions)

Virulence
The measure of the severity of the disease.

INFECTION CONTROL RESOURCES

ORGANIZATIONS

Association for Professionals in Infection Control and Epidemiology Inc (APIC)

Address: 1275 K Street NW, 10th Floor
Washington DC 20036
Phone: 202-789-1890
Fax: 202-789-1899
URL: **http://www.apic.org**
Email **apicinfo@apic.org**

APIC Listserve-moderated listserve for the discussion of infection control practice issues.

To subscribe to the APIClist, send an e-mail message to the following address with "SUBSCRIBE APIC" as the body of the message.
URL: **www.listserv@peach.ease.lsoft.com**

Agency for Healthcare Research and Quality (AHQR)

Address: PO Box 8547
Silver Springs MD 20907-8547
Phone: 800-358-9295 or 1-202-512-1800
Instant Fax: 301-594-2800
URL: **www.ahrq.gov/**

American Assn for Respiratory Care (AARC)

Contact: AARC
Address: 11030 Ables Lane
Dallas, TX 75229
Phone: 972-243-2272
Fax: 972-484-2720
URL: **http://www.aarc.org**

American Hospital Association
Contact: AHA
Address: 1 N. Franklin Suite 27
Chicago IL 60606
URL: **http://www.aha.org**

American Institute of Architects, Academy of Architecture for Health

1997 Guidelines for Design and construction of Hospitals and Healthcare Facilities
Price: about $90.00
Order: 1735 New York Ave, NW
Washington DC 20006
Phone: 202-626-7300
URL: **http://www.e-architect.com/pia/health/home.asp**

American Society for Gastrointestinal Endoscopy
Address: 13 Elm Street
Manchester, MA 01944-8330
Phone: 978-526-8330
Fax: 978-526-4018
URL: **http://www.asge.org**

American Society for Parenteral and Enteral Nutrition
Contact: ASPEN
Address: 8639 Fenton, Ste 412
Silver Springs MD 20910-3805
Phone: 301-587-6315

Association for the Advancement of Medical Instrumentation (AAMI)
Contact: AAMI
Address: 3330 Washington Blvd, Ste 400
Arlington VA 22101-4598
Phone: 703-5350-4890
URL: **http://www.aami**

Association of Operating Room Nurses, Inc.

Address: 2170 S Parker Rd., Ste 300
Denver CO 80231
Phone: 303-755-6300
URL: **http://www.aorn.org**

CENTERS FOR DISEASE CONTROL AND PREVENTION (CDC)

An agency of the Dept of Health and Human Services.

Info: **Centers for Disease Control and Prevention**
Atlanta GA
Phone: 404-639-3311

CDC Epidemiology Program Office

EPI INFO Computer Program for Surveillance,

Data Management and EPI Analysis

Price: Free (download from CDC)
About $85.00 with manual if ordered
Order: USD Inc.
Stone Mountain GA
Phone: 770-469-4098
URL: **http://www.cdc.gov/epo/epiinfo.htm**

CDC National AIDS Hotline

Phone: 800-342-AIDS (2437)
URL: **http://www.ashastd.org/**
Note: Anonymous, confidential HIV/AIDS info, referrals, free publications

CDC National Immunization Information Hotline

Phone: 800-232-2522
URL: **http://www.ashastd.org**

CDC National Prevention Information Network

Address: PO Box 6003
Rockville, MD 20849-6003
Phone: 800-458-5231
Fax: 888-282-7681
URL: **http://www.cdcpin.org**
Note: Info and publications on HIV/AIDS Reference Services, Educational Material, AIDS Clinical Trials, and HIV Surveillance Report

National Center for Infectious Diseases

CDC Publications Activity, NCID Office of Planning and Health
Address: 1600 Clifton Rd., Mailstop C-14
Atlanta, GA 30333
URL: **http://www.cdc.gov/ncidod/ncid.htm**
Note: NCID provides publications and videos for the public and health professionals on infectious diseases. Internet site links to CDC hospital infection control guidelines, courses, and topics.

National Center for HIV, STD and TB Prevention

Phone: 800-639-1819
Note: Recording for STD publications, summary stats and hotline #'s available 24hrs/7days for healthcare professionals and educators, and lists state/local health dept numbers.

National Herpes Hotline: 919-361-8488

URL: **http://www.ashastd.org**

National Center for TB Elimination

Information Services, NCPS
Address: 1600 Clifton Rd., NE, MS E-06
Atlanta, GA 30333
Phone: 404-639-1819
Fax: 404-639-8268
URL: **http://www.cdc.gov/nchstp/tb/default.htm**

Centers for Medicare and Medicaid Studies
(formerly the Healthcare Financing Administration [HCFA])

Address:	7500 Security Blvd. Baltimore, MD 21244
URL:	**http://www.hcfa.gov/**
URL:	**http://www.hcfa.gov/pubforms/htlmtoc.htm**
Note:	HCFA Standards, including Medicaid and Medicare Certification are available.

International Executives Housekeepers Assn (IEHA)

Contact:	IEHA
Address:	1001 Eastwind Dr., Suite 301 Westerville, OH 43081-3361
Phone:	800-200-6342

Joint Commission on Accreditation of Healthcare Organizations (JCAHO)

Address:	1 Renaissance Blvd Oakbrook Terrace IL 60181
Phone:	630-792-5000
Fax:	630-792-5005
URL:	**http://www.jcaho.org**

Latex Allergy Information Service (LAIS)

Contact:	LAIS
Address:	176 Roosevelt Ave. Torrington, CT 06790
Phone:	860-482-6869
Fax:	860-482-7640
Note:	Publication, "Latex Allergy News" 11 times annually ($40). Bibliography of articles and lists of treating physicians available to members.

National Association of Home Care (NAHC)

Address: 228 7th Street SE
Washington, DC 20003-4306
Phone: 202-547-7424
Fax: 202-547-3540
URL: **http://www.nahc.org**
Note: NAHC publishes a free resource catalog of publications, audiotapes, videotapes, software, and related home care products.

National Coalition for Adult Immunizations (NCAI)

Address: 4733 Bethesda Ave., Suite 750
Bethesda, MD 20814-5228
Phone: 301-656-0003
Fax: 301-907-0878
URL: **http://www.medscape.com/affiliates/ncai**
Note: One free copy available of *The Resource Guide for Adult Immunization.*

National Foundation for Infectious Diseases (NFID)

Address: 4733 Bethesda Ave., Suite 750
Bethesda, MD 20814-5228
Phone: 301-656-0003
Fax: 301-907-0878
URL: **http://www.medscape.com/affiliates/ncai**

National Health Information Center (NHIC)

Contact: NHIC, Referral Specialist
Address: PO Box 1133
Washington, DC 20013-1133
Phone: 800-336-4797
Fax: 301-984-4256
URL: **http://nhic-nt.health.org**
Note: Via Internet provides health info resource database that includes 1,100 organizations and government offices.

National Institutes of Health (NIH)

Prices:	vary
Order:	NIH
Address:	Editorial Operations Branch Office of Communications Bethesda MD 20892
URL:	**http://www.nih.gov**
Note:	Location of National Library of Medicine; world's largest medical library and MEDLINE.

National Technical Information Services—research and technical information

Price:	Reasonable, varies with product
Order:	703-487-4142
Address:	NTIS 5285 Port Royal Rd. Springfield VA 22161
Phone:	703-487-4650
URL:	**http://www.fedworld.gov**
Note:	NTIS distributes free lists of scientific, technical and business info requested most.

National Tuberculosis Center

National Tuberculosis Center at NJ Med School
Univ. of Medicine and Dentistry of NJ

Address:	Executive Office, Suite GBI 65 Bergen Street Newark, NJ 07107-3001
Phone:	800-4TB-DOCS (483-3627)
Fax:	973-972-3268
URL:	**http://www.umdnj.edu/ntbc/**

Resident (Long-Term Care) Assessment Users Manual Version 2.0

Price:	\$29.95 plus \$3.00 shipping and handling (# 5011)

continues on next page

Order: American Healthcare Association
AHCA Publications
Dept. C1
P.O Box 96906
Washington DC 20090-6906
Phone: 800-321-0343
URL: **http://www.hcfa.gov/medicare/hsqb/mds20/default.htm**

Society of Gastroenterology Nurses and Associates, Inc. (SGNA)

Address: 401 North Michigan Ave.
Chicago, IL 60611-4267
Phone: 800-245-7462
Fax: 312-527-6658
URL: **http://www.sgna.org/**

Society of Healthcare Epidemiology of America (SHEA)

Address: 19 Mantua Road
Mt. Royal, NJ 08061
Phone: 856-423-7222 Ext 350
FAX: 856-423-3420
E-mail: sheamtg@talley.com
URL: **http://www.shea-online.org**
Note: SHEA publishes a monthly journal: *Infection Control and Hospital Epidemiology* and also, offers physician focused Hospital Epidemiology course and other seminars.

United States Environmental Protection Agency (EPA)

Address: 1200 Pennsylvania Ave., NW
Washington, DC 20460
URL: **http://www.epa.gov**
Note: This site is an excellent source for Medical Waste information. Maintains links to each states medical waste regulations.

World Health Organization

Address: 525 23rd Street NW
Washington, DC 20037
Phone: 202-974-3000
Fax: 202-974-3663
URL: **http://www.who.org**
Note: Via Internet, info on all 44 major program offices is available, including Public Information and Newsletters; Outbreak; Travel and Health Info etc.

For catalogues of publications and videos write:

Address: World Health Organization
Distribution and Sales
1211 Geneva 27
Switzerland

JOURNALS

(AJIC) American Journal of Infection Control

Official Journal of the Association for Professionals in Infection Control and Epidemiology, Inc. (APIC)

AJIC is a recognized, reliable source for peer-reviewed articles on infection control, epidemiology, infectious diseases, quality management, occupational health, and disease prevention.

Editor: Elaine L. Larson RN, PhD, FAAN, CIC
Publisher: Mosby Inc.
Address: 11830 Westline Industrial Drive
St. Louis, MO 63146-9988
Phone: 800-453- 4351 or 314-432-1158
URL: **http://www.mosby.com/ajic** or
URL: **http://www.apic.org/ajic/**

(CID) Clinical Infectious Diseases

CID is the second official publication of the Infectious Disease Society of America, which publishes clinically relevant articles for the Infectious Disease physician.

Editor:	Sherwood L. Gorbach, MD
Publisher:	University of Chicago Press
Phone:	773-753-3347
Fax:	773-753-0811
URL:	**http://www.journals.uchicago.edu/CID**
Note:	Free access to full text articles is available on the CID Web site

(EID) Emerging Infectious Diseases

EID communicates public health info about emerging infectious diseases.

Editor:	Joseph P. McDade, PhD
Publisher:	Centers for Disease Control and Prevention, Inc. (CDC) 1600 Clifton Rd., NE;Atlanta, GA 30333
URL:	**http://www.cdc.gov/ncidod/eid.**
Note:	Journal is free and available online.

(JAMA) Journal of the American Medical Association

JAMA features both clinically oriented and laboratory-based articles covering all practices of medicine.

Editor:	Catherine D. DeAngelis, MD, MPH
Publisher:	American Medical Association
Phone:	800-262-2350
Fax:	312-464-5831
URL:	**http://www.jama.ama-assn.org**
Note:	Full access to online articles is available until April 2000 with registration-only AMA members and paid subscribers after April 2000.

Journal of Hospital Infection

Journal seeks as international audience to provide comprehensive coverage of infection control measures globally.

Editor:	Stephen Barrett, MD
Publisher:	Harcourt International
Phone:	877-839-7126
URL:	**http://www.harcourt-international.com/journals/jhin**
Note:	Abstracts of articles are available online.

(JID) Journal of Infectious Disease

Official publication of the Infectious Disease Society of America - geared to the physician with a special interest in infectious diseases.

Editor:	Marvin Turk
Publisher:	University of Chicago Press
Phone:	773-753-3347
Fax:	773-753-0811
URL:	**http://www.journals.uchicago.edu/JID**
Note:	Free online access to full text articles.

(ICHE) Infection Control and Hospital Epidemiology

Official Journal of the Society of Healthcare Epidemiology of America (SHEA)

ICHE is a monthly peer reviewed scientific journal for infection control and epidemiology programs in hospitals or healthcare facilities.

Editor:	Michael D. Decker MD MPH
Publisher:	Slack Incorporated 6900 Grove Road Thorofare NJ 08086-9447
Phone:	800-257-8290 or 609-848-1000
URL:	**http://www.slackinc.com**
URL:	**http://www.Medscape.com/Affiliates/SHEA/Journals.htm**

(MMWR) Morbidity Mortality Weekly Report

MMWR reports weekly U. S. public health data and includes reports on infectious and chronic diseases, environmental hazards, natural or human-generated disasters, occupational diseases and injuries, and intentional and unintentional injuries. Also publishes recommendations and reports from the Advisory Committee on Immunization Practices (ACIP) and the Healthcare Infection Control Practices Advisory Committee (HICPAC).

Editor:	John Ward, MD
Publisher:	Centers for Disease Control and Prevention, Inc.
Phone:	202-512-1800 request #017-022-0178-1
URL:	**http://www.cdc.gov/mmwr**
Note:	Electronic subscriptions and full text articles are available free online.

(NEJM) New England Journal of Medicine

NEJM covers all specialties of medicine and publishes major reports in all area of medicine.

Editor:	Marcia Angell, MD
Publisher:	Massachusetts Medical Society
Phone:	800-THE-NEJM (842-6356)
Fax:	781-893-0413URL:
URL:	**http://www.nejm.org**
Note:	Online subscription available to subscribers only.

Pediatric Infectious Diseases

Journal publishes original reports and review articles covering infectious diseases in children.

Editors:	John D. Nelson, MD and George H. McCracken, Jr., MD
Publisher:	Lippincott Williams and Wilkins, Ltd.
Phone:	800-638-3030
Fax:	301-824-7390
URL:	**http://www.pidj.com**

The Lancet

Considered the most reputable medical journal in the world, publishes articles that concern global issues in all area of medicine.

Editors: Richard Horton (London) and David H. Frankel (North America)
Fax: 212-633-3850
URL: **http://www.thelancet.com**

BOOKS

APIC Handbook of Infection Control

Editors: Jan Jennings, BSMT (ASCP), MS, CIC and Joan Wideman, BSMT(ASCP), MS, CIC
2002; approx 550 pages (pocket size);
Price not set at time of this printing
Publisher: APIC
Phone: 202-789-1890
URL: **http://www.apic.org/html.cat/handbook.html**

Pocket-sized paperback serves as a quick reference for infection control professionals, nursing staff, physicians, administrators, healthcare students, and other ancillary healthcare providers.

A Practical Handbook for Hospital Epidemiologists

Editors: Loreen A. Herwaldt MD and Michael Decker MD
1997; 448 pages; $60 plus shipping and handling
Publisher: Slack Incorporated (see above) with SHEA
Phone: 800-257-8290
URL: **http://www.orders@slackinc.com**

A complete source for practical advice on hospital epidemiology

APIC Text of Infection Control and Epidemiology

Editor: Jeanne A. Pfeiffer, RN, MPH, CIC
2000; Publication consists of two separate binders
Publisher: APIC and Mosby, Inc.
Phone: 202-789-1890
Fax: 202-789-1899
URL: **http://www.apic.org/html/pubs/text.2000.html**

Text reflects current infection control and epidemiological practices.

Also contains all official APIC documents as well as infection control guidelines from CDC and OSHA.

Note: CD-ROM version also available and subscription for annual supplements available.

APIC Infection Control in Home Care

Editors: Emily Rhinehart, RN, MPH, CIC, CPHQ and Mary McGoldrick Friedman, MS, RN, CRNI
1999; 225 pages.
Publisher: APIC (see above for numbers) $44 members/ $55 non-members
URL: **http://www.apic.org/html/cat/hcicbook.html**

Practical applications of Infection Control in Home Care setting—includes sample tools to implement and Infection Control program.

CDC Guidelines for Prevention and Control of Nosocomial Infections—compiled by SHEA

1998; 325 pages;
$99 Regular Price
$70.00 (DISCOUNT PRICE FOR Attendees at SHEA/CDC Epidemiology Course)
Publisher: ETNA Communications
3023 N. Clark, Suite 744
Chicago, IL 60657-5200
Phone: 800-552-0076 or 414-634-0806

continues on next page

URL: **http://www.etnacomm.com**

Contains CDC guidelines on UTI, Handwashing and Environmental Control, HIV and HBV-Exposure Prone Invasive Procedures, Tuberculosis, IV Device-related Infections, HIV Postexposure Chemoprophylaxis, Surgical Site Infections, Healthcare Personnel, Pneumonia, VRE, Isolation, HCV postexposure follow-up.

Control of Communicable Diseases Manual

Editor: James Chin, MD, MPH
2000; Paperback 579 pages; $30
Publisher: American Public Health Association
800 I Street, NW Washington, DC 20001-3710

An accurate, informative text for public health information with 137 short chapters, each chapter devoted to a single infectious disease or pathogen.

Disinfection, Sterilization, and Antisepsis in Healthcare, Conference Proceedings

Editor: William Rutula, PhD, MPH
1998; 292 pages $58 members/$73 non-members
Publisher: APIC
Phone: 800-840-5870 or 202-789-1890
URL: **http://www.apic.org**

This book contains proceedings of the International Symposium on Disinfection, Sterilization and Antisepsis in Healthcare held at the 1998 APIC Educational Conference. It includes information on low temperature sterilization technologies and chemical germicides.

Guidelines for Design and Construction of Hospital and Healthcare Facilities

From: American Institute of Architects and US Department of Health and Human Services
1996; 300 pages; $60; Item number J-189-96
Publisher: American Institute of Architects
Phone: 888-272-4115 or 415-421-3627
URL: **http://aiaonline.com**

Hospital Epidemiology and Infection Control (2nd **Ed**)

Editor: C. Glen Mayhall, MD
1999; 1656 pages; $169
Publisher: Lippincott Williams and Wilkins
Phone: 800-638-3030
Fax: 301-824-7390
URL: **http://www.lww.com**

A comprehensive, 100 chapter, reference book for hospital epidemiologists and infection control practitioners.

Note: This book is also available in the icanPREVENT Resource Center (see web sites).

Hospital Infections (Fourth Edition)

Editors: John V Bennett MD and Philip P Brachman MD
1998; 759 pages; $149
Publisher: Lippincott Williams and Wilkins
Phone: 800-638-3030
URL: **http://www.lww.com**

This test is divided into 3 sections: Part I reviews the general considerations of hospital infections; Part II discusses the functional areas of concern; and Part III focuses on specific endemic and epidemic hospital infections.

Immunization of Healthcare Workers: A practical approach

Editors: Gregory A Poland MD, William Schaffner MD, and Gina Pugliese RN, MS
320 pages Hardcover
Publisher: Slack Incorporated (see above) with SHEA
Phone: 800-257-8290
URL: **http://www.orders@slackinc.com**

A complete resource for establishing or update immunization programs.

Infections and Nursing Practice

Editors: Barbara Soule RN, MPA and Elaine Larson RN, PhD
1994; 384 pages; $46.95

Clinical reference with infection prevention and control techniques in a variety of care settings exploring the social, cultural, and economic environment in which infection occurs.

Publisher: CV Mosby
URL: **www.mosby.org**

Infection Prevention with Limited Resources: A Handbook for Infection Control Committees

Authors: Patricia Lynch RN MBA, Marguerite Jackson RN PhD, Gary Preston PhD, and Barbara Soule RN MPA
1998; 180 pages; $50
Publisher: ETNA Communications
3023 North Clark, Suite 744
Chicago, IL 60657-5200
Phone: 800-552-0076 or 414-634-0806
URL: **http://www.etnacomm.com**

A framework for nosocomial infection prevention and control when resources are limited. Issues such as organizational strategies, infection prevention priorities and proven methods for risk reduction strategies are discussed.

Prevention and Control of Nosocomial Infections

Editor: Richard P Wenzel MD
1997; 1227 pages; $139
Publisher: Lippincott Williams and Wilkins
Phone: 800-638-3030
URL: **http://www.lww.com**

A comprehensive updated and well referenced information for preventing and controlling nosocomial infections.

Quick Reference to Outbreak Investigation and Control in Healthcare Facilities

Author: Kathleen Meehan Arias, MS, CIC
2000; 329 pages; $51 member/$63 non-member

Publisher: APIC and Aspen Publications

Phone: 202-789-1890

URL: **http://www.apic.org/html/pubs/pubsmain.html/**

Contains guidelines for recognizing, investigating and controlling outbreaks and clusters of infection in healthcare facilities.

Saunders Infection Control Reference Text

Editors: Elias Abrutyn, Donald Goldmann, William Scheckler
1998; 1269 pages; $310

Publisher: WB Saunders Philadelphia PA
Book Order Fulfillment
6277 Sea Harbor Drive;
Orlando, Florida 32887-4430

Call: 1-800-545-5222 or 407-345-3800

URL: **http://customerservice.wbsaunders.com**

This book is divided into seven sections: Introduction, Key Components of Infection Control Programs, Infection Control Guidelines by Facility Size, Location of Service, Infection Control Guidelines by Site of Infection, Infection Control Guidelines for Selected Clinical Problems, Facility-Based Infection Control Guidelines, and Information Resources.

Sharps Injury Prevention Program: A Step by Step Guide

Editor: Gina Pugliese, RN, MS
1999; 77 pages; $25 American Hospital Association Members (AHA) $70 Non AHA Members

Publisher: American Hospital Association

Phone: 800-AHA-2626

URL: **http://www.aha.org**
catalog #196311

Designed to help develop a sharps injury prevention-program and as a step-by-step guide for improving the health and safety of healthcare workers, patients and the community.

Sterilization Technology for Healthcare Facilities

Editors:	Jack Young and Marimargaret Reichert 1997; 307 pages; $95.00
Publisher:	Aspen Publishers
Phone:	800 638-8437
Fax:	301 417-7550
Phone:	301 417-7543
URL:	www.aspenpub.com
E-mail:	**webmaster@aspenpubl.com**

Vancomycin-Resistant Enterococci: Issues and Controversies in Prevention and Control

Editors:	Gina Pugliese, RN, MS and Robert A Weinstein, MD 1998; 310 pages; $79.00
Publisher:	ETNA Communications 3023 North Clark, Suite 744 Chicago IL 60657-5200
Phone:	800-552-0076 or 414-634-0806
URL:	**http://www.etnacomm.com**

Essential resource covering control of VRE in special settings, sample policies from state health departments, reprints of guidelines from CDC and AHA and answers to frequently asked questions.

ISOLATION AND INFECTION CONTROL SIGNS

Isolation Signs consistent with CDCs revised 1996 isolation guidelines

Custom isolation and infection control signage

To Order: ETNA Communications

Phone: 800-552-0076 or 414-634-0806

URL: **http://etnacomm.com**

To Order: Brevis Corporation

Phone: 800-383-3377 or 801-466-6677

Fax: 801-485-2844

URL: **http://info@brevis.com**

INTERNET/WORLD WIDE WEB SITES - free access

Agency for Healthcare Policy and Research:
URL: **http://ahcpr.gov**

AIDS Clearinghouse (CDC):
URL: **http://cdcnac.org**

APIC—Association for Professionals in Infection Control and Epidemiology:
URL: **http://apic.org**

AJIC-American Journal of Infection Control
URL: **http://www.mosby.com/mosby/catalogs/periodicals/medical/4.html**

APIC North Carolina Chapter Newsletter "Bugline"
URL: **http://www.sandhills.org/org/bugline**

CDC:
URL: **http://www.cdc.gov**

Department of Health and Human Services:
URL: **http://www.os.dhhs.gov**

Disease Prevention News (Texas Dept of Health):
URL: **http://tdh.state.tx.us/phpep/dpnhome.html**

Emerging Infectious Diseases:
URL: **http://www.cdc.gov/ncidod.EID**

Food and Drug Administration:
URL: **http://www.fda.gov**

Federal Register:
URL: **http://www.access.gpo.gov/su_docs/aces/aaces140.html**

Handwashing Compliance Control Center:
URL: **http://www.users.aol.com/comcontrol/comply.htm**

Health A to Z (medical info search engine):
URL: **http://www.healthatoz.com**

Hepatitis Foundation International:
URL: **http://www.hepfi.org**

Infectious Disease Links Directory:
URL: **http://www.pages.prodigy.net/pdeziel**

Infectious Disease Web-Site Directory:
URL: **http://www.gen.emory.edu/medweb.html**

Joint Commission on Accreditation of Healthcare Organizations (JCAHO):
URL: **http://www.jcaho.org**

Johns Hopkins School of Public Health:
URL: **http://www.phweb.sph.jhu.edu**

Journal of Hospital Infection:
URL: **http://www.hbuk.co.uk/wbs/jhi**

Library of Congress:
URL: **http://www.lcweb.loc.gov**

Long-term care infection prevention:
URL: **http://www.broadstreetsolutions.com**

Medscape: On-line Resource for Better Patient Care
URL: **http://www.medscape.com**

National Antimicrobial Information Network
(sterilants and disinfectants
URL: **http://ace.ace.orst.edu/info/nain**

National Center for Health Statistics (CDC):
URL: **http://cdc.gov/nchswww/nchshome.htm**

National Center for HIV, STD, and TB:
URL: **http://www.cdc.gov/nchstp/od/nchstp.html**

National Center for Infectious Diseases:
URL: **http://cdc.gov/ncidod/ncid.htm**

National Coalition for Adult Immunization (NCAI):
URL: **http://www.medscape.com/affiliates/ncai**

National Foundation for Infectious Disease:
URL: **http://www.medscape.com/Affiliates/NFID**

National Immunization Program:
URL: **http://www.cdc.gov/nip**

National Institute for Occupational Health and Safety (NIOSH):
URL: **http://www.cdc.gov/niosh/homepage.html**

National Institute of Allergy and Infectious Diseases:
URL: **http://www.niaid.nih.gov**

National Institute of Health:
URL: **http://www.nih.gov**

National Library of Medicine:
URL: **http://www.nlm.nih.gov**

NNIS Semi-annual Report:
URL: **http://www.cdc.gov/ncidod/diseases/hip/nnis/**

National Technical Information Service (NTIS)
URL: **http://www.fedworld.gov**

Nuclear, Biological and Chemical Medical Web Page:
URL: **http://www.nbc-med.org**

Occupational Safety and Health Administration (OSHA):
URL: **http://www.osha.gov**

Outbreak Info:
URL: **http://www.outbreak.org**

Pan American Health Organization:
URL: **http://www.paho.org**

Postexposure Prophylaxis Protocol:
URL: **http://www.epi-center.uscf.edu**

ProMED: discussions and monitoring of emerging diseases
URL: **http://www.fas.org/promed**

Travelers' Health Information:
URL: **http://www.cdc.gov/travel**

Tropical Medicine-Tulane:
URL: **http://www.tropmed.tulane.edu**

Tuberculosis Elimination Division (CDC):
URL: **http://www.cdc.gov/nchstp/tb/dtbe.html**

Vaccine Safety:
URL: **http://www.cdc.gov/nip/vacsafe**

White House (U.S. Health Statistics:
URL: **http://www.whitehouse.gov/fsbr/health.html**

Society for Healthcare Epidemiology of America:
URL: **http://www.medscape.com/affiliates/SHEA**

World Health Organization:
URL: **http://www.who.ch**

LIST SERVES

AIDSNEWS - AIDS treatment news, abstracts from medical journals, discussion of ethical/social issues
URL: **http://www.listserv@rutgers.edu**

APIC - information and discussion on infection control issues
URL: **listserv@peach.ease.lsoft.com**

INCLEN-L-A forum for posing questions to an expert in clinical epidemiology
URL: **http://www.listserv@mcmvm1.bitnet**

MMWR - Receive weekly notification of contents of MMWR (Morbidity and Mortality Weekly Report) through email:
URL: **http://www.listserve@list.cdc.gov**

NIHGUIDE - List of available NIH grants and contracts
URL: **http://www.listserv@umab.bitnet**

OCC-ENV-MED-L- Occupational Health Physicians, Nurses, Public health Professionals, Industrial Hygienists discuss regulatory issues, case presentations and share expertise
URL: **http://www.listserv@mc.duke.edu**

PROMED - Electronic network for communication about emerging infectious diseases globally.
URL: **http://www.promed-request@usa.healthnet.org**

SAFETY - Environmental health and safety issues including laboratory safety and hazardous waste disposal
URL: **http://listserv@uvmvm.uvm.edu**

GUIDELINES

SHEA Position papers (See listing in this resource section of SHEA position papers published in SHEA's journal, Infection Control and Hospital Epidemiology

CDC Guidelines for Prevention and Control of Nosocomial Infections (Most recent guidelines can be downloaded at CDC web site; SHEA has compiled all CDC Guidelines for Surveillance, Prevention and Control of Infections and they are available from ETNA Communications- see ordering information above under books)
URL: **http://www.cdc.gov**

APIC Guidelines for Infection Control Practice have been published in the APIC Journal: American Journal of Infection Control (AJIC) and are also available from APIC (see above) Guidelines include:

A Consensus Panel Report: Requirements for Infrastructure and Essential Activities of Infection Control and Epidemiology in Hospitals; April 1998 AJIC

APIC/SHEA Position Paper: Infection Prevention and Control in the LTC Facility; December 1997 AJIC

CDC Guideline for Isolation Precautions in Hospitals; February 1996 AJIC

CDC Guideline for Preventing the Transmission of Mycobacterium Tuberculosis in Healthcare Facilities, 10/28/94 Federal Register

CDC Guideline for Prevention of Nosocomial Pneumonia; August 1994

Guideline for Selection and Use of Disinfectants; August 1996 AJIC

Guideline for Handwashing and Hand Antisepsis in Healthcare Setting; August 1995 AJIC

Guideline for Infection Prevention and Control in Flexible Endoscopy; February 1994 AJIC

HICPAC Guideline for Prevention of Intravascular Device-Related Infections; August 1996 AJIC

Recommended Practices for Surveillance AJIC June 1998

Guidelines can also be ordered from APIC
URL: **http://www.cdc.gov http://www.apic.org**

OTHER EDUCATIONAL RESOURCES

Construction: Infection Control Issues During Construction and Renovation Tool Kit

Author:	Judene Bartley, MPH, CIC
	1999; $56 member/$64 non-member
Publisher:	APIC
Phone:	800-789-1890
URL:	**http://www.apic.org**

Hepatitis: CDC Hepatitis: Epidemiology and Prevention of Viral Hepatitis A to E: An Overview

Presents an overview of the clinical and epidemiological features of Hepatitis A thru E, a slide set is available to downloading.

URL: **http://www.cdc.gov/ncidod/diseases/hepatitis/slideset/hep.htm**

Tuberculosis: CDC Tuberculosis (TB) Core Curriculum, 4th Ed. What the Clinician Should Know

	2000; available for downloading on the web -144 pages
Publisher:	Centers for Disease Control and Prevention, Inc
Phone:	404-639-3311
URL:	**http://www.cdc.gov/nchstp/tb/pubs/corecurr/default.htm**

Contains basic information about TB for health professionals. It is intended as a reference manual and is has excellent information for educational programs.

Tuberculosis: CDC: Division of Tuberculosis Elimination - Slide Set Core Curriculum on Tuberculosis - slide set to accompany written material-focus on recommendations for the diagnosis, treatment and control of tuberculosis.

URL: **http://www.cdc.gov/nchstp/tb/pubs/slidesets/core.htm**

Guidelines for Preventing the Transmission of Mycobacterium tuberculosis in Healthcare facilities-slide set based on 1994 MMWR supplement. Used to train healthcare professionals on implementation of the guidelines.
URL: **http://www.cdc/gov/nchstp/tb/pubs/slidesets/transmission.htm**

Controlling TB in Correctional Facilities-slide set with recommendations for jails and prisons.
URL: **http://www.cdc.gov/nchstp/tb/pubs/slidesets/corrections/html**

INTERNATIONAL ORGANIZATIONS INVOLVED IN INFECTION PREVENTION BASED OUTSIDE OF THE US—SELECTED LIST

AIDS — UNAIDS

As the main advocate for global action on HIV/AIDS
URL: http://gpawww.who.ch/unaids/unaids.htm

Communicable Disease Surveillance Centre

The Communicable Disease Surveillance Centre (CDSC) in England and in Wales. CDSC participates in several international surveillance networks and is the coordinating center for some of these including SALM-NET, the network for the surveillance of human salmonella infections in Europe and EWGLI, the European surveillance scheme for travel-associated Legionnaires Disease.
URL: **http://www.open.gov.uk/cdsc/cdschome.htm**

International Federation of Infection Control (IFIC)

IFIC is an umbrella organization of societies, associations, and other organizations of healthcare professionals in infection control and related fields. Active members of IFIC are organizations, which are represented by working delegates elected or appointed by each association. Goals include development of a network of infection control (IC) organizations for communication, consensus building, education, and sharing of expertise; liaison to WHO, providing information and educational resources to those in countries without IC organizations; and assisting in establishing IC associations where needed. For more information, refer to: Hambraeus A, Paardekooper C, White MC. IFIC: the first 10 years. American Journal of Infection Control 1997; 25:297-302.

International Federation of Environmental Health

	Eric Foskett, OBE, FCIEH Vice president and directory editor
Address:	26 Grebe Close, Poynton Stockport, Cheshire SK12 1HU United Kingdom
Phone/Fax:	+44 (0) 1625 876670
URL:	http://www.cieh.org.uk/cieh/ related/ifeh.html

International Institute of Parasitology

Address:	International Institute of Parasitology 395A Hatfield Road St Albans, Hertfordshire, AL4 0XU United Kingdom
Phone	+44-(0) 1727-833151
Fax	+44-(0) 1727-868721
E-mail	cabi-iip@cabi.org
URL:	http://www.cabi.org/institut/iip/iip.htm

International Union Against Tuberculosis and Lung Disease

Address:	68, Boulevard Saint-Michel 75006 Paris, France
Phone	33.1.44.32.03.60
Fax	33.1.43.29.90.87
E-mail	101370.370@compuserve.com
URL:	http://iuatld.vjf.inserm.fr/IUATLD/iuatldhome.shtml

European Salmonella Surveillance Network

The European Salmonella Surveillance Network (SALM-NET) national Salmonella surveillance from 14 participating European countries.

URL: Internet http://www.open.gov.uk/cdsc/salmnet.htm

European Surveillance Scheme for Travel Associated Legionnaires' Disease (EWGLI)

Compiled by: Linda Scott, RN, BSN, CIC, Judene Bartley, MS, MPH, CIC, and Gina Pugliese, RN, MS; June 2000; rev. Oct. 2002.

URL: http://www.open.gov.uk/cdsc/ewgli2.htm

INDEX

AAFP 458
AAP 212, 458
Abscess 83, 84, 107, 108, 261, 262, 325, 345, 396, 437, 443
Accreditation 3, 6, 18, 23, 67, 157, 353, 360, 364, 377, 434, 566, 584
ACH 172, 178
Acid-fast stain 523
Acinetobacter 174, 307, 327, 522, 527, 534, 547
ACIP 212, 218, 230, 243, 248, 371, 458, 494, 518, 574
Acquired immunodeficiency syndrome 29, 262
Actinomycosis 262
Action plans 18, 25, 69, 70, 88, 98, 365, 377
Acute dialysis 400
Acute Physiology and Chronic Health Evaluation 347
Acyclovir 31, 539, 544, 549
Adenovirus 262, 270
Adenoviruses 173
Administration sets 325, 332
Administrative controls 251
Adult day care 380, 386
Adult Intensive Care Units 344
Aerobic 437, 444, 522, 546, 549
Aerosol 63, 65, 140, 143, 157, 173, 174, 179, 180, 183, 186, 187, 194, 284, 387, 497
AIA 155, 156, 403
AIDS 29, 45, 223, 230, 416, 417, 503, 505, 508, 564, 583, 587, 591
AII 152, 171, 178, 179, 180, 429, 431, 432
Air 20, 138, 139, 153, 156, 165, 167, 171, 172, 173, 177, 178, 179, 183, 189, 190, 194, 200, 254, 255, 276, 285, 306, 308, 316, 317, 336, 345, 354, 384, 390, 391, 392, 419, 421, 428, 474, 475, 485
Air changes per hour 172, 316, 498
Air conditioning 172
Air handling 154, 178, 256, 308, 363, 411, 466
Air-fluidized beds 191, 192
Airborne infection isolation 152, 171
Airborne Precautions 63, 179, 187, 189, 249, 254, 276, 278, 283, 293, 353, 370, 384, 397, 398, 401, 412, 414, 461, 468, 475, 497, 513
Alcohol-based handrub 207, 208, 210
Alcohol-based waterless antiseptic agent 206, 207
Allergens 176, 297
ALT 407, 499
Ambulatory care 458
Amebiasis 262
American Dental Association 389, 395
American Institute of Architects 156, 194, 316, 403, 477, 562, 578
Americans with Disabilities Act 301, 511
Amikacin 539
Amikin® 539
Amoxicillin 539
Amoxicillin-clavulanate 539
Amoxil® 539
Amphotericin B 539
Ampicillin 539, 540
Ampicillin-sulbactam 540
Anaerobic 304, 522

Anaphylactic 215, 217, 218, 219, 223, 238, 240, 243, 244
Ancef® 540
Ancylostomiasis 267
Anesthesia 168, 288, 318, 449, 468, 469, 471
Angiographies 396
Animals 66, 171, 176, 192, 297, 301, 373, 459
Anthrax 29, 30, 137, 140, 148, 150, 151, 228, 262
Anti-HAV IgM 528
Anti-HBc 407, 528
Anti-HBc IgM 528
Anti-HBs 215, 407, 500, 501, 528
Anti-HCV 407, 499, 517, 528
Anti-HDV 529
Anti-HEV 529
Antibiotic susceptibility 433, 524
Antibiotic-associated colitis 262
Antibiotics 37, 38, 144, 275, 304, 346, 354, 437, 462, 496, 524, 534, 553
Antigen test 72, 73
Antimicrobial prophylaxis 310, 311, 315, 333, 389, 398, 467, 469, 553
Antimicrobial soap 199, 206, 208, 209
Antisepsis 170, 205, 206, 209, 210, 211, 290, 314, 578, 589
Antiseptics 132, 133, 209
AORN 293, 294, 295, 320, 477, 563
APACHE II 347, 350
Apnea 73, 74, 75, 79
ARO 434, 536
Arthropod-borne 262
Artificial fingernails 209
ASA class 320
Ascariasis 262
Asepsis x, 132, 136, 318, 388, 390, 395, 402, 412, 429, 457, 469, 471, 475
Aspergillosis 173, 262, 308
Aspergillus 156, 173, 408, 417, 539, 540, 544, 545
Aspiration pneumonia 461, 469
Assessment Worksheet 25
Asymptomatic Bacteriuria 81, 92, 322, 422, 434
Asymptomatic Patient Precautions 30, 31, 32, 33, 35, 36, 37, 38, 39, 40, 41, 42, 43, 44, 45, 46, 47, 48, 49, 50, 52, 53, 54, 55, 56, 57, 58, 59, 60, 61, 62, 63, 64, 65, 66
Attack rate 16, 139
Augmentin® 539
Avelox 546
Azactam® 540
Azithromycin 543
Aztreonam 540

B. fragilis 546
B. subtilis 161
Babesiosis 262
Bacillus 72, 96, 110, 522
Bacteremia 52, 300, 304, 322, 326, 340, 350, 408, 409, 417, 422, 436, 437, 442, 443, 444
Bacterial spores 160, 161, 287, 555
Bacteriostatic 553
Bacteroides fragilis 312, 540
Bactrim® 548
Barriers 127, 156, 166, 310, 318, 392, 463, 553
Baseline 18, 20, 22, 23, 96, 110, 431, 499, 517, 553
bDNA 527
Bedding 55, 176, 190
Behavioral Health 362, 365
Benign inoculation lymphoreticulosis 263

Biaxin® 543
Bicillin® 546
Bilharziasis 272
Bio Safety level 146
Bioburden 159
Biosafety 195, 521, 531
Biosafety level 172, 193
Bioterrorism 129, 137, 139, 140, 141, 142, 145, 146, 147, 150
Bioterrorism Readiness Plan (BRP) 138
Birthing tanks 175, 185
Blastomyces 545
Blastomycosis 262
Bloodborne 154, 499
Bloodborne pathogens 253, 292, 294, 295, 329, 358, 368, 372, 397, 405, 424, 478, 495, 497, 511
Bloodstream infection 20, 325, 326, 327, 339, 409
Body substance isolation 553
Booster 37, 214, 215, 216, 217, 219, 220, 221, 222, 226, 237, 243, 407, 500
Bordetella pertussis 261
Borrowed/loaner instruments 161
Botulism 29, 137, 262, 265
Bradycardia 73, 74, 76, 79
Branched DNA 527
Breast infection 449
Breast milk 384, 436, 438, 440, 450, 452, 453
Bronchiolitis 261, 262, 456
Broviac 326, 345
BRP 138, 142, 144, 145, 147
Brucella 148
Brucellosis 29, 137, 263
BSI 174, 325, 333, 340
Burkholderia 174, 270
C. botulinum 263
C. difficile 164, 263, 526, 543, 546, 549
C. krusei 544
C. perfringens 263
Campylobacter 92, 104, 198, 263, 266
Cancidas 540
Candida 327, 408, 417, 437, 443, 539, 540, 545
Candida albicans 312, 539, 544, 545
Candidiasis 263, 367
Capsofungin 540
Care plan 413, 418
Caregivers 22, 208, 238, 255, 276, 304, 322, 323, 349, 359, 365, 380, 381, 382, 383, 385, 395, 409, 412, 413, 414, 415, 419, 455, 458, 459, 461, 462, 464, 465
Carpeting 155, 171, 182, 187, 188, 419
Carpets 176
Case-control study 14, 350
Cat-scratch fever 263
Catheter insertion 329, 330, 334, 335, 338, 339, 340, 430
Catheter site dressing 330, 337
Catheter site maintenance 330
Catheter tip 326, 328, 340
Catheter-related bloodstream infection 326
Catheter-related infections 336, 339, 398
Catheterization 77, 322, 323, 413, 430, 449, 451, 469
Cedax® 541
Cefazolin 540
Cefepime 541
Cefizox® 541
Cefotan® 542

Cefotaxime 542
Cefotetan 542
Cefoxitin 542
Cefpodoxime proxetil 541
Cefprozil 541
Ceftazidime 542
Ceftibuten 541
Ceftizoxime 541
Ceftriaxone 52, 542
Cefuroxime 542
Cefzil® 541
Cellulitis 93, 105, 263
Central venous catheter 334
CFU 326
Chancre 263, 367
Chancroid 29, 263
Chemotherapy 65, 218, 327, 370
Chest radiography 396
Chickenpox 263, 497, 507
Childbed fever 453
Children 41, 57, 212, 226, 244, 245, 248, 380, 455, 456, 457, 458, 484
Chlamydia 264, 270, 447, 543, 548
Chlamydia trachomatis 29, 263, 442
Chloramphenicol 543
Chloromyctin® 543
Cholera 29, 263, 266
Chronic dialysis 400
Cilastatin 544
Ciprofloxacin 30, 52, 543
Cipro® 543
CJD 160, 163, 189, 194, 473
Claforan® 542
Clarithromycin 543
Class I Medical Device 286
Class II Medical Device 287
Class III Medical Device 287
Clean linen 119, 191, 284, 357
Cleaning 114, 116, 125, 140, 141, 142, 159, 161, 162, 164, 165, 176, 178, 182, 185, 186, 187, 189, 198, 200, 253, 282, 287, 288, 301, 317, 347, 354, 355, 356, 363, 367, 377, 382, 383, 388, 389, 390, 391, 397, 402, 405, 406, 412, 418, 419, 423, 430, 438, 450, 452, 457, 459, 462, 468, 471, 496, 498, 554
Cleaning brushes 164
Cleocin® 543
CLIA 358
Clindamycin 543
Clinical exit site infection 326
Clinical sepsis 72, 111
Closed-cavity infection 263
Clostridium botulinum 197
Clostridium difficile 32, 92, 189, 197, 260, 262, 265, 266, 422, 525
Clostridium perfringens 198
Clostridium perfringens or welchii 265
Clusters 8, 23, 128, 129, 137, 139, 156, 349, 355, 395, 409, 419, 427, 445, 581
CMS 86, 424
Coagulase-negative staph 72, 96, 110, 312, 436, 443, 444
Coccidioidomycosis 29, 263
Cohort 4, 14, 24, 56, 58, 138, 140, 255, 256, 257, 258, 276, 277, 308, 423, 457, 554
Cold sores 94, 109
Colonization 69, 88, 98, 174, 261, 271, 296, 300, 301, 303, 311, 326, 333, 345, 346, 434, 436, 446, 456, 462, 467, 521, 524, 534, 554
Colorado tick fever 262, 263
Common cold 90, 100
Common vehicle 249

Communicable 48, 51, 61, 353, 354, 359, 363, 383, 387, 462, 554
Communicable disease 6, 7, 13, 21, 27, 28, 30, 31, 32, 33, 34, 35, 36, 37, 38, 39, 40, 41, 42, 43, 44, 45, 46, 47, 48, 49, 50, 51, 52, 53, 54, 55, 56, 57, 58, 59, 60, 61, 62, 63, 64, 65, 66, 114, 115, 150, 352, 364, 365, 366, 367, 374, 376, 377, 378, 385, 387, 397, 398, 401, 409, 415, 432, 458, 459, 465, 497, 516, 530, 578, 592
Companion Animals 192, 297
Competencies 112, 161, 176, 477, 496
Compliance 3, 6, 21, 290, 329, 346, 348, 358, 368, 376, 378, 394, 409, 425, 429, 433, 469, 513, 584
Condom catheter 323
Congenital 218, 223, 235, 246, 273, 308, 436, 439, 440, 513, 515, 518, 556
Congenital disease 439, 555
Congenital rubella 264, 271
Conjunctivitis 33, 34, 95, 109, 263, 264, 363, 380, 422, 442, 487
Construction 127, 152, 153, 154, 155, 156, 157, 171, 178, 179, 183, 194, 308, 346, 347, 355, 364, 368, 383, 390, 398, 402, 403, 412, 414, 418, 423, 438, 450, 457, 462, 469, 477, 562, 578, 590
Construction and renovation policy 153, 154
Contact 8, 30, 31, 33, 34, 35, 36, 39, 40, 41, 44, 46, 48, 51, 53, 54, 55, 56, 57, 58, 59, 60, 61, 62, 64, 138, 143, 160, 161, 162, 165, 174, 186, 187, 198, 199, 200, 207, 209, 217, 220, 223, 233, 241, 244, 249, 252, 257, 258, 260, 261, 275, 278, 279, 294, 301, 319, 359, 364, 370, 382, 385, 391, 418, 422, 429, 432, 435, 441, 450, 455, 456, 468, 471, 472, 473, 481, 485, 487, 488, 490, 492, 493, 495, 497, 513, 514, 515, 518, 556, 561
Contact precautions 33, 34, 35, 37, 44, 46, 56, 252, 257, 276
Contamination 132, 134, 141, 142, 143, 155, 156, 175, 176, 185, 188, 189, 190, 197, 198, 199, 202, 209, 210, 258, 278, 279, 280, 281, 282, 283, 284, 292, 293, 304, 314, 317, 332, 333, 346, 357, 383, 404, 406, 429, 452, 453, 461, 463, 464, 470, 472, 473, 475, 521, 524, 555
Continuous Ambulatory Peritoneal Dialysis (CAPD) 401
Continuous quality improvement 304, 320, 555
Contraindications 31, 37, 47, 50, 51, 52, 54, 213, 214, 215, 216, 217, 218, 220, 221, 222, 223, 231, 237, 238, 239, 240, 241, 243, 244, 245, 247, 452, 481
Control measures 8, 18, 23, 130, 171, 179, 180, 189, 329, 347, 354, 363, 367, 375, 376, 382, 389, 390, 397, 402, 412, 418, 423, 426, 427, 438, 450, 457, 462, 468, 484, 513, 521, 572
Cooling of foods 197, 201
Cooling tower 172
Correctional settings x, 366, 369, 372, 376
Corynebacteria 327
Coryza 260
Cost-benefit analysis for reprocessing 289
Cover gown 278, 279, 280, 281, 282, 292

Coxsackie virus 35, 441
CR-BSI 326, 331, 332, 335, 337, 338, 339
Creutzfeldt-Jakob Disease 160, 473
Critical 2, 4, 141, 157, 163, 168, 169, 178, 196, 203, 300, 350, 351, 363, 391, 478, 534, 535, 536, 558
Cross-contamination 133, 251, 457
Croup 261, 264
CRP 153, 154
Cryptococcosis 264
Cryptococcus 539, 540, 544, 545
Cryptosporidiosis 29, 264
Cryptosporidium 175, 198, 266
CSF Testing 530
CT 396, 397
Cuffed central venous catheter 335
CVC 326, 330, 331, 334, 335, 336
Cystic fibrosis 270
Cysticercosis 264
Cytomegalovirus 264, 438, 487, 513, 539, 543
Cytovene® 544

Dalfopristin 547
Data collection tools 25
Data elements 21, 23
Data sources 4, 22, 23, 68, 87
Day care 41, 214, 228, 245, 380, 455, 459
Decubitus ulcer, infected 264
Definitions of infections 72, 73, 74, 75, 76, 77, 78, 79, 80, 81, 82, 83, 84, 85, 89, 90, 91, 92, 93, 94, 95, 96, 99, 100, 101, 102, 103, 104, 105, 106, 107, 108, 109, 110, 111, 426
Delirium 87
Delta antigen 529
Demolition 155, 171, 179
Dengue 262, 264
Dental healthcare personnel 387
Dental lab 388, 393
Dentistry 185, 387, 394, 395, 568
Dermatomycosis 271, 273
Dermatophytosis 271, 273
Device related 72, 73, 96, 325, 349, 413
Device utilization ratio 16
Diagnostic services x, 396, 397
Dialysis 87, 175, 183, 184, 230, 335, 346, 355, 400, 401, 403, 404, 405, 406, 407, 408, 409, 410
Dialysis station 405, 406
Dialyzer ports 407
Dialyzer reuse 402
Diapering 381, 383, 384
Diarrhea 30, 32, 39, 60, 62, 92, 104, 196, 197, 258, 260, 264, 354, 363, 369, 372, 380, 387, 422, 432, 481, 487, 506, 525
Diflucan® 544
Diphtheria 29, 36, 37, 38, 212, 221, 222, 226, 237, 264, 431, 432, 487, 516
Diphtheroids 72, 96, 110
Directly observed therapy 370
Dirty linen 357
Disaster Preparedness 137
Disinfection 21, 114, 116, 129, 140, 141, 142, 159, 160, 161, 162, 163, 165, 169, 170, 176, 185, 189, 211, 253, 287, 290, 307, 317, 347, 354, 355, 360, 363, 367, 377, 382, 388, 389, 390, 391, 393, 394, 397, 402, 405, 409, 412, 413, 416, 418, 423, 429, 438, 450, 451, 452, 457, 462, 464, 468, 472, 473, 555, 578
Donovanosis 266

DOT 147, 370
Drapes 176, 318
Droplet 249, 260, 261, 275, 353, 468
Droplet nuclei 173, 254, 256, 497
Droplet precautions 40, 256
Dust 125, 127, 155, 173, 177, 178, 186, 187, 191, 414, 474
Dusting 186
Dysentery 62

E. coli 39, 198, 322, 437, 444, 522, 527, 534, 539, 540, 541, 547, 548
E.E.S.® 543
Ebola 264, 267, 276
Ebola viral hemorrhagic fever 264
Echinococcosis 264
Echovirus 264, 441
Ectoparasites 297, 301, 363
Education and training 3, 8, 112, 329
EEE 149
EFV 517
EKC 34
Emergency power 178
Empiric 555
Empiric Isolation 250
Empiric precautions 259, 260, 261
Employee health 3, 6, 7, 347, 355, 356, 357, 364, 367, 382, 390, 398, 402, 412, 418, 423, 424, 425, 431, 432, 438, 450, 457, 462, 468
Encephalitis 29, 137, 149, 231, 262, 265, 267, 439
Encephalomyelitis 262, 265
Encopresis 362
End stage renal disease 400
Endemic 18, 26, 139, 242, 243, 274, 275, 374, 437, 438, 480, 484, 534, 553, 555, 579
Endogenous 67, 250, 345, 417, 555
Endometritis 265, 272, 448, 451, 453
Endoparasites 297
Endophthalmitis 325, 437, 442
Endoscopic reprocessors 175
Endoscopy 164, 166, 167, 170, 175, 281, 562, 589
Endotoxin formation 133
Endotoxin testing 184
Endotracheal tube 471
Enemas 279, 280, 316
Entamoeba histolytica 546
Enteral feeding bags 415
Enteral Nutrition 202, 204, 562
Enteral/Parenteral Nutrition 197
Enteric pathogens 260, 301, 381
Enterobacter 174, 307, 312, 322, 327, 437, 522, 527, 534, 539, 540, 541, 542, 544, 546, 547
Enterobiasis 265
Enterococci 312, 322, 437, 444, 527, 534, 544, 545, 582
Enterococcus 265, 312, 434, 526, 539, 540, 541, 542, 543, 544, 545, 546, 547, 548, 549
Enterocolitis 265, 272
Enteroviral infection 264, 266, 267, 269
Enuresis 362
Environment 44, 46, 112, 137, 140, 142, 154, 167, 254, 257, 258, 308, 366, 376, 388, 428, 437, 455, 473, 474, 485, 487, 488, 489, 491, 493, 580
Environment of care 152, 153, 157, 355, 356, 484, 485
Environmental Controls 253
Environmental Protection Agency 163, 570
Environmental sampling 176, 189, 190, 317

Environmental surfaces 141, 159, 163, 171, 175, 176, 185, 189, 252, 253, 257, 258, 317, 346, 387, 458, 485
Enzymatic detergent 164
EPA 141, 163, 173, 186, 187, 317, 475, 570
Epidemic 34, 95, 109, 128, 130, 139, 243, 274, 422, 480, 536, 555, 557, 579
Epidemiology ix, 8, 9, 11, 12, 17, 26, 28, 71, 89, 99, 113, 130, 135, 136, 150, 153, 156, 157, 170, 194, 204, 211, 247, 249, 257, 277, 285, 290, 295, 304, 309, 320, 324, 340, 349, 360, 364, 365, 379, 386, 395, 398, 410, 416, 434, 445, 454, 460, 465, 477, 482, 486, 507, 509, 510, 511, 518, 520, 521, 530, 531, 536, 537, 555, 559, 561, 563, 569, 571, 573, 576, 577, 579, 583, 586, 587, 588, 590
Epidural catheters 345
Epiglottitis 265
Episiotomy 448
Epstein-Barr virus 265, 525
Eryc® 543
Erythema infectiosum 40, 265, 515
Erythromycin 37, 54, 442, 543
Escherichia coli 29, 259, 265, 266, 312, 539
ESRD 400, 401
Ethyl alcohol 162
Ethylene oxide 160
EtO 160, 168
Exanthem subitum 271
Exanthems 260
Exit Site Infection 326
Exogenous 67, 304, 556
Experimental/clinical study 14
Exposure 31, 32, 41, 42, 43, 45, 47, 50, 51, 53, 55, 59, 61, 65, 66, 115, 137, 138, 142, 143, 144, 147, 148, 162, 164, 167, 168, 169, 187, 214, 216, 224, 230, 235, 240, 241, 242, 245, 263, 276, 283, 292, 294, 295, 301, 368, 369, 370, 371, 387, 405, 424, 429, 436, 447, 471, 472, 478, 481, 484, 485, 488, 489, 491, 492, 493, 495, 496, 497, 498, 499, 502, 504, 506, 507, 508, 509, 513, 514, 515, 516, 517, 528, 554, 577
Eye protection 252, 429, 470
Eyewear 167, 470

Face shield 252
Facility assessment 355
Famciclovir 543
Famvir® 543
Faucet aerators 183
FBI 138, 147
FDA 165, 166, 204, 286, 288, 290, 508, 584
FEMA 150
Ferrets 301
Fetal death 515
Fetal electrodes 448, 451
Fever 29, 72, 73, 74, 77, 79, 81, 83, 90, 91, 93, 96, 100, 102, 103, 107, 110, 111, 139, 148, 149, 196, 260, 261, 263, 274, 326, 331, 336, 339, 345, 408, 443, 444
Fifth disease 380, 515
Filters 153, 172, 177, 178, 179, 186, 203, 316, 333, 404, 406, 471, 481
Flagyl® 546
Flavobacterium 549
Flooding 171, 175, 181
Flowers 188, 419

Floxin® 543
Fluconazole 544
Fluorochrome stain 523
Fluoroscopy 396, 397
Food and Drug Administration 196, 204, 286, 290, 291, 508, 584
Food handling x, 46, 60, 62, 129, 196, 199, 204, 356, 372, 376, 383, 384, 415, 424, 459, 463, 487, 488, 491, 492
Food poisoning 263, 265
Food preparation 200, 203, 301, 363, 372, 381, 384, 414, 461, 463
Food workers 197
Food-related illness 196
Foodborne illness 196, 197, 198, 372, 415, 463
Fortaz® 542
Foscarnet 544
Foscavir® 544
Fungi 160, 161, 173, 521, 523, 539, 544, 545
Fungizone® 539
Fungus 57
Fungus infection dermatophytosis 273
Furunculosis 265

Ganciclovir 544
Gangrene 265
Garamycin® 544
Gas gangrene 263, 265
Gastric tubes 345
Gastroenteritis 92, 104, 175, 263, 264, 265, 266, 271, 272, 274, 275, 422
Gastrostomy tubes 345
Gatifloxacin 544
Gentamicin 544, 548
German measles 217, 266, 271
Giardia lamblia 266, 546
Giardiasis 29, 266
Gloves 30, 31, 32, 33, 34, 35, 36, 37, 38, 39, 40, 41, 42, 43, 44, 45, 46, 47, 48, 49, 50, 51, 52, 53, 54, 55, 56, 57, 58, 59, 60, 61, 62, 63, 64, 65, 66, 116, 167, 180, 199, 207, 208, 209, 251, 252, 257, 258, 278, 279, 280, 281, 282, 284, 303, 307, 308, 314, 318, 329, 330, 336, 337, 355, 384, 402, 405, 429, 451, 463, 470, 496, 553
Glutaraldehyde 162, 163, 164, 165, 167, 168
Gonococcal ophthalmia neonatorum 266
Gonorrhea 29, 266, 367, 370, 442, 526, 540, 543
Gown 30, 31, 32, 33, 34, 35, 36, 37, 38, 39, 40, 41, 42, 43, 44, 45, 46, 47, 48, 49, 50, 51, 52, 53, 54, 55, 56, 57, 58, 59, 60, 61, 62, 63, 64, 65, 66, 116, 252, 253, 258, 278, 279, 280, 281, 282, 308, 314, 318, 336, 451, 469
Gram-stain 522, 523
Granuloma inguinale 266
Granuloma venereum 266
Group A Streptococcus 261, 315, 524
Group B streptococcus 272, 442, 525
Group D streptococci 312
Guidewire exchange 336
Guidewire techniques 332
Guillian-Barré syndrome 266

H. influenzae 72, 73, 229, 265, 525, 539, 540, 541, 542, 543, 544, 545, 546, 547
HACCP 196, 200, 203

Haemophilus influenzae 29, 212, 226, 268, 270, 522
Hair 313, 318, 367, 451, 469
Hand antisepsis 205, 206, 209, 210, 211, 589
Hand hygiene 113, 135, 140, 180, 205, 207, 208, 209, 210, 211, 301, 329, 347, 354, 363, 367, 382, 389, 390, 397, 402, 412, 418, 423, 438, 450, 457, 462, 468, 470, 496
Hand, foot, and mouth disease 35, 266
Hand/forearm antisepsis 314
Handpieces 388, 391
Handwashing 120, 129, 135, 136, 140, 142, 180, 190, 202, 205, 206, 209, 210, 211, 251, 257, 258, 278, 279, 280, 281, 282, 283, 284, 301, 323, 327, 329, 346, 347, 354, 359, 363, 367, 372, 377, 378, 381, 382, 383, 389, 390, 397, 402, 403, 412, 413, 417, 418, 423, 424, 428, 429, 432, 438, 450, 452, 457, 458, 459, 462, 468, 470, 474, 495, 496, 497, 498, 577, 584, 589
Handwashing agents 132, 133
Handwashing sink 120, 403, 474
Handwashing station 153
Hantavirus pulmonary syndrome 29, 266
HAV 41, 246, 247, 528
HAVRIX® 246
Hazard Analysis and Critical Control Point 196
Hazardous Communications Standard 167
HBeAg 528
HBIG 42, 215, 226, 232, 233, 236, 440, 496, 500, 501, 517
HBsAg 224, 226, 227, 242, 243, 267, 407, 408, 440, 499, 500, 501, 528
HBV 42, 162, 163, 164, 215, 242, 387, 405, 407, 408, 432, 440, 495, 497, 500, 501, 508, 514, 517, 518, 528, 529, 577
HBV DNA 528
HCFA 86, 424, 565, 569
HCWAG 511
HDV 529
HDV RNA 529
Healthcare environment ix, 2, 152, 171, 310
Heating, Ventilation, Air Conditioning 172
Helicobacter pylori 266
Hemodialysis (HD) 400
Hemodialysis catheter 335, 336
Hemorrhagic fever 137, 194, 264, 267
HEPA filter 172
HEPA filtration 153
Hepatitis A 198, 214, 226, 227, 228, 231, 233, 246, 247, 248, 259, 405, 438, 488, 525, 590
Hepatitis A virus 161, 528
Hepatitis B 42, 167, 212, 213, 215, 216, 224, 226, 227, 228, 229, 231, 233, 242, 367, 368, 374, 405, 407, 440, 447, 452, 488, 489, 499, 500, 501, 514, 516, 517, 528
Hepatitis B virus 42, 161, 243, 440, 528
Hepatitis C 43, 488, 499, 514, 517, 528
Hepatitis D virus 529
Hepatitis, viral 29, 267
Hepatitus A 41
Herpangina 267

Herpes simplex 44, 94, 109, 267, 447, 489, 514, 524, 526, 539, 543, 544, 549
Herpes simplex virus 161, 439
Herpes zoster 267, 276, 516
Herpesvirus hominis 267
HEV 529
HEV RNA 529
Hickman 326, 345
HICPAC 3, 113, 135, 157, 177, 195, 205, 211, 248, 249, 250, 262, 263, 264, 265, 266, 267, 268, 269, 270, 271, 272, 273, 274, 275, 285, 295, 298, 309, 312, 321, 328, 340, 365, 395, 398, 410, 420, 478, 485, 486, 512, 518, 531, 574, 589
High efficiency filter 172
High Efficiency Particulate Air filter 172
High-level disinfection 160, 164, 165, 166, 168, 183, 391
Histoplasmosis 267
HIV 29, 45, 161, 162, 163, 164, 167, 215, 218, 219, 223, 226, 229, 230, 235, 239, 240, 245, 260, 261, 267, 367, 368, 369, 370, 371, 372, 374, 378, 387, 417, 432, 440, 447, 452, 489, 495, 497, 499, 502, 503, 504, 505, 506, 507, 508, 509, 510, 512, 514, 515, 517, 518, 525, 526, 527, 531, 564, 565, 577, 585, 591
Holding temperature 197
Home care x, 13, 97, 100, 101, 102, 103, 104, 105, 106, 107, 108, 109, 110, 111, 142, 300, 411, 412, 413, 414, 415, 418, 423, 438, 450, 457, 462, 469, 566, 577
Home care provider bag 414
Hookworm 267
Hot tubs 175
Hot water 180, 181, 182
Housekeeping 175, 186, 356, 368, 376, 377, 378, 405, 428, 475, 476, 485, 498
HTLV I/II 452
Human immunodeficiency virus 45, 416, 420, 440, 445, 499, 510, 517, 527
Humidity 172, 178, 355, 474
Hungarian measles 40
HVAC 172, 177, 178, 179
Hydatidosis 264
Hydrogen peroxide 162, 168
Hydrotherapy pools 175
Hygienic practices 97, 283, 381, 383, 413, 415, 462
Hymenolepis nana 273
Hypothermia 74, 79, 96, 110
Hypothesis 13, 130, 556

IAIS 448
IC program 2, 6, 9, 12, 24, 250, 348, 358, 364, 366, 376, 385, 394, 408, 415, 419, 423, 424, 425, 445, 452, 464, 476
Ice 175, 184, 185
Ice-making 175, 185
Ice-storage 175, 184
ICRA 153, 154
ICU setting 344, 345, 349
ICUs 22, 70, 174, 329, 339, 344
IGIV 232, 234
IHCW 510, 511
Imipenem 544
Immune globulin 31, 51, 59, 144, 213, 218, 224, 226, 229, 232, 233, 234, 235, 237, 241, 276, 440, 480, 496, 501, 517

Immunization 7, 30, 63, 129, 143, 212, 213, 222, 226, 227, 237, 240, 241, 243, 247, 248, 301, 359, 371, 381, 382, 405, 430, 431, 432, 458, 479, 480, 481, 484, 486, 498, 508, 513, 516, 518, 564, 567, 574, 579, 585
Immunocompromised x, 51, 58, 129, 156, 175, 178, 179, 187, 198, 199, 213, 214, 215, 216, 217, 218, 219, 221, 222, 229, 233, 245, 267, 271, 275, 277, 297, 301, 371, 401, 412, 417, 419, 420, 487, 510
Impetigo 46, 93, 108, 267, 380, 456
Implantable access device 335
Implants 161, 168, 310
In utero 435, 438, 439, 440, 441, 443, 556
Incidence 8, 15, 139, 196, 325, 331, 337, 347, 364, 379, 399, 419, 436, 534, 555, 556
Incidence rate 16
Incubation period 30, 31, 32, 33, 34, 35, 36, 37, 38, 39, 40, 41, 42, 43, 44, 45, 46, 47, 48, 49, 50, 51, 52, 53, 54, 55, 56, 57, 58, 59, 60, 61, 62, 63, 64, 65, 66, 250, 275, 556
Indwelling catheterization 323
Infected or colonized surgical personnel 315
Infected patient precautions 30, 31, 32, 33, 34, 35, 36, 37, 38, 39, 40, 41, 42, 43, 44, 45, 46, 47, 48, 49, 50, 51, 52, 53, 54, 55, 56, 57, 58, 59, 60, 61, 62, 63, 64, 65, 66
Infection control program 6, 10, 252, 259, 277, 348, 361, 419, 424, 425, 426, 433, 577, 581
Infection control resources 9, 385, 394, 395, 561
Infection Control Risk Assessment 153
Infection risk factors 450
Infectious agent 19, 28, 69, 88, 98, 112, 132, 152, 167, 171, 205, 212, 250, 424, 438, 468, 480, 485, 495, 496, 513, 556, 558, 559
Infectious mononucleosis 265, 267
Infectious parotitis 269
Inflammation 69, 88, 98, 303, 328, 556
Influenza 47, 90, 100, 150, 173, 216, 217, 226, 227, 228, 229, 230, 231, 238, 248, 267, 276, 309, 371, 380, 405, 422, 431, 432, 493, 494, 495, 496, 497, 507
Influenza-like 90, 100
Infusaport 345
Infusate-related bloodstream infection 326
INH 65, 516
Injury Severity Score 347
Inmate assessment 367
Integrated pest management 356
Intensive care units 188, 214, 344, 443, 445
Intermediate disinfection 160
Intermittent catheterization 323, 430
International travelers 223, 242, 480
Intraamniotic infection syndrome 448
Intracranial pressure monitoring 345
Intraoperative area 466, 469, 474
Intraoperative ventilation 316
Intrapartum 435, 438, 439, 440, 441, 442, 443, 444, 447, 556
Intrapartum (natal) infection 556
Intravascular catheters 325
Intravenous injection ports 332
Intubation 52, 281, 306, 444
Iodophor 169
IPV 226, 243, 244

Isolation 74, 75, 76, 140, 145, 179, 180, 193, 194, 249, 250, 277, 278, 279, 280, 281, 282, 301, 370, 390, 402, 414, 419, 420, 424, 426, 428, 429, 468, 484, 495, 496, 507, 524, 526, 536, 553, 557, 559, 577, 583, 588
Isopropyl alcohol 162, 165, 169
ISS 347, 350
Itraconazole 545
IV therapy 331, 334

Jails 366, 379, 591
JCAHO 3, 112, 153, 157, 181, 424, 434, 566, 584
Jewelry 315, 470

Kawasaki syndrome 267
Ketoconazole 545
Kinyoun 523
Kirby-Bauer 524
Klebsiella 322, 327, 437, 522, 534, 540, 541, 547, 548
Klebsiella pneumoniae 312
Klebsiella species 307

Laboratory 72, 73, 146, 228, 244, 246, 358, 520, 521
Laboratory waste 192
Laminar flow 172
Laser plume 172
Lasers 389, 394
Lassa 267
Lassa fever 268
Latex 387, 419, 456, 458, 468, 566
Laundry x, 171, 176, 190, 191, 283, 284, 285, 363, 368, 372, 375, 376, 378, 412, 428, 506
Laundry facilities 190
Laundry handling 284
Leak testing 164
Legionella 174, 180, 182, 270, 308, 498, 526, 527, 543, 545, 547, 548
Legionnaires' disease 158, 182, 268, 308
Leprosy 268
Leptospirosis 268
Levaquin® 545
Levofloxacin 545
Lice 268
Line list 23, 129
Linezolid 545
Listeria 444, 447, 539
Listeria monocytogenes 198, 268, 445, 548
Listeriosis 268, 443
Localized catheter colonization 326
Lomafloxacin 545
Long-Term Care 86
Lorabid® 546
Loracarbef 546
Low-level disinfection 160, 169
LTCF 421, 422, 424, 425, 426, 427, 428, 429, 430, 431, 432, 433
Lyme disease 29, 268
Lymphocytic choriomeningitis 268
Lymphogranuloma venereum 268

M. catarrhalis 539, 540, 541, 542, 543, 544, 545, 546, 548
M. chelonae 175
M. gordonae 175
M. tuberculosis 160, 161, 164, 523, 526, 534, 547
M. xenopi 175
Maculopapular rash 93, 108
Mad cow disease 160
Magnetic resonance imaging 396

Maintenance 141, 171, 347, 355, 364, 368, 383, 390, 398, 402, 412, 418, 423, 438, 450, 457, 462, 464, 469, 486, 498
Malaria 29, 268, 481
Malassezia 437
Mammography 396, 397
Managing critical data 2, 4
Mantoux 167, 367, 430, 431
Manufacturer's recommendations 134, 161, 179, 208
Marburg virus 268
Mask 252, 256, 278, 279, 280, 281, 282
Mastitis 453
Mattress 191
Maxaquin® 545
Maxipime® 541
MDR 286
Mean 13
Means of exposure 30, 31, 32, 33, 34, 35, 36, 37, 38, 39, 40, 41, 42, 43, 44, 45, 46, 47, 48, 49, 50, 51, 52, 53, 54, 55, 56, 57, 58, 59, 60, 61, 62, 63, 64, 65, 66
Measles 29, 50, 221, 226, 232, 233, 234, 235, 236, 240, 268, 489
Measurement process 23, 25
Mechanical ventilation 306
Median 13
Medical device 159, 161, 286, 287, 288, 290, 291, 476
Medical Device Reporting 286
Medication refrigerators 134
Medications 132, 133, 196, 250, 333, 346, 354, 357, 358, 362, 389, 394, 405, 406, 422, 481
Mefoxin® 542
Meloidiosis 268
Meningitis 260, 268, 373
Meningococcal 230, 231, 268, 373, 374
Meningococcal disease 231
Meningococcal pneumonia 268
Meningococcemia 269
Meropenem 546
Merrem 546
Metronidazole 546
MIC 524
Microbiological sampling 191
Microbiological testing 183, 184
Microorganism proliferation 133, 175
Minocin® 548
MMR 50, 213, 217, 218, 219, 220, 226, 227, 228, 229, 230, 231, 232, 236, 480
Mode 13, 174
Molecular biology 525
Molluscum contagiosum 269
Mononucleosis 265, 267
Moxifloxacin 546
MRI 396, 397
MRSA 189, 345, 408, 433, 434, 436, 534, 536, 539, 540, 541, 542, 543, 544, 545, 546, 547, 548, 549
MRSE 539, 540, 541, 542, 543, 544, 545, 546, 547, 548, 549
MSSA 408, 541
Mucormycosis 269
Multi-use patient items 133
Multidose vial 333
Multidrug-resistant bacteria 270
Mumps 50, 53, 212, 217, 219, 221, 226, 241, 354, 363, 371, 387, 517
Mushrooms 198
Mycobacteria 161, 174, 409, 523, 543, 547
Mycobacteria, nontuberculosis (atypical) 269
Mycobacterium tuberculosis 261, 591

Mycoplasma 270, 543, 548
Mycoplasma pneumonia 269

Nafcillin 546
Nail polish 315, 470
Nails 209, 211, 314, 470
Nasal canula 471
Nasogastric tubes 345
National Commission on Correctional Healthcare 377, 379
Natural nails 209
NCCHC 368, 369, 377
NCCLS 524
Nebcin® 548
Necrotizing enterocolitis 269, 444
Needleless intravascular devices 332
Needles 42, 43, 45, 133, 168, 191, 192, 253, 254, 284, 334, 359, 390, 403, 429, 495, 497, 506, 508, 515
Negative predictive value 15
Neisseria meningitidis 260, 268, 373
Neonatal host factors 436
Neonatal infection 436, 557
Neonatal sepsis 442
Neutropenic patients 179
Newborn nursery 443
Nizoral® 545
NNIS risk index 320
No-touch technique 133
Nocardiosis 269
Non-antimicrobial soap 206
Non-tuberculous mycobacteria 174, 409
Noncritical 163, 169
Norwalk agent 269
Norwalk Virus 198
Nosocomial infection 4, 9, 13, 17, 18, 19, 24, 26, 68, 69, 70, 71, 87, 88, 94, 98, 346, 347, 348, 350, 365, 377, 415, 426, 427, 436, 454, 459, 465, 577, 580, 588
Nosocomial infection rate 15, 427
Nosocomial pneumonia 305, 309
NTM 174, 175
Nuclear medicine 396
Nucleic acid probes 525
Null hypothesis 13

Obstetrics 447, 454
Occupational health 129, 143, 154, 253, 315, 484, 486, 510, 511, 571, 585, 587
Occupational therapy 463
Odds 16
Odds ratio 16
Ofloxacin 543
Oliguria 72, 111
Omnipen® 539
Opened-but-unused device 287
Operating room ventilation 311, 468
Operative associated 467
OPIM 187, 278, 279, 280, 281, 282, 287, 368, 394, 495
Opportunistic 420, 521
OPV 243, 244
Oral/nasal endotracheal tube 345
Orf 269
Organ transplant patients 179
OSHA 158, 292, 294, 295, 329, 358, 369, 376, 424, 577, 586
Outbreak 128, 130, 248, 428, 437, 443, 453, 554, 557, 570, 581, 586
Outcomes 20
Oxacillin 539, 540, 541, 544, 546, 547, 548
Oxyuriasis 265

Pandemic 150, 557
Parainfluenza 261, 269
Parenteral 197, 203, 204, 332, 562
Parvovirus B19 265
Pasteurella 524, 546
Pasteurized 199, 201
Pathogenicity 557
Patient assessment 395
Patient care equipment 253, 258
Patient contact 44, 51, 220, 251, 487, 488, 489, 490, 491, 493
Patient placement 140, 254, 255, 257
PCR 149, 526, 527
PE 153, 173, 178, 179, 188, 308, 465
Pediatrics 188, 247, 359, 380, 386, 445, 455, 458, 459, 460, 530
Pediculosis 268, 269, 367, 373, 382, 490
Penal institutions 366
Penicillin 37, 534, 541, 542, 544, 546, 547
PenVee K® 546
PEP 496, 502, 503, 504, 505, 506, 508, 509, 517, 584
Perfusion 345, 472, 473
Perinatal infection 448, 557
Period of communicability 30, 31, 32, 33, 34, 35, 36, 37, 38, 39, 40, 41, 42, 43, 44, 45, 46, 47, 48, 49, 50, 51, 52, 53, 54, 55, 56, 57, 58, 59, 60, 61, 62, 63, 64, 65, 66, 557
Perioperative 294, 310, 313, 467, 469, 470, 474, 477
Peripartum 442
Peripheral venous catheters 331, 333, 334
Peritoneal dialysis (PD) 400
Peritonitis 408
Personal protective equipment 143, 167, 180, 190, 283, 284, 292
Personnel restrictions 30, 31, 32, 33, 34, 35, 36, 37, 38, 39, 40, 41, 42, 43, 44, 45, 46, 47, 48, 49, 50, 51, 52, 53, 54, 55, 56, 57, 58, 59, 60, 61, 62, 63, 64, 65, 66
Pertussis 29, 54, 55, 212, 226, 259, 261, 269, 274, 490
Pests 176, 193
Pets 30, 60, 176, 301, 414
Pharmacy 22, 133, 333, 348, 357, 469, 535
Pharyngitis 37, 38, 64, 100, 272, 367
Phenolics 162, 164
PHF 197
Phycomycosis 275
Physical therapy 428, 461, 465
Physiotherapy tanks 175
Pica 362
PICC 334, 335, 336
Pillow 61, 191
Pink Eye 95, 109
Pinworm 55, 265, 269
Piperacillin 547
Pipracil® 547
Plague 29, 137, 140, 148, 228, 269
Plague - Bubonic 269
Plague - Pneumonic 269
Plants 171, 188, 419
Plasmid profile analysis 526
Pleurodynia 269
Plume 172, 475, 497
Pneumocystis carinii 270, 548
Pneumonia 74, 75, 76, 90, 91, 101, 102, 149, 174, 263, 268, 269, 270, 272, 276, 305, 308, 309, 380, 417, 422, 430, 436, 437, 439, 442, 443, 444, 456, 476, 577, 589
Pocket Infection 327

Policies and procedures 3, 5, 6, 7, 161, 196, 348, 356, 357, 371, 385, 402, 425, 428, 429, 430, 431, 433, 465, 469, 470, 472, 473, 474, 477, 484, 535
Polio 229, 231, 243
Poliomyelitis 29, 212, 243, 248, 270
Poliovirus 161, 226
Polymerase chain reaction 526
Pools 175, 185, 382, 385, 461, 464
Positive predictive value 15, 328
Post-mortem care 142
Postexposure prophylaxis 7, 31, 142, 143, 215, 243, 368, 484, 489, 490, 491, 492, 493, 495, 496, 498, 500, 501, 502, 503, 504, 505, 506, 507, 508, 517, 518, 577, 586
Postnatal (postpartum) infection 557
Postoperative area 467
Postpartum 219, 443, 449, 452, 453, 557
Potable water 174, 175
Potentially hazardous foods 197, 200, 201
Power 13, 77, 80, 103, 138, 178
PPD 65, 227, 230, 367, 492, 507, 516
PPE 116, 120, 140, 161, 292, 294, 346, 368, 390, 392, 394, 495, 496, 497, 498, 513
PPV 226, 239
Pregnancy 44, 52, 59, 213, 214, 215, 216, 217, 218, 219, 221, 222, 223, 236, 238, 239, 241, 246, 247, 375, 440, 481, 498, 506, 508, 513, 515, 516, 517
Pregnant employee 447, 513, 516, 518
Prenatal 374, 435, 447
Preoperative area 466
Preoperative preparation of the patient 313, 314, 469
Preoperative shaving 311, 467
Preoperative skin prep 311, 467
Prepartum 447, 450
Pressure ulcers x, 300, 303, 304, 422
Prevalence rate 16, 23
Prevent transmission of infectious diseases 3, 8
Primaxin® 544
Prion 160, 163
Prisons 366, 369, 591
Processes 5, 21, 112, 144, 154, 159, 162, 166, 189, 355, 409
Prolonged rupture of membranes 439, 448
PROM 448, 449, 450
Prophylaxis 7, 30, 31, 32, 33, 34, 35, 36, 37, 38, 39, 40, 41, 42, 43, 44, 45, 46, 47, 48, 49, 50, 51, 52, 53, 54, 55, 56, 57, 58, 59, 60, 61, 62, 63, 64, 65, 66, 143, 215, 231, 233, 243, 309, 316, 366, 370, 374, 388, 391, 451, 469, 480, 484, 490, 496, 498, 499, 500, 501, 502, 503, 504, 505, 506, 508, 515, 517, 518, 547, 577, 586
Prospective 8, 14, 19, 21, 319, 349, 557
Protective Equipment Task Matrix 250, 278, 279, 280, 281, 282
Protective or protected environment 153
Protective/protected environment 173
Proteus mirabilis 312
Ps. aeruginosa 161
Pseudallescheria 539
Pseudomonas 174, 307, 327, 437, 522, 534, 539, 540, 541, 542, 543, 545, 546, 548

Pseudomonas aeruginosa 174, 312, 540
Pseudomonas cepacia 270, 544
Psittacosis 29, 270
Psychological aspects 145
Puerperal fever 453
Pulse field gel electrophoresis 526
Purulent sputum 74, 75, 76, 101
Pyelonephritis 274

Q fever 29, 137, 148, 270
Quality control 24, 161, 333
Quaternary ammonium 163, 169
Quinupristin 547

Rabies 29, 228, 229, 231, 233, 248, 270, 301
Raccoons 301
Radioactive substances 396
Ralstonia 174
Range 9, 13, 135, 161, 177, 275, 352, 353, 366, 511
Rat-bite fever 270, 272
Recall 161, 286, 357, 403
Recall process 289
Recreation therapy 461
Refrigeration of foods 201
Refrigerator 121, 122, 123, 134, 200, 201, 356, 357, 358, 404, 473, 476
Regulated medical waste 176, 192, 193
Regulations 3, 4, 6, 27, 86, 119, 141, 147, 177, 180, 192, 203, 206, 249, 250, 289, 293, 313, 328, 358, 364, 368, 369, 372, 374, 376, 380, 385, 405, 415, 424, 425, 426, 428, 465, 476, 479, 488, 570
Rehabilitation x, 2, 185, 355, 451, 461
Relapsing fever 271
Relative risk 16
Renovation 127, 152, 153, 154, 155, 156, 171, 179, 308, 346, 347, 355, 364, 368, 383, 390, 398, 402, 412, 414, 418, 423, 438, 450, 457, 462, 469, 590
Reprocessing 117, 124, 159, 162, 165, 167, 254, 286, 287, 288, 289, 290, 291, 355, 391, 404, 407, 408, 458, 496
Reservoir 173, 174, 176, 180, 346, 387, 392, 404, 417, 473, 521, 558
Resident care 429, 432
Resident health program 425, 430
Resistant bacteria 259, 261, 270, 271, 277, 422, 433
Respiratory care 22, 281, 348, 413, 416, 561
Respiratory infections 260, 261, 305, 457, 493
Respiratory infectious disease 271, 274
Respiratory protection 158, 255, 414
Respiratory syncytial virus 56, 173, 271, 308, 456
Respiratory tract infections 64, 90, 100, 305, 418, 422, 443
Resterilization 287
Restriction endonuclease analysis 526, 527
Retrospective 14, 19, 426, 554
Reusable medical devices 159, 290
Reuse 134, 156, 286, 287, 289, 290, 291, 392, 397, 404, 406, 472
Reye syndrome 271
Rheumatic fever 271
Rhinoviruses 173

Ribotyping 527
Ricin 148
Rickettsia 543, 548
Rickettsial fever 271
Rickettsialpox 271
Rifadin® 547
Rifampin 52, 547
Ringworm 57, 271, 273
Risk ix, 3, 4, 5, 9, 12, 14, 15, 16, 18, 19, 21, 27, 40, 42, 44, 56, 60, 62, 66, 67, 68, 69, 70, 85, 87, 88, 97, 98, 112, 128, 132, 133, 136, 137, 139, 140, 145, 152, 153, 154, 155, 159, 161, 167, 173, 174, 175, 176, 177, 179, 180, 182, 186, 188, 197, 198, 199, 202, 203, 205, 212, 213, 214, 215, 217, 223, 224, 226, 227, 228, 229, 230, 231, 236, 238, 239, 240, 241, 242, 243, 245, 247, 250, 258, 261, 276, 283, 284, 287, 288, 293, 294, 297, 300, 302, 303, 305, 307, 308, 310, 311, 316, 320, 322, 325, 327, 331, 332, 334, 335, 336, 337, 344, 345, 346, 347, 348, 349, 350, 353, 362, 365, 366, 367, 368, 369, 370, 371, 374, 377, 378, 380, 381, 385, 387, 388, 391, 395, 397, 401, 409, 411, 412, 415, 416, 417, 418, 419, 421, 423, 424, 427, 430, 435, 436, 437, 438, 439, 440, 441, 444, 445, 447, 448, 449, 450, 451, 453, 455, 456, 457, 458, 459, 461, 462, 463, 465, 466, 467, 469, 472, 473, 479, 480, 484, 485, 486, 487, 489, 493, 494, 495, 496, 498, 507, 510, 511, 513, 514, 515, 516, 517, 518, 521, 535, 536, 553, 554, 557, 558, 559
Risk assessment 112, 154, 178, 431
Risk management 153, 166, 289, 359, 510
Risk stratification 4, 24, 347, 558
Risks for outbreaks 129
Ritter's disease 271, 272
RNA load 527
Rocephin® 542
Rocky Mountain spotted fever 29, 271
Rodents 271, 301
Room air humidifiers 183
Roseola infantum 271
Rotavirus 58, 259, 266, 271, 437
RSV 56, 173, 271, 308, 437, 456, 457, 493
Rubella 29, 50, 59, 69, 212, 217, 219, 220, 226, 227, 232, 236, 241, 266, 271, 354, 363, 371, 380, 387, 439, 453, 491, 513, 516, 517
Rubeola 50, 51, 219, 255, 260, 268, 513, 516, 517

S. aureus 46, 161, 272, 315, 327, 436, 443, 444, 456, 526, 527, 540, 541, 543, 544, 545, 546, 547, 548, 549
S. epidermidis 327, 444, 547
S. maltophilia 548
S. pneumoniae 72, 73, 525, 536, 542, 543, 544, 545, 546, 547
Salmonella 20, 60, 92, 104, 197, 198, 266, 487, 539, 592, 593
Salmonella typhi 274
Sanitary sewer 193
Sanitation 97, 356, 372, 381, 414, 457, 458, 459, 558
Sanitizer 200, 381, 383, 413, 463, 481

Scabies 61, 93, 94, 108, 115, 271, 363, 367, 373, 387, 422, 432, 461, 491
Scalded skin 271, 272
Scarlet fever 272
Schistosomiasis 272
Scombroid toxin 198
Scoring models 347
Scrofula 274
Scrub suits 176, 292, 318
Scrubs x, 124, 292, 293, 294, 295, 469, 477
Semicritical 163, 164, 165, 168, 169
Sensitivity 15, 214, 222, 223, 237, 419, 456, 458, 558
Septra® 548
Serratia 327, 522, 534
Service animals 297, 298, 301
Sewage system 181, 182
Sharps 20, 21, 42, 43, 45, 120, 192, 282, 295, 359, 389, 390, 414, 429, 472, 473, 475, 514, 515, 582
Sharps disposal 193, 473, 475, 503, 506
Shigella 62, 92, 104, 198, 259, 266, 359
Shigellosis 29, 272
Shingles 94, 109, 493
Shoe covers 318, 470
Simplified Acute Physiology Score II 347
Single-use device 287, 288, 290
Single-use unit dose 133
Sinusitis 90, 100, 345
SIR 14, 16
Skin antisepsis 311, 467
Skin care 209
Skin cleansers 132, 133
Skin closure 318
Skin contaminant 72, 73, 82, 105, 106
Skunks 301
Smallpox 63, 137, 140, 149
Sodium hydroxide 163
Sodium hypochlorite 162, 168, 169, 187, 394
Soiled linen 141, 190, 282, 283, 284, 285
Spacing of vaccines 236
Spaulding 159
Specificity 15, 328, 558
Specimen collection 358, 521
Specimen packaging 147
Specimen transport 147
Speech therapy 461
Sphingomonas 174
Spills 141, 171, 186, 187, 188, 282, 383, 419, 429
Spirillum minus 270, 272
Sporanox® 545
Sporotrichosis 272
SSI 16, 17, 83, 84, 107, 108, 310, 312, 313, 314, 315, 316, 318, 319, 320, 466
SSI rate 16, 320
Standard deviation 14
Standard precautions 30, 31, 32, 33, 34, 35, 36, 37, 38, 39, 40, 41, 42, 43, 44, 45, 46, 47, 48, 49, 50, 51, 52, 53, 54, 55, 56, 57, 58, 59, 60, 61, 62, 63, 64, 65, 66, 140, 141, 142, 146, 249, 250, 251, 254, 256, 257, 258, 259, 346, 347, 354, 363, 367, 368, 372, 375, 378, 382, 385, 389, 390, 397, 402, 412, 415, 418, 423, 438, 450, 457, 462, 465, 468, 473, 488, 495, 496, 513, 516, 536, 558, 559
Standardized infection rate 14

Standards 5, 6, 11, 18, 23, 135, 153, 155, 157, 164, 170, 173, 177, 183, 206, 250, 287, 295, 320, 328, 353, 356, 360, 363, 377, 403, 424, 434, 451, 476, 477, 565
Staphylococcal 265, 272
Staphylococcal disease 272, 273
Staphylococcal enterotoxin B 137, 149
Staphylococcus 78, 80, 96, 110, 444, 522, 526, 527, 539, 540, 543, 546, 549
Staphylococcus aureus 198, 261, 270, 307, 312, 322, 408, 456, 457, 491, 534, 536, 537
Steam sterilization 163, 193
Stenotrophomonas 174, 544, 546
Sterilization 21, 116, 129, 140, 141, 159, 160, 161, 162, 163, 164, 165, 168, 170, 185, 189, 211, 287, 288, 290, 307, 310, 311, 317, 320, 347, 354, 355, 360, 363, 367, 377, 378, 382, 388, 389, 390, 391, 397, 402, 412, 418, 423, 429, 438, 450, 451, 457, 462, 464, 468, 472, 473, 476, 558, 578, 582
Storage 119, 132, 133, 161, 167, 175, 177, 183, 184, 192, 202, 283, 284, 301, 346, 356, 357, 358, 372, 377, 389, 393, 394, 404, 406, 430, 452, 473, 474
Streptobacillus moniliformis 270, 272
Streptococcal disease 29, 272, 273
Streptococcus pyogenes 46, 522
Streptococcus, group A 270
Strongyloidiasis 273
Subglottic secretions 348
Suctioning 52, 87, 348, 413, 471
SUD 141, 286, 287, 288, 289
Surgical apparel x, 292, 293, 469
Surgical attire 295, 318, 477
Surgical drain 311, 345, 468
Surgical hand antisepsis 208
Surgical instruments 168, 317, 555
Surgical mask 180, 256, 280, 318, 354, 402, 414, 418, 458, 470
Surgical personnel 208, 292, 315
Surgical procedures 16, 176, 208, 310, 392, 466, 475, 476
Surgical scrub 136, 311, 314, 467, 470, 471
Surgical site infection 98, 108, 293, 310, 311, 321, 361, 448, 452, 453, 466, 471, 558, 577
Surgical team 314, 318, 320, 466
Surgical technique 310, 311, 318, 348, 452, 468
Surgical wound classification 320
Surveillance x, 4, 8, 9, 12, 13, 18, 19, 20, 21, 22, 24, 25, 26, 27, 28, 67, 68, 69, 70, 71, 86, 87, 88, 97, 98, 112, 132, 181, 276, 287, 308, 319, 320, 339, 349, 350, 360, 361, 364, 365, 366, 369, 376, 377, 385, 395, 408, 409, 415, 416, 419, 424, 426, 427, 445, 453, 464, 465, 476, 477, 535, 536, 554, 555, 559, 563, 564, 588, 589, 592, 593
Surveillance approaches 26
Surveillance data 5, 70, 128, 427, 428, 477
Surveillance process 4, 19, 69
Susceptible 30, 31, 32, 33, 34, 35, 36, 37, 38, 39, 40, 41, 42, 43, 44, 45, 46, 47, 48, 49, 50, 51, 52, 53, 54, 55, 56, 57, 58, 59, 60, 61, 62, 63, 64, 65, 66, 129, 155, 173, 199, 219, 223, 226, 245, 255, 276, 407, 408, 476, 489, 490, 491, 492, 493,

494, 516, 524, 537, 559
Swan-Ganz 344
Synercid® 547
Syphilis 29, 273, 367, 370, 379, 441, 442, 446, 497, 515, 518

T. glabrata 544
Taenia solium 273
Tanks 169, 175, 183, 184, 185, 404, 464
Tap water 165, 174, 181, 393, 394, 413, 415
Tapeworm 273
Tazobactam 547
TB 65, 66, 152, 158, 171, 173, 223, 241, 245, 277, 354, 363, 367, 369, 370, 372, 387, 397, 422, 424, 428, 430, 431, 432, 443, 452, 456, 457, 458, 468, 496, 497, 507, 516, 565, 568, 585, 590, 591
TB skin test 21, 154
Tequin 544
Tetanus 29, 212, 221, 222, 226, 229, 233, 236, 237, 273, 431, 432, 498, 516
Tetracyclines 548
Thawing of frozen foods 200
Therapeutic 67, 133, 316, 344, 396, 398, 469, 510, 535, 559
Therapeutic Intervention Scoring System 347
Therapists 133, 364, 415, 452, 464, 485
Therapy pools 175
Thermometer 96, 110, 121, 122, 123, 169, 200, 201, 419
Third-party Reprocessor 288
Ticarcillin-clavulanate 548
Tick-borne 271
TIG 222, 232, 233, 237
Timentin® 548
Tinea 271, 273
Tobramycin 548
Torulopsis 539, 545
Tourists 479
Toxic shock syndrome 29, 272, 273
Toxoplasmosis 273, 441
Toys 353, 382, 383, 459
TPN 203, 335, 339
Trachoma 273
Transmission-Based Precautions 249, 250, 398, 496, 516
Transplacental 69, 435, 439, 441, 443, 453, 515
Transport 124, 140, 141, 147, 154, 177, 191, 192, 193, 253, 254, 255, 256, 257, 258, 278, 282, 284, 285, 358, 393, 398, 401, 407, 428, 468, 473, 523
Travel 28, 223, 231, 233, 238, 240, 242, 243, 374, 479, 480, 481, 482, 570, 586, 592, 593
Trench mouth 273, 274
Triage 114, 140, 143, 144, 146, 353, 354, 363, 387
Trichinella 198
Trichinosis 29, 198, 273
Trichomoniasis 273
Trichophyton 161
Trichuriasis 273
Trimethoprim-sulfamethoxazole 548
Trovafloxacin 548
Trovan® 548
Tuberculosis 7, 29, 65, 66, 115, 140, 167, 179, 255, 256, 261, 268, 274, 276, 277, 354, 363, 369, 379, 414, 417, 422, 443, 456, 457, 460, 468, 492, 495, 507, 513, 530, 568, 577, 586, 588, 590, 591, 593

Tularemia 29, 137, 140, 149, 274
Tunnel infection 326
Tunneled central venous catheter 335
Turtles 60, 301
Type I (alpha) error 13
Type II (beta) error 13
Typhoid 29, 231, 274
Typhus 274
Typhus fever 271

Ultraclean air 316
Ultrasound 183, 279, 396, 399
Umbilical catheters 338, 339
Unasyn® 540
Uncinariasis 267
Uniform 176, 190, 292, 293
Unipen® 546
Universal precautions 559
Unpasteurized 199, 418
Unvaccinated 63, 220, 235, 242, 244, 500
Urinalysis 92, 103, 520
Urinary catheter 67, 274, 322, 345, 348, 412, 422, 447, 461, 468
Urinary tract infection 261, 322, 323, 324, 380, 417, 449, 461, 469, 476
Urine specimens 103, 323
USAMRIID 146
UTI 77, 78, 79, 80, 91, 92, 103, 119, 174, 261, 274, 322, 323, 422, 430, 437, 444, 449, 577
UV radiation 316

Vaccine 7, 28, 31, 37, 47, 50, 51, 54, 63, 144, 213, 214, 215, 216, 217, 218, 219, 220, 221, 222, 223, 224, 226, 227, 228, 229, 230, 231, 232, 233, 234, 235, 236, 238, 239, 240, 241, 242, 243, 245, 246, 247, 248, 358, 368, 371, 405, 407, 431, 432, 440, 480, 481, 484, 496, 500, 501, 516, 517, 536, 586
Vacuums 186
Valacyclovir 549
Valcyte 549
Valganciclovir 549
Valley fever 263
Valtrex® 549
Vancocin® 549
Vancomycin 259, 265, 434, 534, 537, 544, 545, 547, 549, 582
Vantin® 541
VAQTA® 247
Varicella 29, 31, 94, 109, 152, 171, 212, 213, 222, 223, 224, 226, 227, 228, 229, 231, 233, 236, 245, 247, 255, 260, 263, 274, 275, 276, 358, 371, 397, 439, 447, 480, 492, 493, 494, 516
Varicella-zoster 31, 32, 267, 275, 276, 439, 492, 493, 513, 516, 539, 543, 544, 549
Variola 63
vCJD 160
Vector-borne 27, 249
VEE 149
Vegetative bacteria 160, 161
Ventilation 32, 50, 51, 63, 65, 66, 116, 119, 124, 138, 153, 157, 171, 172, 173, 178, 179, 194, 254, 256, 310, 316, 354, 355, 376, 384, 412, 428, 471, 474, 498
Ventilation grills 125
Ventilation systems 139, 172, 177, 382
Ventilator circuit changes 306
Ventilator tubing 307

Ventilator-associated pneumonia 348, 351
Ventriculostomy 345
Vesicular rash 94, 109
vesicular rickettsiosis 271
Vibramycin 548
Vibrio parahaemolyticus 266, 274
Vincent's angina 273, 274
Viral encephalitides 262
Viral hemorrhagic fever 137, 194, 264
Viral pneumonia 270
Virulence 65, 223, 521, 559
Viruses 160, 161, 173, 189, 218, 443, 444, 521, 523, 524, 525, 531, 539, 543, 544, 549
VRE 189, 433, 434, 534, 536, 577, 582
VZIG 31, 32, 224, 233, 276, 492, 493
VZV 173, 179, 224

Water-damage 173
Waterborne microorganisms 165, 174, 180
WEE 149
Whipworm 273
Whirlpools 175, 185, 448, 451, 461, 464
Whooping cough 269, 274
Workflow 116, 162, 355
Wound infections 136, 274, 361, 476

X-rays 68, 279, 389, 394

Yellow fever 29, 231, 262, 480
Yersinia enterocolitica 198, 266, 275

Z test 14
Ziehl-Neelson 523
Zinacef® 542
Zithromax® 543
Zosyn® 547
Zovirax® 539
Zyvox 545

EVALUATION FORM

APIC Handbook of Infection Control, 2002

Instructions: Using the scale below, please circle the number that best represents your assessment of this publication.

1 = Strongly Disagree 2 = Somewhat Disagree 3 = Neutral
4 = Mostly Agree 5 = Strongly Agree

Needs

My objectives in purchasing the publication were met.	1 2 3 4 5
My expectations for the publication were met.	1 2 3 4 5

Format

The format made the publication easy to use.	1 2 3 4 5
Format was clear and concise.	1 2 3 4 5

Content

The content was current and accurate.	1 2 3 4 5
The content was well organized.	1 2 3 4 5
References were helpful.	1 2 3 4 5

Quality

The quality of production showed attention to details.	1 2 3 4 5
I would recommend this publication to my colleagues.	1 2 3 4 5

Cost

The cost of this publication was what I expected to pay.	1 2 3 4 5
My employer paid for this purchase.	1 2 3 4 5
The price was a value for the product.	1 2 3 4 5

Are there additional components to this publication that would enhance it? If so, please indicate.

____

____

What future publications would you like from APIC?

____

____

If you discovered any bugs/errors that need correcting, please make a note to help us correct this in the next printing/edition.

____

____

Other comments:

____

____

Thank You! Please mail/fax your completed evaluation form to the APIC National Office:

Association for Professionals in Infection Control and Epidemiology

1275 K St. NW, #1000, Washington DC 20005-4006,
(202) 789-1899 (fax)